Teledermatology

Teledermatology

Edited by

Richard Wootton

Centre for Online Health, University of Queensland, Australia

Amanda M. M. Oakley

Department of Dermatology, Health Waikato, Hamilton, New Zealand

Foreword by
Douglas Perednia
Association of Telemedicine Service Providers, Portland, Oregon, USA

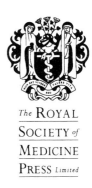

The ROYAL
SOCIETY *of*
MEDICINE
PRESS *Limited*

© 2002 Royal Society of Medicine Press Ltd
1 Wimpole Street, London W1G 0AE, UK
207 Westminster Road, Lake IL 60045, USA
www.rsmpress.co.uk

The publisher has used its best endeavours to ensure that the URLs for external websites referred to in this book are correct and active at the time of going to press. However, the publisher has no responsibility for the websites and can make no guarantee that a site will remain live or that the content is or will remain appropriate.

British Library Cataloguing in Publication Data
A catalogue record for this book is available from the British Library

ISBN: 1-85315-507-1

Typeset by Phoenix Photosetting Ltd, Chatham, Kent

Printed in Great Britain by Bell & Bain Ltd, Glasgow

Contents

List of Contributors

David C. Balch Telemedicine Center, Center for Health Sciences Communication, Brody School of Medicine at East Carolina University, Greenville, North Carolina, USA

Andrea Bauer Department of Dermatology and Allergology, University of Jena, Jena, Germany

Trine S. Bergmo National Centre of Telemedicine, University Hospital of Tromsø, Norway

Ashish Bhatia Medical College of Virginia Hospitals, Richmond, Virginia, USA

Carl R. Blesius Unit for Cybermedicine, Department of Clinical Social Medicine, Heidelberg Medical School, Germany

Ralph Peter Braun Pigmented Skin Lesion Unit, Department of Dermatology, University Hospital Geneva and DHURDV Geneva, Lausanne, Switzerland

Nancy A. Brown Telemedicine Research Center, Portland, Oregon, USA

Günter Burg Department of Dermatology, University Hospital, Zürich, Switzerland

Timothy K. Chartier Department of Dermatology, Harvard Medical School, Boston, Massachusetts, USA

Christopher Clay Department of Dermatology, Royal Perth Hospital, Perth, Australia

Greg R. Day University of Waikato, Hamilton, New Zealand

Thomas Diepgen Unit for Cybermedicine, Department of Clinical Social Medicine, Heidelberg Medical School, Germany

Prosper Doe Regional Dermatology Training Centre, Kilimanjaro Christian Medical College, Moshi, Tanzania and Dermatology Unit, Komfo Anokye Teaching Hospital, Kumasi, Ghana

Peter Elsner Department of Dermatology and Allergology, University of Jena, Jena, Germany

Henry Foong Boon Bee Foong Skin Specialist Clinic, Fair Park, Ipoh, Malaysia

Jennifer Geras The Wound Center, Akron General Medical Center, Ohio, USA

Olaf Götz Department of Dermatology and Allergology, University of Jena, Jena, Germany

Paul Greenwood McGuire VA Medical Center, Richmond, Virginia, USA

Bill Grigsby Department of Agricultural Economics and Rural Sociology, Pennsylvania State University, University Park, Pennsylvania, USA

Michael Haney Prevention and Interventions, Children's Medical Services, Florida Department of Health, Florida, USA

Gisli Ingvarsson Department of Dermatology and Venereology, University Hospital of Tromsø, Norway

Uli Klein Unit for Cybermedicine, Department of Clinical Social Medicine, Heidelberg Medical School, Germany

Paul Kostuchenko Medical College of Virginia Hospitals, Richmond, Virginia, USA

Lorenz Kuehnis Arpage Systems AG, Switzerland

Joseph C. Kvedar Department of Dermatology, Harvard Medical School and Partners Telemedicine Inc., Boston, Massachusetts, USA

Heikki Lamminen Digital Media Institute, Tampere University of Technology and Department of Ophthalmology, Tampere University Hospital, Tampere, Finland

Ruthild Linse Department of Dermatology and Allergology, University of Jena, Jena, Germany

Maria Loane Centre for Online Health, University of Queensland, Australia

Eric R. Menn Partners Telemedicine Inc., Boston, Massachusetts, USA

Laura Milesi Roche Pharmaceuticals, Switzerland

Karen Morse Children's Medical Services, Florida Department of Health, Florida, USA

Dagfinn Moseng Department of Dermatology and Venereology, University Hospital of Tromsø, Norway

Eliot N. Mostow Northeast Ohio University College of Medicine, Ohio, USA

Amanda Oakley Department of Dermatology, Health Waikato, Hamilton, New Zealand

Margretta A. O'Reilly Department of Dermatology, University of Utah School of Medicine, Salt Lake City, Utah, USA

Jörn Paessler Unit for Cybermedicine, Department of Clinical Social Medicine, Heidelberg Medical School, Germany

Hon S. Pak Dermatology Clinic, Wilford Hall Army Medical Center, Lackland Air Force Base, Texas, USA

Marta J. Petersen Department of Dermatology, University of Utah School of Medicine, Salt Lake City, Utah, USA

Howard Rogers Department of Pediatrics, University of Florida, USA

Jean-Hilaire Saurat Pigmented Skin Lesion Unit, Department of Dermatology, University Hospital Geneva and DHURDV Geneva, Lausanne, Switzerland

Peter Schmid-Grendelmeier Department of Dermatology, University Hospital, Zürich, Switzerland and Regional Dermatology Training Centre, Kilimanjaro Christian Medical College, Moshi, Tanzania

Hugues Talbot CSIRO, Sydney, Australia

Jörg Tittelbach Department of Dermatology and Allergology, University of Jena, Jena, Germany

Ville Voipio University of Technology, Metrology Research Institute, Helsinki, Finland

Vivian L. West Telemedicine Center, Center for Health Sciences Communication, Brody School of Medicine at East Carolina University, Greenville, North Carolina, USA

Richard W. Whitehouse Department of Diagnostic Radiology, Manchester Royal Infirmary, Manchester, UK

J. M. Whitworth Department of Pediatrics, University of Florida, Florida, USA

Betsy Wood Unit for Special Technologies, Children's Medical Services, Florida Department of Health, Florida, USA

Richard Wootton Centre for Online Health, University of Queensland, Australia

Gabriel Yihune Unit for Cybermedicine, Department of Clinical Social Medicine, Heidelberg Medical School, Germany

Foreword

Teledermatology is, without doubt, one of the most useful, rewarding and frustrating telehealth applications. There is no question about its potential utility. Skin diseases are extraordinarily common, accounting for roughly 25% of all visits to medical practitioners. They are also diverse. Many skin problems are manifestations of systemic disease, and can be the first clues to the presence of debilitating or life-threatening conditions. Others are important for their role in human suffering by causing pain, itching or disfiguration. Nearly all skin problems come with psychological costs – 'Is it serious?' 'I look terrible.' 'Is it contagious?' Anything that can help in the accurate diagnosis, treatment and management of these problems should be welcomed.

There is also no question that the presence or absence of a dermatologist is a crucial component of the evaluation and management process for any serious skin condition. Study after study has shown that dermatologists are substantially more skilled than non-dermatologists in the diagnosis of skin problems. This should hardly be a surprise. One study found that the average physician receives fewer than 40 hours of dermatology training by the end of medical school and residency. (I myself had to choose between rotating through radiology or dermatology in medical school. I picked radiology . . .) The trick then is getting a dermatologist to look at the right skin problem at the right time when no dermatologist happens to be handy. This is what teledermatology is all about.

When it all comes together, teledermatology can be very rewarding. Anyone who has done it for a little while will have their own stories to tell. One story is about the 50-year-old white female who had been treated for a thumb lesion for 18 months, only to have it correctly diagnosed remotely as a melanoma. Another story is about the 42-year-old aircraft mechanic who lived in a remote community and was about to go on disability for a 30-year blistering disorder that had been unresponsive to treatment. He was diagnosed with eczema herpeticum using store-and-forward teledermatology, and has since been symptom-free on antiviral drugs. And then there is my favourite – the 14-year-old son of a rural physician who after three years had his abdominal rash diagnosed from a single image. It was an allergic contact dermatitis to the nickel in his trouser fastener. He was cured by placing a piece of duck tape over the offending pant stud. (Yet another excellent use for duck tape.)

None of these diagnoses would have been made for years, if ever, had teledermatology not been used to make the connection. The fact is that millions of people, even in industrialized countries, do not have ready access to a dermatologist. This is a direct result of a permanent and unremediable fact of life – specialists will always tend to cluster in large metropolitan areas. Anyone wishing to see them in person will have to travel. Those who cannot or will not travel for their health care will have to suffer or make use of telehealth instead. Given the high time and opportunity cost of hauling specialists over hill and dale, there are simply no alternatives.

So where's the frustration? It can be found in nearly every aspect of a new way of conducting healthcare transactions. Teledermatology is no exception, and also adds a few twists that are missing in other clinical telehealth applications.

One important problem lies in sorting out what constitutes a 'gold standard' for diagnosis and treatment in dermatology. People continually ask whether teledermatology is accurate and reliable for the purposes of clinical diagnosis and management, but in many cases we have no idea whether our face-to-face assessment of a case is truly correct. It is neither appropriate nor best practice to biopsy every skin lesion, yet the alternative is often to live with a best guess or differential diagnosis. As a result, a dozen different ways have been tried to answer the original question, usually by comparing the differential diagnosis or the order in which the diagnoses are listed by remote and in-person physicians. Unfortunately these evaluations are generally unable to take into account the various degrees of diagnostic difficulty which may be encountered, the 'value' of making a given diagnosis and many other factors. There may never be a satisfactory solution to this problem for those who wish to remain teledermatology sceptics, but that does not necessarily mean that the technique is any less valuable as a healthcare tool.

Another problem encountered in teledermatology practice is the difficulty of valuing the care provided. As an almost purely outpatient specialty that rarely deals in disorders that are fatal because of their cutaneous manifestations, dermatology tends to be associated with relatively low reimbursement schedules. This makes the economics of teledermatology more difficult than those of teleradiology, orthopaedics or a number of other specialties. The problem of value is most difficult to assess in health systems which do not allow patients to pay out-of-pocket for specific services, since a relatively trivial problem for society in general may be a valuable malady to a specific individual. The lack of free market economics in most healthcare systems is socially accepted, but makes it more difficult for us to measure teledermatology's overall economic value.

Finally, it is quite frustrating that the pace of deployment of telehealth in general and teledermatology in particular continues to be slow everywhere in the world. This can be attributed to many factors, including technological complexity, inadequate telecommunications services, low awareness, economic, social and other causes.

All this said, probably one of the best long-term remedies to teledermatology frustration is this book itself. If I were starting work in this field today, then this book is surely where I'd begin. The best way to learn about telehealth is to read all you can, and then meet and talk with those working in the particular clinical application of interest. A great deal of telemedicine knowledge is still consigned to the 'grey literature' consisting of notes, messages, informal articles, anecdotes, descriptions and conversations. It can be difficult to become oriented. Until now, there has not been a single book that covers most of the areas of interest to the teledermatology practitioner. I am pleased to say that this book largely fills that gap. Newcomers to telehealth and teledermatology will welcome the information provided herein as an introduction. Meanwhile, 'old timers' and those of us trying desperately to keep a hand (or even finger!) in the field will be glad at last to have a reference worthy of the name.

The best way to use this book is to absorb it gradually. If you can, read one chapter, let it sink in, and then read another. Given the diverse nature of the content it is not particularly important that the chapters are read sequentially. Above all, keep an open mind with respect to everything that you see and hear in this field. Teledermatology is far from its ultimate place in medical practice, and there is much work and learning still to be done. Your results will be needed for the second edition.

Douglas A. Perednia
Portland, Oregon, 2001

Preface

This is the third book in the Royal Society of Medicine's telemedicine series. Its predecessors are:

The Legal and Ethical Aspects of Telemedicine, BA Stanberry, 1998
Introduction to Telemedicine, R Wootton and J Craig (eds), 1999

The present volume describes how telemedicine applies to dermatology. It does not represent the definitive textbook on the subject, which is unlikely to be written for some years yet, because teledermatology is an evolving field and its parameters remain largely undefined. Instead, the book represents the collective experience of practitioners in different parts of the world practising a wide range of teledermatology applications. We think that anyone involved in telemedicine will find the material interesting because much of it is relevant to other applications than simply teledermatology.

The aim of the book is principally to permit those who are involved in dermatology to begin to assess how telemedicine might be applied to their working practice. Clinicians should find it particularly useful, of course, but many chapters are also of relevance to health service managers, imaging and information technology staff.

The book is an eclectic collection of essays. Contributors have come from Europe, North America, Asia and Australasia, and work in a variety of medical, technical and administrative specialties. The majority are practising dermatologists with substantial practical experience of telemedicine and health informatics.

The book is divided into four sections:

1. An introductory section dealing with background matters, with an emphasis on digital imaging.
2. A section describing the global experience of teledermatology consultations of various forms.
3. A section concerning distance education in dermatology, for the patient, the doctor and the student.
4. A final section about techniques which look promising for the future, but which are currently experimental. This includes the development of standards in teledermatology, a topic that is still in its infancy in telemedicine generally.

We hope you enjoy reading it.

Richard Wootton
Brisbane, Australia
Amanda Oakley
Hamilton, New Zealand

November 2001

Section 1: Background and Technical Matters

▶ 1

Introduction

Amanda Oakley and Richard Wootton

What is telemedicine?

In the introductory book in this series, telemedicine was defined as the delivery of health care and the exchange of health care information across distances.[1] In general terms, telemedicine is access to specialist knowledge by means of telecommunications and information technology. Teledermatology is a subspecialty of telemedicine. The term encompasses consultations between a patient with a skin disease (and/or the primary healthcare provider) and a dermatologist for diagnosis and management advice. It also covers dermatological education for health professionals and for consumers.

How is telemedicine performed?

'Access to specialist knowledge' implies that a telemedicine interaction occurs between an information provider and a client. The fundamental components of a telemedicine system required to bring about this interaction comprise:

1. a means of information capture
2. a means of information transport
3. a means of information display.

The interaction is almost always a two-way process, i.e. having conveyed the information to an expert, the referring doctor needs to know what the expert's opinion is.

The communication process (e.g. information capture/transmission/display and the reply), i.e. the telemedicine interaction, can be done either in real-time, or by pre-recorded means (often called 'store-and-forward'). In real-time teledermatology, at least two individuals are communicating synchronously. This may be during a videoconference or a simple telephone call. Store-and-forward teledermatology refers to the transfer of pre-recorded information in a time-independent fashion. Many teledermatology episodes include video or still images of the skin condition under discussion.

What equipment is required for teledermatology?

Teledermatology can be practised almost anywhere given the right equipment. Patients in private residences, rest homes, ships, aeroplanes, battlefields, up mountains or in Antarctica can access specialist expertise when required. Satellite systems enable access from the most remote locations on the planet, while DSL (digital subscriber line) connections enable fast downloads via the ordinary telephone system. The teledermatology systems described in this book use the telephone network, digital networks (e.g. ISDN, integrated services digital network), T1 leased lines, LANs (local area networks), GSM (global system for mobile communications) mobile phones, microwave links, ATM (asynchronous transfer mode) on fibreoptic cables and the Internet.

Fast, sophisticated and automated telemedicine is now possible, employing intuitive interfaces and powerful information management systems. However, quite simple systems are also described in these pages and have proved effective aids to dermatological practice.

The use of teledermatology has the potential to improve the care of the patient, particularly if there are low referral rates to a specialist, as in rural or remote areas or when the patient is institutionalized.[2]

What is in the literature?

There are a small but increasing number of publications on the subject of teledermatology. A PubMed search (http://www.ncbi.nlm.nih.gov/entrez/ [last checked 26 July 2001]) carried out in June 2001 with the keyword 'teledermatology' in the title field listed 55 papers. The first was published in 1995.[3] Twenty papers were published after January 2000. The keyword 'telemedicine' listed 1345 papers since 1974. Useful review articles have recently been published in British,[4] American[5] and Australasian[6] dermatology journals.

Essential components of clinical teledermatology

Dermatologists were early adopters of telemedicine because their consultations are primarily about taking a careful history and visual inspection – perfectly possible if the history and images contain all the clues to diagnosis and management. The method of communication may use conventional or advanced forms of technology.

Requirements for history

In order to make a diagnosis, certain demographic details are required, including the patient's age, sex, ethnicity and geographic residence. The referral should outline the suspected diagnosis, location/distribution of the lesion/eruption, duration, size, features, aggravating and relieving factors, and any previous treatment. General medical information should include significant concurrent and past health problems, prescribed and non-prescribed medications and allergies, and the family history. Results of investigations such as mycology and skin biopsy may be important. In addition, the reason for referral should be indicated. The dermatologist should be able to obtain further information if required.

The standard referral from a general practitioner to a dermatology clinic rarely includes all relevant information. By further interrogation – whether face to face, by telephone or by videoconference – an experienced dermatologist can frequently make a diagnosis without requiring an examination. Although there has yet to be a published study of the relative importance of history compared with images in teledermatology, diagnostic accuracy appears adequate even when image quality is poor. Successful interactive teledermatology systems described in this book include those depending on relatively low bandwidth communication (basic rate ISDN lines) as well as those based on more expensive broadband communication (e.g. T1 leased lines).

Store-and-forward teledermatology systems frequently require the referring practitioner to complete standardized templates in order to reduce error due to inadequate data. The information can then be stored in a database for retrieval later. Teledermatology consultations between experts assume that a good history has been taken, so that referrals may be less formal, but this reduces the ability to retrieve data later. A variety of store-and-forward teledermatology techniques are described in this book.

Requirements for images

Inappropriate images may result in no diagnosis or a wrong diagnosis being made during a teledermatology session. As yet there are no standards for photographic technique and referring practitioners receive little or no training in clinical photography.[7] Modern digital cameras are easy to use and attention to detail can result in excellent images of skin diseases. Three chapters of the book are devoted to images, underlining their importance to the dermatologist. Diagnosis may require a general view to show the distribution/location of the skin problem (the 'scout image') as well as close-up views for morphological detail, with plain background, good lighting, correct exposure and sharp focus. Images taken with a digital camera are generally of higher quality than snapshots of video images, but the latter may be more informative if taken at the direction of the specialist. For example, a general practitioner may not realize that correct diagnosis of a rash on the hand may require a view of the patient's feet. Images taken at high resolution initially should remain of diagnostic quality after correction of brightness/contrast, magnification, cropping and compression to reduce file sizes and speed up file transfers.

Requirements for consultation

Whether using interactive or store-and-forward teledermatology, it is essential to ensure privacy, security of data and technology that is accurate, reliable and simple to use. In general, the patient's express informed consent is necessary, particularly if identifiable information such as a recognizable photograph is transferred. It is of course worth keeping a sense of perspective, as case presentations are often held in a closed academic setting without the knowledge of the subject of the discussion.

Teledermatology protocols should be carefully prepared and followed to protect the patient. During a video session, the patient needs someone to explain the process beforehand and to facilitate the consultation, in effect acting as the consultant's hands and the patient's ears. The personnel involved should be adequately trained, but they do not have to be medical practitioners; remote consultations involving nurses and other non-medically qualified health workers are described in the book.

Not all teledermatology consultations will complete a healthcare episode. Ideally, health systems should be able to back up teledermatology with face-to-face consultations to verify diagnosis and to perform diagnostic tests or surgical treatment. However this may be impractical; for example when the patient is on a battlefield, in the Antarctic or in a space vehicle.

Suitable cases for teledermatology

Each practising teledermatologist is likely to have his or her list of preferred clinical presentations. Some of these are discussed elsewhere in the book. Patients suitable for real-time teledermatology, where interactive discussion is necessary (such as follow-up during phototherapy as described in Chapter 6), may have quite different characteristics from those suitable for store-and-forward consultation (such as wound care as described in Chapter 10).

Unsuitable cases for teledermatology

Which cases are unsuitable for teledermatology may depend on the technology being used. It may be possible to diagnose melanoma at a distance if the consultant is supplied with digital dermoscopic images (as described in Chapter 18), but it would be unwise to do so in other circumstances. Privacy issues may limit the examination of genital rashes, and it may not be possible to obtain an image of adequate quality of a small child's skin problem.

Teledermatology for education

There has been a vast increase in the quantity of health information over the last few years, and much of it is accessible to health consumers as well as experts. By use of the Internet, dermatologists can keep up with the latest medical advances, consult online textbooks and share clinical problems with other experts. Increasing numbers of hospital departments and universities arrange regular interactive tutorials and case discussions by videoconference.

Patients can be directed to reliable online information about hospital facilities, their disease and its management, research trials and support groups. This book includes chapters about a teledermatology teaching programme for medical students, an impressive dermatology online atlas, and patient information on the Internet.

Patient self-help

There is evidence that patients are themselves using the Internet to seek further information or advice regarding their illness. Increasingly patients search databases themselves, or send email messages to physicians for advice.[8] Many patients who sent unsolicited email messages for advice to a dermatology department expressed frustration or lack of trust in their own physician or healthcare service; some patients were embarrassed or wanted to remain anonymous yet seek expert advice. Dealing with such unsolicited messages poses a number of problems, including privacy, confidentiality, security and medicolegal issues.[8] Furthermore, patients getting advice via the Internet may increase their level of anxiety or reach spurious conclusions leading to poor outcome. There is, however, evidence that patients can obtain relevant advice, in a way in which they will understand, by accessing sites such as the patient information leaflets provided by the American Academy of Dermatology (AAD) website.[8] As an indication of the public interest in such sites the AAD website received 800 000 'hits' from approximately 86 000 users in July 1998.[9]

Legal aspects of teledermatology

Dermatologists have expressed concerns that teledermatology is risky in a medicolegal sense.[10] The legal implications of telemedicine have been extensively debated and are not specific to dermatology. Most legal and ethical issues are the same as those of medicine in general. Security of data, confidentiality and risk must be considered. The reader is referred to reviews by Stanberry[11] and Jacobson and Selvin.[12]

Cross-boundary consultations have given rise to particular concern because a licence to practice medicine is limited to a specific jurisdiction. In the USA, many consider that statutes limiting medical licensure to individual states are outdated.[13] Several examples of international teledermatology consultation are described in this book; a system of universal licensure may therefore need to be developed. The American Academy of Dermatology has proposed minimum standards for credentialing (as well as for clinical, technical and administrative matters) in its Position Statement on Telemedicine, approved in December 1999.[14] See Chapter 16 for further details.

The current scene

Despite the lack of published literature, teledermatology consultations have been reported by many multispecialty telemedicine programmes to be particularly successful, as outlined by Grigsby and Brown in their survey of teledermatology in the USA (see Chapter 5). Diagnostic accuracy seems acceptable. Patients and at least some doctors are satisfied.

The Telemedicine Information Exchange (TIE) (http://tie.telemed.org/ [last checked 26 July 2001]) lists 36 programmes (out of 256 on the database) where dermatology is the top-ranked application. These are mainly in the USA, as this is the TIE's primary coverage area, but Swedish, South African, Canadian, Japanese and British interactive and still image services are also listed.

International collaboration

Evidence for the growth of interest in teledermatology is shown by the emergence of international teledermatology organizations, which include the European Confederation of Telemedical Organizations in Dermatology (ECTODerm) (http://www.ectoderm.org/ [last checked 26 July 2001]), the Internet Dermatology Society (http://www.telemedicine.org/ids.htm [last checked 26 July 2001]), the International Society for Skin Imaging (http://www.issi.de/ [last checked 26 July 2001]) and the KSYOS Research Foundation (http://www.ksyos.nl/ [last checked 26 July 2001]). The electronic mailing list rxderm-l@ucdavis.edu has about nine hundred dermatologist members (Professor Art Huntley, personal communication) practising in many different countries. It has proved an effective and educational discussion forum for clinical dermatology, sometimes posting dozens of messages each day.

The development of low-cost, fast and reliable data communication has resulted in numerous effective international collaborations, including this book.

Conclusion

Teledermatology can be used in many different ways to improve the delivery of dermatological care. The experience reported in this book demonstrates that there is no single 'correct answer' to any given problem – often a number of different solutions are possible. We suggest that you read the work reported in this book and benefit from the experience of others.

References

1 Wootton R, Craig J, eds. *Introduction to Telemedicine*. London: Royal Society of Medicine Press, 1999.
2 Perednia DA, Wallace J, Morrisey M, et al. The effect of a teledermatology program on rural referral patterns to dermatologists and the management of skin disease. *Medinfo* 1998;**91**:290–293.
3 Perednia DA, Brown NA. Teledermatology: one application of telemedicine. *Bulletin of the Medical Library Association* 1995;**83**:42–47.
4 Eedy DJ, Wootton R. Teledermatology: a review. *British Journal of Dermatology* 2001;**144**:696–707.
5 Whited JD. Teledermatology: current status and future directions. *American Journal of Clinical Dermatology* 2001;**2**:59–64.
6 Lim AC, Egerton IB, Shumack SP. Australian teledermatology: the patient, the doctor and their government. *Australasian Journal of Dermatology* 2000;**41**:8–13.
7 Vidmar DA. Plea for standardization in teledermatology: a worm's eye view. *Telemedicine Journal* 1997;**3**:173–178.
8 Eysenbach G, Diepgen TL. Patients looking for information on the Internet and seeking teleadvice: motivation, expectations, and misconceptions as expressed in e-mails sent to physicians. *Archives of Dermatology* 1999;**135**:151–156.

9   Huntley AC. The need to know – patients, e-mail, and the internet. *Archives of Dermatology* 1999;**135**:198–199.

10   Stanberry B. Telemedicine: barriers and opportunities in the 21st century. *Journal of Internal Medicine* 2000;**247**:615–628.

11   Stanberry B. *The Legal and Ethical Aspects of Telemedicine.* London: Royal Society of Medicine Press, 1999.

12   Jacobson PD, Selvin E. Licensing telemedicine: the need for a national system. *Telemedicine Journal and E-health* 2000;**6**:429–439.

13   Perednia DA. Fear, loathing, dermatology, and telemedicine. *Archives of Dermatology* 1997;**133**:151–155.

14   Telemedicine Task Force, American Academy of Dermatology. Position Statement on Telemedicine, 2000 (http://www.aad.org/Members/telemedicine.html available only to members of the American Academy of Dermatology).

▶2
Digital Imaging

Richard W. Whitehouse

Introduction

A recent survey related to the introduction of teledermatology found that 50% of general practitioners felt that they were complete novices with computers.[1] The development of teledermatology is still in its early stages,[2] with published studies based on the use of a variety of commercially available equipment.[3,4] This chapter describes the basics of digital imaging from that perspective. Detailed descriptions of the technology and software advances in digital imaging and digital image processing are beyond the scope of this chapter – up-to-date textbooks covering these aspects are available.[5,6]

A digital image is the display of a set of electronically stored numbers as a matrix of colours on a display unit (such as a computer monitor). Digitization of an image is consequently the process of converting a picture into a matrix of numbers representing colour values, which can be stored electronically and then redisplayed on appropriate equipment. The matrix is a map of blocks, called pixels, each of which has a single colour value. It is usual (though not strictly necessary) for pixels to be square and arrayed in aligned rows and columns so that each can be located by its Cartesian co-ordinates. Digital images are consequently displayed as maps of individually localized pixels, each with its own colour value (often known as 'bit-maps'; see Figure 2.1). The digital image data may be stored on some electronic medium as a 'bit-map file' but can also be stored in other computer file formats.

Bits and Bytes

Computer information is represented internally as binary numbers, i.e. those using only zeros or ones. This is an electronic requirement so that simple on/off switches can be used to represent the numbers. A single switch can represent 0 or 1 (off or on), whilst two switches can represent values between 0 and 3, i.e. 0 (both off), 1 (switch 1 on, switch 2 off), 2 (switch 1 off, switch 2 on) or 3 (both switches on). For larger numbers, more switches are used, the first counting in 1's, the second in 2's the third in 4's, the fourth in 8's and so on. In computer parlance, each switch carries one 'bit' of data. As this is a very small information storage quantity, it is usual for data capacity to be measured in 'Bytes', each Byte being composed of 8 bits. Thus a Byte can store 256 values including zero (0–255). This is a common source of confusion when data-

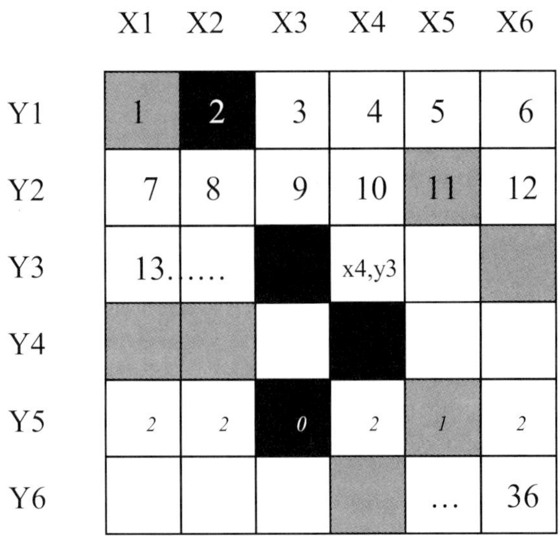

	X1	X2	X3	X4	X5	X6
Y1	1	2	3	4	5	6
Y2	7	8	9	10	11	12
Y3	13.	....		x4,y3		
Y4						
Y5	2	2	0	2	1	2
Y6					...	36

Fig. 2.1. To illustrate the digital representation of an image, a simple greyscale image is shown, consisting of 36 square pixels in a 6 × 6 matrix, containing black, white and grey pixels. To locate each pixel, the x direction is across the image and the y direction is down, from the top left corner (a true Cartesian reference system would give this y direction a negative value, but it is conventional to read from the top left corner, across and downwards, so that image coordinates are positive from the top left corner). The first two rows of pixels have been enumerated, thus for example, pixel number 9 is located at X3, Y2. Pixel 16 has been labelled by its coordinate location. In row 5 (Y5), the pixels have been labelled with their colour values, 0 = black, 1 = grey and 2 = white. It is not necessary to digitally encode each coordinate location. Identifying the image as a 6 × 6 matrix, a series of 36 numbers for each colour value in turn will digitize this image – the first two lines would code as 1,0,2,2,2,2,2,2,2,2,1,2. (This can be compressed to 1,0,8 × 2,1,2 – producing a method of lossless data compression.)

transmission speeds are discussed. Care should be taken when a speed is described as '56 kbps' – does this mean 56 kbit/s or 56 kByte/s?

Another potential source of confusion are the terms kiloByte and megaByte, which are used for describing larger data-storage capacities. Strictly, these remain in the binary numbers system, so kiloByte actually means 2^{10} (1024) Bytes, not 1000 Bytes, and megaByte means 2^{20} (1048 576) Bytes, not 1000000.

Black and white images, text files and vector graphics

Images composed of only black or white pixels are stored as bit-maps at one bit per pixel. Such images may be 'line drawings' such as cartoons, composed only of black lines on a white background. Shades of grey can also be represented by a method analogous to that used for the printed images in newspapers, where shades of grey are represented by black dots of different sizes and/or packing densities. This may not seem very relevant to dermatological images, but it is important to the understanding of the techniques used in many colour printers. Black text on a white background could be stored as a 1 bit per pixel bit-map, but it is much more efficient to code each character separately (at 1 Byte per character) and save these codes as a 'text file'. The size, style, pitch, layout and other parameters relevant to a text document can then be separately encoded and varied independently of the text characters. An analogous method can be applied to images comprised of lines – a bit-map requires a list of all the pixels in the image, but a line can be described by its vectors. The position of the line endpoints, its thickness and a formula describing its curvature are all that is necessary. These 'vector graphics' files can be considerably smaller than equivalent bit-map files and can also be infinitely rescaled to give magnified images that still have smooth edges. This contrasts with magnified bit-map images, which simply show the individual pixels (Fig. 2.2). Colour vector graphics files use uniform colours to fill in between the lines, again requiring less data storage. Vector graphics files are not appropriate for very heterogeneous colour images such as those produced by digital cameras.

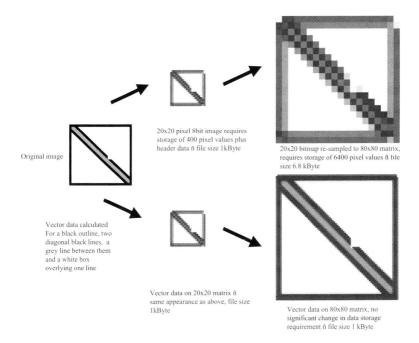

Original image

20x20 pixel 8bit image requires storage of 400 pixel values plus header data ñ file size 1kByte

20x20 bitmap re-sampled to 80x80 matrix, requires storage of 6400 pixel values ñ file size 6.8 kByte

Vector data calculated For a black outline, two diagonal black lines, a grey line between them and a white box overlying one line

Vector data on 20x20 matrix ñ same appearance as above, file size 1kByte

Vector data on 80x80 matrix, no significant change in data storage requirement ñ file size 1 kByte

Fig. 2.2. Comparisons of vector and bit-map representations of a simple line image. The top row of images demonstrates the increase in file size that occurs when a bit-map is resampled to a larger matrix. Image smoothing can be performed during resampling without further increase in file size but reacquisition from the original image at the higher matrix size would be required to reproduce the improved resolution of the vector image. The lower row of images are reproduced from one vector file at the same pixel resolutions as the bit-maps above.

Greyscale images

For greyscale images, only shades of grey need to be recorded. As the human eye can distinguish about 250 different shades of grey between pure white and pure black, the pixel values of greyscale images can be conveniently stored at 8 bits (1 Byte) per pixel, allowing 256 shades. Consequently an uncompressed 8-bit greyscale bit-map image file has approximately as many Bytes as there are pixels in the image. This is approximate because image files contain additional data, such as the image file name and other data related to the file, for example the date and time it was generated. Greyscale images with larger numbers of shades of grey are routinely used in medicine and some photographic applications. Computed tomography and magnetic resonance images are usually 12-bit images, with 4096 shades of grey, whilst 16-bit greyscale images with over 65 500 shades of grey are occasionally used in photography. A 16-bit greyscale image can be converted into an 8-bit greyscale image, thus producing an image file only half the size, and an image that looks identical to the eye. However, if the image is manipulated (e.g. by changing the contrast or brightness, or edge enhancement), then the 8-bit image will quickly begin to show visible steps between the fewer remaining shades of grey. The 16-bit image, on the other hand, will retain smooth gradations generated from shades of grey that were too close together to be distinguished in the original 16-bit image file. Thus the more shades of grey in the original dataset, the more image manipulation is possible before an unacceptably degraded image results.

Colour images

For colour images, the data can be stored as a single number per pixel, each number representing a different colour from a 'palette' of available colours. Alternatively, several separate numbers can be stored for each pixel, one for each 'colour channel'. The commonest colour image formats use three colour channels: red, green and blue (RGB). Different combinations of brightness of each of these colours are used to reproduce all visible colours. With 256 possible steps for each colour channel, a typical colour bit-map will have three 8-bit channels for each pixel (giving a 24-bit colour image) and consequently 3 Bytes per pixel. This gives 2^{24} (approximately 16.8 million) possible colours.

The 'single number' per pixel colour files may have a fixed palette of available colours. An 8-bit fixed palette colour image will have 256 colours available. An image composed of more colours, or colours not represented in this palette, will, when converted to that file format, have those colours changed to the nearest available colour in the palette, with consequent degradation of the image. Many images are, however, composed of several shades of a similar colour, with many other colours not present at all – a clinical photograph of a skin rash will have many pixels of skin tone, some redder than others (i.e. the rash), but will probably have no large areas of blue or green (particularly if a single colour or white background was used when the photograph was taken). Modern software for producing 8-bit colour images can prepare a 'custom palette' which identifies the predominant colours in the image and saves a copy of this palette with the image file. Even so, an 8-bit colour file is severely limited in the colours that can be represented. However, a 16-bit colour image (often called 'high colour') with a customized palette of 65 000 colours, usually looks indistinguishable from a 24-bit colour image, whilst being 33% smaller. Because of the reduced file size, it can be processed and transmitted more quickly. High colour is in practice most commonly used for driving the image display of the computer, rather than saving the image file.

Image size, shape and resolution

The size of a digital image can be expressed in different ways. The most common is the number of pixels along the x and y axes of the image because this defines both the number of pixels in the entire image (the product of these numbers) and the shape of the rectangle in which they lie (the aspect ratio). Images may be expected to be a particular size when viewed, consequently image file headers contain data on the pixel resolution required to achieve these dimensions. For example an image of 1000 by 750 pixels which is expected to be 4 by 3 inches in size has a resolution of 250 pixels per inch. When displayed on a computer monitor, software programs ignore the resolution in pixels per inch and initially display digital images using a 1 : 1 relationship between the image pixels and the monitor pixels. Consequently, a monitor with a display resolution of 1024×768 pixels will display an image of 1000×750 pixels as almost completely filling the screen (the edges of the image may be obscured by 'toolbars' and borders used by the software program).

When printed, however, the default settings for most software and printers is to print the image to the size specified by the header, which may not be appropriate for the printer. As above, an image of 1000×750 pixels with a resolution of 250 pixels per inch would print as an image of 4×3 inches. However, if the resolution in the file header were set to 1000 pixels per inch it would print at a size of 1×0.75 inches, with the pixel data averaged to suit the printer resolution (e.g. 72 lines per inch). Furthermore, the printed image would have only 72 by 54 (3888) printer pixels in it. To suit the printer resolution, the image would have to be printed at 72 pixels per inch and would measure 13.9×10.4 inches. The resolution of an image file in pixels per inch can be changed by changing the data in the file header, with no change to the actual image data.

In order to decide what image size and shape parameters are appropriate for a teledermatology system, the available hardware and its intended use should be considered beforehand. As computer-related devices are constantly under development any description of the current state of the art quickly becomes out of date, but extrapolation from the following observations should be helpful. The numbers of pixels per image in digital cameras costing under £1000 (US$1500) has increased from about 1.5 million pixels to 3.3 million pixels (2100×1575 pixels) over a two-year period. Most digital cameras use an aspect ratio of 4 : 3, chosen because it is equal to that of computer monitors. Some digital cameras use an aspect ratio of

3 : 2, corresponding to that of 35-mm film. Computer monitors have variable display resolutions but in order for text, program tool bars and icons to remain legible it is not usual to exceed 1024×768 pixels on 15-inch monitors, 1280×1024 on 19-inch monitors and 1600×1200 on 21-inch monitors, i.e. the best 'consumer' digital cameras exceed the display resolution of most popular monitors by up to two times in linear dimensions. What screen and image resolution is required for adequate diagnosis is under investigation, with image resolutions of 1490×1000 pixels not being significantly better than 720×500 pixels in one study.[7] Video cameras produce still images of even lower resolution (typically 640×480 pixels or less), and have not been compared directly with still digital cameras. However, a teledermatology study comparing different video cameras showed that better quality cameras produced better results.[8]

Computer monitors

The difference between a fixed and a customized colour palette is just as important for the computer display as it is for the image file. In a computer, the image data are sent to the monitor via a 'graphics card'. The graphics card requires its own memory, with sufficient space to store the colour data for all the pixels in the display. Consequently a monitor running at SVGA resolution (800×600 pixels) has 480 000 pixels which will require 1.4 MBytes of video memory for 24-bit colour. Older graphics cards running at 4 bits (16 colours), 8 bits (256 colours) or 16 bits (65 000 colours) used fixed palettes but newer cards not only have considerably more memory but can also use customized palettes, changing the palette to suit the image being displayed. In practice a new computer should have a graphics card specified which is capable of driving the monitor at its highest resolution in full (24-bit) colour.

If it is intended to use the monitor at its highest resolution routinely, then a further consideration is the 'refresh rate' of the monitor, which is often lower at high resolution. Monitors which refresh the screen image less than 60 times per second (60 Hz) will produce an image with visible flicker which rapidly becomes tiring to view.

Printers

If 'hard copy' prints of digital images are required, then further complications ensue. Colour printers can be divided into two broad categories – the cheapest and most widely available are those that fill each image pixel with small dots of fixed density colour, the darker shades of each colour being produced by placing more dots within the pixel boundaries (ink-jet printers use this method). This is the same idea as that used to create greyscale images from black and white 1-bit images (see above). The other type of printer homogeneously fills each pixel with different thicknesses of ink to create each colour (dye sublimation printers use this method).

The resolution of ink-jet printers is commonly stated in 'dots per inch', which relates to the number of very small dots of fixed density that the ink-jet can generate.

As between none and 255 dots of colour are required to cover the range of colour densities needed to fully represent the image data in an 8-bit colour channel, it requires a matrix of 16×16 dots to reproduce all the possible shades for a single colour channel. The other colour channels use separate ink nozzles which spray the ink on to the same pixel so no more area is required. Consequently an ink-jet printer with a 'resolution' of 1440 dots per inch will reproduce full colour images at a resolution of 90 pixels per inch (just as care needs to be taken to distinguish bits from Bytes, so too for dots and pixels per inch).

Dye sublimation printers commonly have resolutions of 150 or 300 pixels per inch (sometimes referred to as lines per inch to distinguish it from dots per inch), giving both a higher true resolution and a very smooth colour within each pixel. This produces a high-quality hard-copy image, of 'near photographic quality'. However, dye sublimation or equivalent printers are expensive, both for the hardware and the inks.

Colour inks are not as stable as black ink and some colours are more stable than others. Colour printing is performed with secondary colour inks (Cyan, Magenta, Yellow and blacK) rather than primary colour inks (Red, Green and Blue), because an ink works by removing the unwanted colours from the light reflected from it (i.e. it is a subtractive process), whilst monitor screens produce colours by adding light of the appropriate colour. In addition, secondary colour inks are more stable. Whereas mixing red, green and blue inks together produces a reasonable black, mixing cyan, magenta and yellow is less successful, so that a true black ink colour is necessary. When printing an RGB colour image file, the computer software automatically recodes the image data into the appropriate CMYK values to send to the printer. The image data can be stored as a CMYK file but the additional black channel increases the data storage requirement by 33% with no increase in the number of colours in the image. Consequently 32-bit CMYK image files may be of interest to colour printers but are not appropriate to teledermatologists.

'Hard-copy' prints of colour images are necessarily limited in the range of colours they can display. The 'whitest white' in the image is determined by the colour of the paper on which the image is printed and the brightness and colour of the illumination, whilst the darkest black is determined by the ink. As the image is seen by courtesy of the light reflected from it, and even black ink will reflect to a significant degree, the ratio of brightest white to darkest black on a print is invariably less than 100 and may be less than 10. By contrast, images seen by transmitted light (e.g. transparencies) or by generated light (e.g. computer monitors) can have far greater ranges of brightness (and colour). The vibrancy of such images is part of their appeal.

Image complexity, file size and compression

One of the principal requirements of teledermatology is the ability to transfer images promptly to other sites for interpretation by a dermatologist. The most convenient way to do this is through the telephone network. The speed of data transmission by telephone wires is limited and although faster transmission speeds can be achieved by a variety of methods, these cost more. Consequently the smaller the image file size for transmission by whatever method, the quicker and more cheaply it can be moved around. Although some techniques that can reduce image file size have been described already (using 8-bit or 16-bit colour with optimized palettes), the reduction in file size from 24-bit colour is relatively modest and degradation of image quality may occur.

Data compression methods perform mathematical manipulations on the image file data to produce encoded data which occupy less storage space but from which the image data can be reconstructed for display. Such data manipulation can be divided into two types, 'lossless' and 'lossy'. Lossless compression means that the reconstructed image data will be identical to the original image data, whilst lossy compression means that some changes will have been introduced into the data by the compression calculations so that the reconstructed data will not be quite the same as the original.

Before further discussion of image compression, there are other considerations of image optimization that may result in smaller image file sizes. Most important of these is the number of pixels in the image. If there is no requirement to magnify regions of the image for closer inspection, then there is little point in having an image that exceeds (in pixels) the size of the display screen being used by the dermatologist. An image of 2048×1536 pixels has twice the number of pixels along each edge of the image than a 1024×768 display but has four times as many pixels and its file size is consequently four times greater than necessary for the identical image appearances on the display. If only a small region of the image is required at higher magnification then two images, both of 1024×768 pixels, one of the whole image and the other of the magnified region, will result in a pair of images with half the total file size of the original. Images should in any case be routinely cropped to remove all unnecessary edge data. The reduction in file size is directly proportional to the reduction in image area.

Image complexity is of direct relevance to image compression. Images that contain large regions of single colour will compress to significantly smaller files using either lossy or lossless compression algorithms. Consequently clinical photographs should be taken against a uniformly illuminated single colour background (Fig. 2.3). A mid grey background may be best to assist the camera in selecting appropriate exposure factors and to allow the easy identification of any unwanted colour cast in the resultant image. For close-up photographs of small lesions, a mid grey card with a central hole is a useful frame for the same reason. An extension of this 'image simplification' would be to replace all parts of an image that were unnecessary with a uniform colour fill before compression for transmission (Fig. 2.3c). A more complex variation of this idea would be to use lossless compression for the important parts of an image and lossy higher compression for the rest.[9]

Digital cameras (and other digitization devices) introduce some random variation into the image that was not present in the original scene (image noise). Image noise is complex in structure and consequently contributes significantly to both overall image complexity and compressed image file size. Noise is removed in parts of the image replaced by uniform colour fills as described above, and can also be reduced by software programs, although the latter results in some blurring of the image which

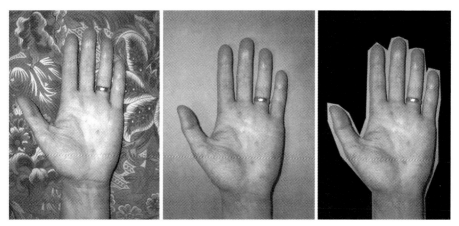

Fig. 2.3. Digital photographs of a hand with mild chronic dermatitis on different backgrounds. For each image the uncompressed file size is 4.6 MBytes. (a) Lossless compression file size 2.9 MByte, JPEG lossy compression file size 0.23 MByte. (b) Lossless compression file size 2.1 MByte, JPEG lossy compression file size 0.13 MByte. (c) Lossless compression file size 1.1 MByte, JPEG lossy compression file size 0.09 MByte.

may not be acceptable. Different digital cameras produce different levels of noise (Fig. 2.4), but there are few published comparisons. In general, image noise created by charged-coupled device (CCD) digitization is greatest in the darker parts of the image. Consequently uniform illumination of the subject to reduce areas of deep shadow and avoiding photographic underexposure will reduce image noise at the time of image acquisition.

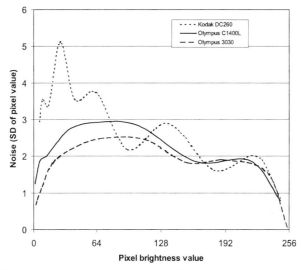

Fig. 2.4. Graph of measured image noise against image brightness for three digital cameras. Note the tendency for higher noise in darker parts of the image.

File names and compression algorithms

Computer files are commonly named by a collection of user-defined characters, followed by a dot (.), followed by a further three characters called the file extension. These latter characters, the file extension, are often used to identify the file type or format. For example, TIFF files (targeted image file format) have the extension .TIF and JPEG (joint photographics expert group) use .JPG. There are many different file formats for images, but TIFF and JPEG are two of the commonest. They also represent the two major groups as TIFF image files support lossless compression methods whilst lossy compression is used for JPEG files.

The advantage of lossless compression is obvious – the image is not corrupted in any way. However, the major limitation of lossless compression is the modest degree of compression that can usually be achieved – typically files are 30–50% of the size of the uncompressed image file. The type of medical image may influence the suitability of the compression algorithm, and the algorithm may itself be modified to improve the compression achieved for selected image types. Consequently lossless compression to 20% of the file size may be achieved by appropriate compression algorithm selection.[10–12] Lossy compression can produce much greater reductions in file size but with higher degrees of compression, greater changes in the image appearances occur. There are no hard and fast rules regarding how much compression can be used before unacceptable image degradation occurs, nor what the resultant file size at any set level of compression will be (Fig. 2.5). This is partly because of the influence of image complexity as described above but also because lossy compression algorithms can be 'optimized' to suit the type of image being compressed.[13]

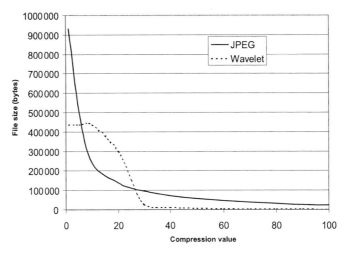

Fig. 2.5. Graph demonstrating the change in file size by choice of image compression 'level' for JPEG and Wavelet methods. The original uncompressed image file size was 2.3 MByte.

As a general rule, lossy compression resulting in image files down to 33% of the size of uncompressed images does not cause any visible image changes. Between 33% and 10% one can detect subtle differences that do not detract from the image, whilst below 5% the images become visually 'simplified'. These observations are generally supported by published studies of a variety of image types (mostly radiological).[14–16] Particularly at these higher compression levels, another lossy compression algorithm, 'wavelet compression', can produce better quality images than JPEG compression.[17–19] Wavelet compression is not currently used in digital cameras and these higher levels of compression may not be appropriate for clinical diagnostic images although they have been considered satisfactory for retinal images.[20] The relative performance of different compression algorithms varies with the degree of compression,[21] the advantage (if any) of wavelet over JPEG compression for dermatological images at lower levels of compression therefore warrants further assessment.

Programs that produce lossy compressed image files from bit-map images on the computer usually allow the level of compression to be set on a sliding scale (0–100). This scale is arbitrary and some programs use an inverted scale of image quality instead of image compression. If the original image file was a high-quality (low-compression) file and the intention is to produce a more compressed file of the same image, then when saved it will replace the original image file on the computer. At the time of saving the more highly compressed image file, the display will still show the original image file, whilst the newly saved file may be of considerably poorer quality. This will not be apparent until the file is reopened, by which time the original image will no longer exist. To avoid this potential catastrophe, always rename files when compressing them and review the new file to confirm its suitability.

The practical advantage of lossy compression over lossless compression has been questioned. As data storage capacity and data transmission speeds increase, the difference between optimized lossless compression (from two to five times compressed) and acceptable quality lossy compression (around 10 times compressed) becomes less important.[22]

Image editing software

All of the adjustments to digital images described in this chapter, including saving them as different file names and with different compression algorithms, are performed by image editing software. There are many different commercially available programs which will provide image editing functions. Some come as part of other software – for example Windows 98 (Microsoft) includes a basic image editing program, 'Microsoft Photo Editor'. Programs can be obtained from the Internet, either for continuing free use ('freeware') or for assessment for a limited period before a registration fee is due ('shareware'). More expensive and more powerful image editing programs can be purchased from software suppliers, e.g. 'Corel Photopaint'.

The image adjustments to be applied to digital clinical photographs prior to transmission should have two aims:

1. to reproduce as closely as possible the appearance of the lesion
2. to reduce the image file size as much as possible without visible image degradation.

The most important steps to achieve the first aims are photographic (e.g. lighting, focus, aperture, exposure time, zoom and colour balance) and are not the subject of this chapter. A colour cast in an image can however be corrected or reduced by appropriate image-editing software, increasing or reducing the brightness of each single colour channel in turn. Many other digital filters for image 'enhancement' are available in image-editing software. Image sharpening, softening or noise reduction may have some value in selected clinical images but the improvements obtained are subjective and excessive application of these filters will significantly degrade the image.

The manipulations to an image to reduce its file size are all described in the preceding sections. The best way to develop a consistent and acceptable final result is to become familiar with the software of your choice by experimentation over a variety of images.

Standards

The preceding sections indicate only some of the wide variety of factors under the control of the designers, developers and users of a teledermatology system using commercially available products. In order to achieve some degree of consistency and a minimum acceptable quality it is important to have internationally agreed standards for the images produced by this equipment.

In medicine generally, and radiology in particular, international standards for digital medical images have been established by the National Electrical Manufacturers Association (NEMA), referred to as the Digital Imaging Communication in Medicine (DICOM) standards. Compliance with DICOM standards goes some way to ensuring that medical images produced by one manufacturer's equipment can be used on equipment from another manufacturer (although an additional electronic interface may be needed).

The DICOM standards have been developed by working groups, one of which is particularly relevant to teledermatology: the WG 19 (Dermatologic Standards) group has been established to extend the DICOM standard with respect to standards for dermatological imaging and digital communications. The Secretariat is the American Academy of Dermatology and the Chairman is Joseph C. Kvedar, MD, of Harvard Medical School. At the time of writing, this working group was in the process of soliciting support for a DICOM-based dermatology image-capture and viewing package (see Chapter 17). The American Academy of Dermatologists has recently developed minimum recommended standards for basic digital image quality, those relevant to the contents of this chapter are reproduced below.

AAD recommendations

The AAD general recommendation about system capabilities (Table 2.1) is that imaging and communications hardware used for telemedicine consultations should possess at least the following minimum capabilities. The colour rendered by the monitor and camera should represent true colours. To ensure this, equipment should be calibrated for colour correction according to their specifications, including such techniques as a 'colour wheel' if appropriate. (A colour wheel is a colour illustration of the range of colours available, arranged in a circle with the three primary colours equally spaced around the circumference, the three secondary colours appropriately interspersed and colours in between these six also graduated between them. The lighter or darker shades of each colour are included in a radial direction. Colours on screen can then be matched or calibrated against the colours on the wheel, Fig. 2.6.)

Table 2.1. AAD recommendations

Item	Specification
Analogue colour display	450 TV lines of resolution
Analogue colour camera output	450 TV lines of resolution
Digital display	0.28 mm dot pitch,
	640 × 480 pixel spatial resolution, 24-bit colour depth
Digital colour output	1000 × 1000 pixel spatial resolution,
Single chip camera	24-bit colour depth
Three chip camera	Output equivalent to spatial resolution of a 1000 × 1000 pixel single chip camera, 24-bit colour depth

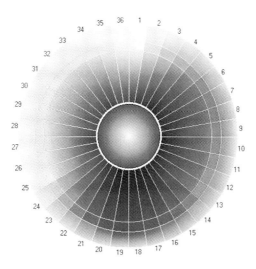

Fig. 2.6. Colour wheel (reproduced here in monochrome).
See http://www.mauigateway.com/~donjusko/jpgcharts.htm (last checked 29 July 2001).

The recommendations for videoconferencing systems are:

► They should adhere to the standards developed by the International Telecommunication Union (ITU).

► They should be capable of providing a resolution of 14 line pairs per millimetre resolution. This should be documented by use of a high-contrast test object such as the 1951 United States Air Force test pattern (this should be obtainable without requiring the use of a contact microscope peripheral device).

► They should be capable of accurately producing a full range of human skin tones.

Adoption of standards for compression is difficult because research in their use for dermatology is limited. Standards for creation and transmission of clinical information are also in a state of flux. No national or international policy has evolved as it relates to transmission of medical information over telecommunication networks, particularly the Internet. For the present it is recommended that at least two layers of security be implemented (including passwords and encryption) for non-dedicated transmission lines. Access to dedicated lines through multipoint control units and other switching devices should also be appropriately protected. The American Medical Informatics Association has developed explicit guidelines for the clinical use of email.[23] Adherence to these guidelines is recommended.

In the light of the current capabilities of digital cameras and computer monitors, it is clear that the hardware standards are easily achievable, but the lack of published research into compression and transmission of dermatology images necessarily leaves some gaps. Maintaining standards of image quality over time (quality assurance) should also be addressed.[24]

Archiving

The long-term storage of digital image data has taxed radiology departments for years with CT and MR data and more recently with computerized radiography systems or their equivalents. Radiologists have also baulked at the concept of lossy compression for diagnostic images and, for example, the image data storage requirements for a CT scanner may exceed 100 MBytes per day. The storage needs of a teledermatology system are likely to be considerably lower, but even so allowance for future changes in workload or digital image file sizes should be made. If lossy image compression is to be used to facilitate file transmission to the central dermatologist for review, then it may be most appropriate to archive the image using lossless compression at the peripheral site. Archived images need to be easily and quickly retrievable, uniquely and robustly identifiable and secure (both from tampering or illicit access and from degradation or corruption in storage). Where the data are stored (temporarily or long term) on hard disk drives, regular backups should be made to avoid loss from disk drive failure. The choices for long-term storage lie between magnetic media and optical media. Examples of each are DAT tape and CD-ROM respectively. In general, magnetic media are cheaper and can be reused, writing new data over old, but are slower as tapes for example have to be wound to the appropriate position for data retrieval. As with all other computer technology, continuous developments will render this description obsolescent within months, but currently a CD-ROM writer costing less than £100, supported by a modern PC, can write 650 MBytes of data to a blank CD (costing less than £1) within 20 minutes. Any single 1-MByte image file can be retrieved from a CD-ROM within seconds. This would appear to be ideal for storage of dermatological digital images.

Conclusion

Digital images are becoming ubiquitous and their use in (tele-)dermatology is inevitable. Users of digital images need to be aware of the relationship between the appearance of the original scene (the patient) and the influence of the subsequent steps that may be taken to provide an image for them to view. Computer and graphics jargon can obscure what are in reality simple arithmetic relationships between the number of pixels in an image, its displayed size, the number of colours and the image file size. The many different image file formats and file compression methods create potential for further confusion. Four simple questions should place the computer aspects of a digital image into clear perspective:

1. What is the image size in pixels?
2. How many colours are represented in the file format?
3. Has the image been adjusted by graphics software or the image file undergone 'lossy' compression; if so, how does it compare with the original image?
4. Is the display accurately reproducing the digital image data?

Understanding the fundamentals of digital imaging will allow better teledermatology to be practised.

References

1   Collins K, Nicolson P, Bowns I, Walters S. General practitioners' perceptions of store-and-forward teledermatology. *Journal of Telemedicine and Telecare* 2000;**6:**50–53.
2   Taylor P. A survey of research in telemedicine. 1: Telemedicine systems. *Journal of Telemedicine and Telecare* 1998;**4:**1–17.
3   Kvedar JC, Menn ER, Baradagunta S, Smulders-Meyer O, Gonzalez E. Teledermatology in a capitated delivery system using distributed information architecture: design and development. *Telemedicine Journal* 1999;**5:**357–366.
4   Krupinski EA, LeSueur B, Ellsworth L, et al. Diagnostic accuracy and image quality using a digital camera for teledermatology. *Telemedicine Journal* 1999;**5:**257–263.
5   Bovik A, ed. *Handbook of Image and Video Processing*. Edinburgh: Harcourt, 2000.
6   Bankman IN, ed. *Handbook of Medical Imaging, Processing and Analysis*. Edinburgh: Harcourt, 2000.
7   Vidmar DA, Cruess D, Hsieh P, et al. The effect of decreasing digital image resolution on teledermatology diagnosis. *Telemedicine Journal* 1999;**5:**375–383.
8   Loane MA, Gore HE, Corbett R, et al. Effect of camera performance on diagnostic accuracy: preliminary results from the Northern Ireland arms of the UK Multicentre Teledermatology Trial. *Journal of Telemedicine and Telecare* 1997;**3:**83–88.

9 Bruckmann A, Uhl A. Selective medical image compression techniques for telemedical and archiving applications. *Computers in Biology and Medicine* 2000;**30**:153–169.

10 Kang KS, Park HW. Lossless medical image compression by multilevel decomposition. *Journal of Digital Imaging* 1996;**9**:11–20.

11 Chen ZD, Chang RF, Kuo WJ. Adaptive predictive multiplicative autoregressive model for medical image compression [letter]. *IEEE Transactions on Medical Imaging* 1999;**18**:181–184.

12 Kivijarvi J, Ojala T, Kaukoranta T, Kuba A, Nyul L, Nevalainen O. A comparison of lossless compression methods for medical images. *Computerized Medical Imaging and Graphics* 1998;**22**:323–339.

13 Abu-Rezq AN, Tolba AS, Khuwaja GA, Foda SG. Best parameters selection for wavelet packet-based compression of magnetic resonance images. *Computers in Biomedical Research* 1999;**32**:449–469.

14 Slone RM, Foos DH, Whiting BR, et al. Assessment of visually lossless irreversible image compression: comparison of three methods by using an image-comparison workstation. *Radiology* 2000;**215**:543–553.

15 Yamamoto LG. Using JPEG image compression to facilitate telemedicine. *American Journal of Emergency Medicine* 1995;**13**:55–57.

16 Good WF, Maitz GS, Gur D. Joint photographic experts group (JPEG) compatible data compression of mammograms. *Journal of Digital Imaging* 1994;**7**:123–132.

17 Harpen MD. An introduction to wavelet theory and application for the radiological physicist. *Medical Physics* 1998;**25**:1985–1993.

18 Schomer DF, Elekes AA, Hazle JD, et al. Introduction to wavelet-based compression of medical images. *Radiographics* 1998;**18**:469–481.

19 Thompson SK, Hazle JD, Schomer DF, et al. Performance analysis of a new semiorthogonal spline wavelet compression algorithm for tonal medical images. *Medical Physics* 2000;**27**:276–288.

20 Eikelboom RH, Yogesan K, Barry CJ, et al. Methods and limits of digital image compression of retinal images for telemedicine. *Investigative Ophthalmology and Visual Science* 2000;**41**:1916–1924.

21 Ricke J, Maass P, Lopez-Hanninen E, et al. Wavelet versus JPEG (Joint Photographic Expert Group) and fractal compression. Impact on the detection of low-contrast details in computed radiographs. *Investigative Radiology* 1998;**33**:456–463.

22 Okkalides D. Assessment of commercial compression algorithms, of the lossy DCT and lossless types, applied to diagnostic digital image files. *Computerized Medical Imaging and Graphics* 1998;**22**:25–30.

23 Kane B, Sands DZ. Guidelines for the clinical use of electronic mail with patients. *Journal of the American Medical Informatics Association* 1998;**5**:104–111.

24 Kocsis O, Costaridou L, Efstathopoulos EP, Lymberopoulos D, Panayiotakis G. A tool for designing digital test objects for module performance evaluation in medical digital imaging. *Medical Informatics and the Internet in Medicine* 1999;**24**:291–308.

3

Lighting and Colour in Digital Photography

Ville Voipio and Heikki Lamminen

Introduction

The most often cited performance figure of a digital camera is its spatial resolution, i.e. the number of pixels in the resulting image. This may give the impression that the most important characteristics of a digital image are resolution and sharpness. While these factors are indeed important, the overall success of a digital photograph also depends very much on colour and lighting.

The significance of colour and lighting can be seen when a professionally shot television broadcast is compared to quick snapshots taken with a digital camera. The former will probably have only one-tenth of the number of pixels of a high-quality digital camera image, but the television image may still look better because its exposure and colour balance have been carefully planned.

There are no quick and easy ways to produce well-exposed and true-colour digital photographs, but knowledge of the technical background will help to avoid problems. Modern digital photography is near to conventional photography and the ability to take good analogue photographs is a valuable aid in digital photography. In the domain of colour and lighting the difference is mostly that digital imaging equipment is much more sensitive to exposure errors than film-based equipment.

Colour perception

Colour is a property of the human eye – there is no absolute physical variable representing colour. The apparent colour of a surface depends on several physical properties of the surface itself and the light sources used to view it. All colour photography equipment is built on the model of human colour vision, and thus the basic mechanisms of colour perception are relevant to all digital colour reproduction.

Colour is detected by the three different types of cone cells in the retina. These cells are called by different names in different fields of study, but essentially one type detects long wavelengths (red), one medium wavelengths (green) and one short wavelengths (blue). Thus the retina acts as a very low resolution spectrometer which measures the relative amounts of long, medium and short wavelength radiation falling on the cones. The sensitivity curves of each type of cones are shown in Figure 3.1. With this model it is possible to describe every possible colour using just three parameters (tristimulus).

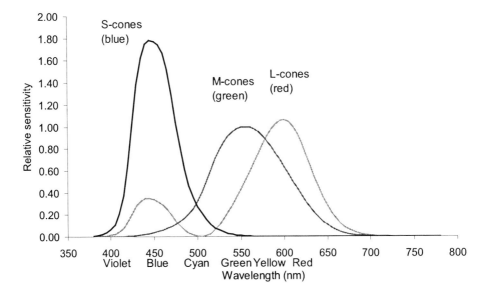

Fig. 3.1. Relative sensitivity of different types of cones.

Colour perception depends on the spectrum of the light entering the eye. When we talk about the colour of a surface, we refer to the spectrum of the light reflected from that surface. A red surface reflects long-wavelength radiation and absorbs shorter wavelengths. A blue surface reflects short-wavelength radiation and absorbs longer wavelengths.

These definitions of surface colour are unfortunately rather inaccurate and may cause confusion. If a red surface is lit with blue light, it absorbs all light and looks black (Fig. 3.2). In the yellow, low-pressure sodium lighting commonly used on highways, all surfaces look either yellow or black, as there is only monochromatic yellow light available.

Due to the way that the human eye handles colour, there can be two different spectra which give exactly the same colour perception. For example, a single spectral line in the yellow region will stimulate both red and green cone cells. The eye interprets the combination of red and green stimulation as yellow. The same cellular response may be achieved by using light with both red and green spectral lines, or even with a very wide spectrum of red and green light.

To illustrate the difference between different yellows, we may think of two yellow surfaces. One of them reflects only a narrow spectrum of yellow light, while the other reflects a wide range of red and green radiation (Fig. 3.3). In white light both surfaces are yellow, but in red light the narrowly yellow-reflecting surface does not reflect anything and looks black. The wide-band-reflecting surface also reflects red, so it looks red in red lighting.

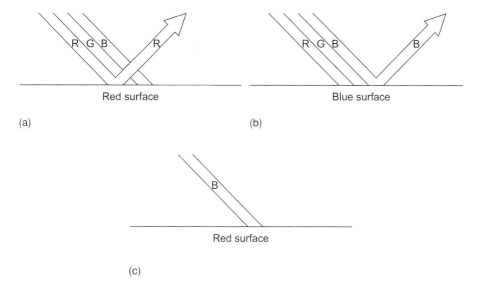

Fig. 3.2. (a) White light reflecting from a red surface; (b) white light reflecting from a blue surface; (c) blue light incident on a red surface (no reflected light).

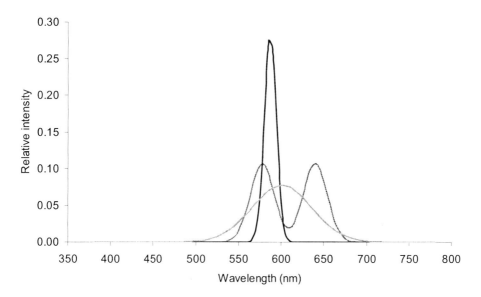

Fig. 3.3. Three different spectra giving the same orange-yellow colour perception.

It should always be borne in mind that the human perception of colour is a rather inaccurate representation of the spectral properties. Colour is not a property of a surface, it is just a perception which results from the interaction of the illumination and the surface colour.

Colour detection in digital cameras

Digital cameras record the colour in much the same way as the human eye. The camera element in the film plane, usually a solid-state charged-coupled device (CCD) or complementary metal-oxide semiconductor (CMOS) chip, is covered with small red, green and blue colour filters. Each pixel is sensitive to all visible light, but because there is a colour filter in front of it, the pixel becomes sensitive to a specific range of wavelengths (Fig. 3.4). Thus there is a very strong analogy between pixels in the camera sensor and cones in the retina.

It should be noted that as each pixel in the sensor senses only one colour, the camera has to interpolate the remaining two principal colour components to each pixel. This process may produce image artefacts in some – fortunately rather rare – situations. These artefacts can sometimes be seen in sharp high-contrast images. For instance, a sharp, high-resolution black and white line pattern may show some other colours on the black and white boundary. The artefacts may disappear or become more pronounced when the angle between the camera and the pattern is changed.

The human eye adapts very flexibly to different lighting conditions.[1] White paper looks white in sunlight, it looks white in indoor fluorescent lighting, and it still looks white in the rather yellowish light from filament lamps.[2] A digital camera has no such automatic adaptation, and if no corrections are made, the paper will appear to be anything from blue to yellow in photographs taken under different lighting.

To correct this problem digital cameras use white balance adjustment. This adjustment may be fully automatic, semi-automatic or manual. Fully automatic white balance adjustment analyses the colours in the photograph and then corrects them according to some algorithm. These algorithms are usually intended for some specific

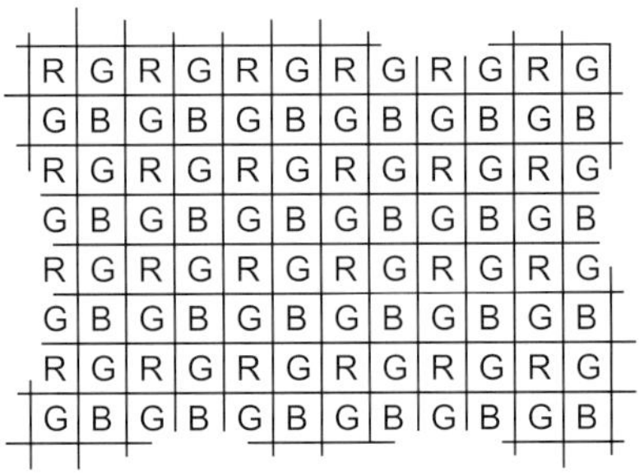

Fig. 3.4. RGB filters in front of camera element pixels (Bayer configuration).

purpose, such as landscape photography. However, it is easy to confuse the automatic adjustment if the picture has some unusual dominant colour. For example, skin pictures with only skin in the view will be of the wrong colour with the automatic adjustment; usually they come out greyish as the algorithm deduces the pink colour to be the result of pink lighting.

All modern digital cameras have different fixed white balance settings to be used with different light sources. These preset values represent the red, green and blue components of light reflecting from an ideal white surface with each light source. However, these preset values are approximations and will not necessarily produce desirable results.

Most cameras allow manual white balance adjustment. The camera is pointed at a white surface (e.g. a piece of white paper) and then the reference white value is recorded from this image. This procedure may give better white balance than preset values, but it should be kept in mind that the tristimulus values are only a three-value representation of the complete spectrum. Adjusting the white to be white does not guarantee that all other colours will be reproduced accurately. If the application calls for accurate colour rendering, it is advisable to add some standard colour patches to the scene.

The way that digital cameras handle colour is intrinsically more accurate than that of conventional cameras using photographic film. All parts of the digital process can be standardized, so that the colour will remain the same from one photography session to another. This is harder to achieve in a film process where there are a number of analogue processing steps which affect the colour reproduction. However, it is much easier to make errors with digital equipment, and so the colour balance settings must always be well documented.

Exposure control

Digital cameras require a lot of light. Inexpensive pocket cameras have very small-diameter zoom objectives whose light-collecting ability is poor. Digital sensors (CCD or CMOS) are smaller in area and less sensitive than conventional film. In all photography the amount of light falling onto the film or image sensor depends on three factors: illumination, the light-collecting power of the optical system and the exposure time.

The light-collecting power of the system may be changed either by using a different objective or by adjusting the aperture of the objective. Most digital cameras have a fixed objective that cannot be changed, and usually these objectives have only one or two different aperture settings. A larger aperture allows more light to enter the objective, while a smaller aperture gives a sharper image with better depth of focus.

Exposure times may be increased to collect more light. There are some practical limits, however. When taking a photograph of a person, the subject may move significantly in a short time. Also, if the camera is held in the hand, the exposure time may not significantly exceed 1/30 s. Longer times will produce motion blur in the image. Blurring effects due to camera shake may be reduced by using tripods; blurring

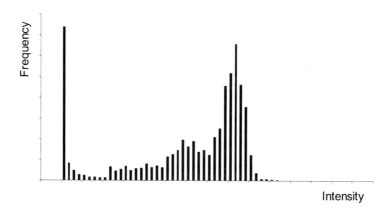

(a)

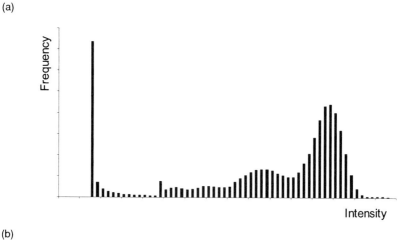

(b)

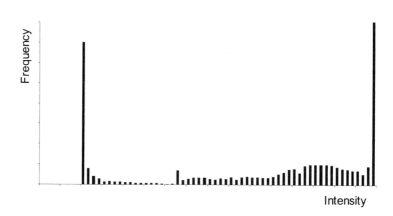

(c)

Fig. 3.5. The effect of incorrect exposure on image quality: (a) is one aperture stop underexposed, (b) is correctly exposed and (c) is one stop overexposed. The highest (rightmost) bin of (c) is truncated to preserve the same vertical scaling with other histograms.

due to object motion may be reduced by supporting the part to be photographed. The ability of a digital camera to use long exposure times varies widely from one model to another. Some cameras produce noisy images with a two-second exposure time, while some can produce acceptable images with a two-minute exposure.

Ordinary film cameras will usually permit an exposure error of one or two aperture stops (i.e. doubling or quadrupling the ideal exposure). Such errors can be corrected in the film development phase. The dynamic range of a CCD sensor is much narrower, and badly exposed images are hard or impossible to correct afterwards without significant deterioration of image quality. Underexposed digital images will look noisy, as the sensor noise will be amplified with the image. Overexposed images cannot be corrected, as the information is irrecoverably lost in the overexposed areas.

It is sometimes very difficult to tell from the integral liquid crytal display (LCD) of a digital camera whether the exposure has been correct or not. Some digital cameras indicate the overexposed parts of the image by colouring them with, for example, flashing red. Also, some cameras offer a histogram display, which shows the intensity distribution in the image. Figure 3.5 shows under- and over-exposed images and their histograms.

In general, the more expensive digital cameras have a better noise-free dynamic range, which allows more post-processing of the image. However, no camera can produce good results with the wrong exposure. Different cameras offer different possibilities for exposure control. Some less expensive cameras may not offer manual adjustment of exposure control, but these cameras are not suited for professional use anyway.

Lighting considerations

Even if the amount of light is correct, the image may be unclear or difficult to interpret if wrong or poorly positioned light sources have been used. The correct use of light requires some experience, but, again, some general understanding will help to prevent problems.

A light source may be point-like or of larger area. Point light sources (e.g. the built-in flash of a camera) produce very clear shadows, whereas more diffuse lighting produces soft shadows (Fig. 3.6). While sharp shadows are usually distracting, some shadows may help in interpreting three-dimensional profiles.

The easiest setup is to use no flashes. This way the camera sees the same view as a human viewer. The lack of light may become a problem with this approach, and not all room lighting is suitable for photography.

Natural light (sunlight) should be blocked out, as its intensity and colour varies over a very wide range. At night there is no light entering from windows, while in the day the intensity and colour of the light depend on the time and the weather. Direct sunlight is extremely bright and produces sharp shadows. The use of direct or indirect sunlight makes it very difficult to achieve reproducible results.

Very often office rooms are lit with fluorescent lighting. This is also difficult for digital photography. Fluorescent tubes produce a series of rather sharp spectral peaks

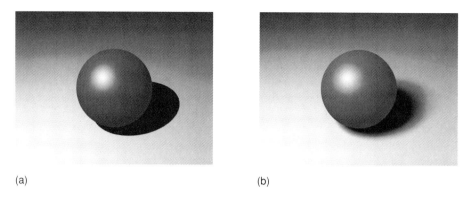

(a)   (b)

Fig. 3.6. The effect of lighting on shadows. Point-like light sources cast sharp shadows (a), whereas larger areas give smooth shadows (b).

instead of a smooth spectrum. This may introduce some colour error in the photographs. There are several different types of fluorescent tubes, and they may have quite different spectral properties. Furthermore, the colour of a fluorescent tube may change as the tube ages, which makes accurate colour reproduction rather difficult.

Fluorescent tubes respond very quickly to variations in their supply voltage. As almost all lighting uses alternating current, fluorescent tubes flicker very quickly. With 50 Hz alternating current (as used in Europe) the fluorescent tube reaches 100 intensity maxima every second. While this rate is so fast that the eye seldom notices it, it is a slow rate for a digital camera. Consequently some cameras will produce images with horizontal or vertical bands when used with fluorescent lighting. Special photographic fluorescent lights are therefore available, which may also be used with digital cameras. They use very high frequency alternating current and have special phosphors in the tube so that their spectral properties are more suitable for photography.

Ordinary incandescent bulbs have a very smooth optical spectrum. Unfortunately, they produce relatively little light and much heat, and so their use in photographic lighting is limited. Also, the colour temperature of an incandescent bulb is relatively low (i.e. the light is yellowish) so that blue shades may not reproduce well. Halogen bulbs may also be used, but in some cases they have undesirable spectral properties. Halogen lamps provide a very intense and easily directed stream of light at a very reasonable price. Incandescent lamps react much more slowly to supply voltage variations than fluorescent tubes, so that flickering is not a problem.

Very often the intensity of light conveniently available from a constant light source is too low and photographic flashes have to be used instead. The easiest solution is to use the flash built in to the digital camera. Unfortunately, this does not usually produce very good results. The light from the flash comes from exactly the same direction as the picture is taken. Thus all reflections normal (perpendicular) to the camera become visible. Also, the camera flash is a point light source, which is not necessarily a good

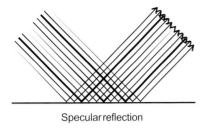

Specular reflection

(a)

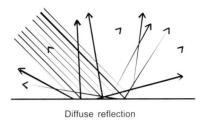

Diffuse reflection

(b)

Fig. 3.7. The surface structure affects reflective properties. Both spheres have the same surface profile. However in (a) the sphere reflects specularly, whereas in (b) the sphere reflects diffusely (non-directionally).

thing in medical imaging. So, if a flash is required, it is preferable to connect an external flash to the digital camera.

One of the challenges of photography is to remove all unwanted reflections from the image. This becomes easier if it is understood where the reflections come from. All surfaces reflect light to some extent. Most natural surfaces are diffuse, i.e. a sharp beam of light is reflected in all directions. Shiny surfaces exhibit specular reflection, and a sharp beam of light reflecting from the surface will reflect as a sharp beam of light so that very little light is seen from other directions (Fig. 3.7). Very few natural surfaces are completely specular, but moist mucous tissue, for example, exhibits considerable specular reflection.

Diffuse surfaces may be lit with sharp directional light, as it is diffused in all directions. Specular surfaces have to be lit with diffuse light if the surface properties are to be shown. It should be noted that very few surfaces are completely diffuse. For example, skin has some directionality, which should be taken into account when setting the lights. Even a small change in light-source position may affect the image quality significantly.

As the lighting setup involves numerous variables, it is advisable to have a professional photographer help with the initial setup of the photographing location. This will save a lot of trouble later in the process.

Picture post-processing

Once digital photographs have been taken, there may be a need for post-processing. Post-processing usually involves brightness, intensity or colour correction. Commonly available image-processing software offers a large number of options for colour correction. However, many image-processing options are aimed at making the image look more natural. This may be in conflict with the desire for accurate and repeatable colour reproduction, and so image post-processing should be kept to a minimum.

No image post-processing can add information to an image. Careful processing may allow certain important details to become visible, but careless processing will destroy potentially important information. All colour balance and exposure errors should be corrected in the photography setup, and post-processing should be left as a last resort. If post-processing is required, then it is very important to document each step taken in the post-processing to ensure reproducibility.

If colour filtering is required it has to be done in the real world rather than the digital domain. If the wavelength of interest is, say, 480–500 nm, then a suitable cyan filter should be used in front of the objective. This filtering cannot be performed by software after the image has been captured. If there is no filter in front of the objective, the camera will record all wavelengths. Post-processing can be used to produce a cyan image, but this is done by switching off the red channel and adjusting the intensities of the green and blue channels. The picture thus formed contains information from the green and blue pixels of the camera, i.e. from a very wide wavelength range. So, while the image looks superficially the same in the two cases, it is only by using the filter that the desired wavelength range can actually be recorded.

Picture viewing

Digital images are usually viewed on a computer monitor. The way that a computer monitor reproduces colour is, again, closely related to the structure of the eye. A computer monitor has three different colours (with cathode ray tube (CRT) monitors these are also called phosphors for historical reasons) for each pixel: red, green and blue. The red stimulates long-wavelength cones, the green stimulates medium-wavelength cones and the blue stimulates short-wavelength cones. This way almost any colour perception may be created. It should be kept in mind, however, that there are certain limitations to the colour reproduction ability of an RGB (red/green/blue) monitor, as the blue colour will always stimulate red or green cones slightly. Fortunately, the missing colours are quite rare, and not very common in medical images (such as some shades of cyan).

Other colour 'models' than RGB are possible. Some can represent all possible colours visible by the human eye.[3] These models, however, are rather laborious to convert into RGB or any other output device model, and their practical use is limited.

Despite the simple principles, calibrating a computer monitor to show accurate colour is difficult. In a monochrome monitor each pixel has only one parameter: intensity. Each digital intensity value will produce some optical intensity value on the screen. The relation between the digital and optical values may not be linear, but it can still be described with a single curve.

With colour monitors the number of parameters is at least three times greater, as each colour component has its own calibration curve.[4] Also, different monitors may have slightly different red, green and blue phosphors, i.e. the red colour produced by two monitors may be of slightly different shades. The intensities may also vary locally over the display screen, they may change over time and they may alter with temperature. Good colour calibration therefore requires skill and the right equipment. After the monitor has been calibrated, any adjustment of contrast or brightness will make recalibration necessary. Any changes in external lighting may also make the calibration invalid.

Fortunately, the human eye is not an absolute measurement instrument. It will adapt to a wide range of colour variation.[5] International standardization is also helping in this respect, and many new computer monitors, printers and digital cameras now recognize the sRGB standard which defines standard RGB colours[6] (Box 3.1). In most applications the level of reproducibility offered by sRGB is satisfactory.

Box 3.1.   The sRGB standard

A digital image-production system has several components that deal with colour. Cameras, scanners, computer monitors and printers may use different colours. A digital photograph will look different when viewed with different monitors or printed on paper. The traditional approach to this problem has been to calibrate the devices to match each other. This is time consuming and difficult to do accurately. To overcome this problem, some large digital imaging companies have introduced a standard-RGB system (sRGB).[6] All devices recognizing the sRGB standard should produce similar colours within the limits of their capabilities.

There are some even more accurate colour systems, for example the CIE Lab colour space. However, these systems are difficult to implement in digital equipment, as they are not directly based on RGB values. sRGB is built on existing standards, such as the HDTV (High Definition Television) standard. Also, sRGB is reasonably compatible with non-sRGB monitors, scanners and cameras.

The main advantage of sRGB is that the user need not care about colour transformation or calibration. This is a big advantage especially with colour printers, because non-sRGB printers may produce very inaccurate colours without calibration. However, sRGB is not as accurate as custom calibration. If exact colour reproduction is needed, sRGB does not remove the need for frequent calibration. However, in most applications the level of reproducibility offered by sRGB is satisfactory.

The lighting of the viewing room should be constant. It is not generally a good idea to position the computer monitor in a room where a lot of natural light can enter. Also, the settings of the monitor should not be touched after satisfactory settings have been found. This makes it possible for picture viewers to gain experience of an individual monitor's colour rendering.

Flat LCD panels use the same colour system as traditional CRT monitors, and they may be used as well. However, their viewing angle may be limited compared to CRT monitors, and colours may become distorted at the extremes of the viewing angle.

Hard copy

Very often a paper copy of a digital image is required. This hard copy can be produced by different methods, which will produce significant variations in the colour range and reproduction.

One of the most accurate methods is direct writing on photographic paper or film. In this method the image is written on photographic film with red, green and blue beams of light. After the writing process the photographs are developed in the ordinary way. Hard copies produced with this method are essentially photographs. They have the same colour reproduction properties, and they will keep their colours over time just like any other photograph. The equipment required for this process is fairly expensive and the material costs may also be significant. However, there is a lot of experience with storage of photographs, which is a well-understood process.

If photographs are printed on paper with a computer printer, then a subtractive colour system is used. A subtractive (CMY) system has three principal colours: cyan, magenta and yellow. Cyan reflects everything else but not red, so it can be called anti-red. Yellow is anti-blue and magenta is anti-green. When green colour is printed, it is printed by overlaying cyan ink and yellow ink. Cyan blocks red and yellow blocks blue, so only green is reflected from the surface (Fig. 3.8). In theory, a black surface is obtained by printing all three colours on top of each other. In practice, the black obtained this way is not completely black, and separate black ink is used. This four-ink process is known as the CMYK system.

The conversion between RGB and CMYK is not a simple one. There are several colours that RGB can reproduce but CMYK cannot. For instance, several shades of blue are difficult to reproduce with CMYK. So, the wider colour 'space' of RGB has to be shrunk to fit CMYK when printing. There are several algorithms to do this, but the result is always a compromise of some sort. Some new ink-jet printers can expand the CMYK colour space by using six inks instead of four. The improvement is mainly in the reproduction of Caucasian skin tones, something that may be useful in dermatology.

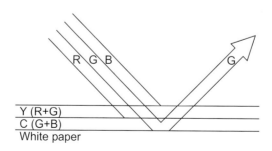

Fig. 3.8. Subtractive colour mixing. Green colour may be obtained by printing cyan and yellow ink on white paper.

Some new colour printers support the sRGB standard so that the image can be sent to the printer as RGB data. The printer can then perform all the necessary transforms to produce accurate colours. The use of such printers is to be encouraged, as they remove the need for calibration in most applications.

The colour range of an ink-jet printer is much wider than that of a colour laser printer. With both printer types optimum colour reproduction requires special coated paper. High-quality photographic ink-jet paper is expensive, whereas coated colour laser paper costs only approximately twice as much as ordinary office paper. Ink-jets usually produce very unsaturated colours on plain paper, and photographic paper has to be used when printing photographs.

If hard copies are to be used for archiving purposes, it should be noted that computer prints may fade rather quickly. Ink-jet prints in particular tend to bleach within a few years. This may be avoided by storing the prints in a dark place and using an ink-jet printer with pigment inks. Colour laser prints do not fade significantly, but due to the better image quality, ink-jet prints are generally preferable. Ordinary photographs printed from digital originals may be a good solution for long-term storage.

Printers are often advertised by giving resolution figures, usually in dpi (dots per inch). These numbers are often of questionable accuracy, and as the colours are formed by using a large number of ink drops per pixel, the real resolution in colour photographs is much lower than these figures (see Chapter 2). The real resolution of a printer can be tested by printing some photographs and comparing the output of different printers visually.

Conclusion

The differences between conventional film photography and digital photography are rather subtle. Conventional lighting principles are valid with digital photography. Perhaps the most important difference is that digital cameras are more sensitive to incorrect exposure than film cameras. However, the photograph is immediately available with digital imaging, which makes it quicker to find the correct values.

Digital cameras allow accurate and repeatable colour reproduction. There is no development process or changing film chemistry. However, there are several factors along the digital imaging chain that may change the colour appearance of the result. The basics of the digital colour have to be understood in order to produce repeatable colour. New colour standards (most notably sRGB) will help to maintain satisfactory colour reproduction in most applications.

References

1   Walsh V. Colour vision. Adapting to change. *Current Biology* 1995;**5**:703–705.
2   Nieves JL, Garcia-Beltran A, Romero J. Response of the human visual system to variable illuminant conditions: an analysis of opponent-colour mechanisms in colour constancy. *Ophthalmic and Physiological Optics* 2000;**20**:44–58.

3   Hunt RWG. *Measuring Colour*, 2nd edn. New York: Horwood, 1991.
4   Shepherd AJ. Calibrating screens for continuous colour displays. *Spatial Vision* 1997;**11**:57–74.
5   Tachakra S. Colour perception in telemedicine. *Journal of Telemedicine and Telecare* 1999;**5**:211–219.
6   Hewlett Packard and Microsoft. http://www.srgb.com/ (last checked 29 July 2001).

4

Digital Cameras: Still Photography and Video Imaging in Teledermatology

Ashish Bhatia, Paul Kostuchenko and Paul Greenwood

Introduction

The traditional practice of dermatology relies heavily on visual information from the patient, as well as tactile information and the clinical history. Although the transmission of tactile information has not yet become practicable, the transfer of visual information and history is a part of all telemedicine systems. The clinical history can be obtained by talking to the patient and/or through the use of case notes completed by other medical personnel. Digital imaging systems capable of capturing high-quality images are readily available, so it is possible to transfer images of the patient's hair, skin, mucosal surfaces or nails to the consultant via real-time video links or still photography. In telemedicine, both techniques have their strengths and weaknesses.

Digital still photography is used with most store-and-forward teledermatology systems. In this technique, the digital images and a report of the patient's history are transmitted to a consultant for subsequent evaluation. The advantages of digital still photography for store-and-forward teledermatology lie in the high-quality images, low bandwidth necessary for transmission and the temporal flexibility for the participants involved. The image quality obtainable with digital still cameras continues to improve, while their cost continues to fall. Spatial resolution, colour range and signal-to-noise ratio are the properties that seem to be improving most rapidly. The data storage capacity of digital cameras is also increasing to accommodate the larger image file sizes associated with higher resolution images. The prices of the requisite storage media continue to drop as well. There is also an increasing availability of digital still cameras with single lens reflex (SLR) bodies. The SLR digital cameras offer the same features which professional medical photographers find necessary for high-quality imaging. One of the biggest advantages of SLR digital cameras is that many accept the same lenses and attachments as their 35-mm film counterparts. Examples of SLR digital cameras include the Canon EOS D-30, the Fuji FinePix S1 Pro, the Olympus E-10 and the Nikon D1.

Digital still images are generally viewed on a computer monitor. These provide a higher pixel density than the standard television monitors that are used with interactive video telemedicine systems. One of the advantages of high-resolution digital still imaging is the ability to see an overview of an area of a patient's body and then to magnify the area of interest while retaining the fine image details. This allows a closer look at the lesion or area of interest. Interactive video telemedicine systems, however, are often limited in resolution by the internationally agreed videoconferencing standards (e.g. H.320). Most television monitors used with real-time video telemedicine have a resolution of 400–550 horizontal lines. In comparison, a high-resolution computer monitor can display 1024 horizontal lines of resolution or more. Also, interactive video transmission requires far more bandwidth over the communication line connecting the two locations.

Another advantage of the store-and-forward teledermatology approach is that the images and history forms are transferred to the consultant's viewing station and the information is stored there. This enables the consultant to view the information at any time after transfer of the data. Neither the consultant nor the patients and staff have to alter their schedules to meet at a time convenient to all parties involved.

Finally, store-and-forward consultations with high-quality digital photography require less time to perform than real-time video consultations.[1] Several factors contribute to this time saving. First, the technique allows the consultant to focus on the material presented via a few images and a predetermined history form. With this information at hand, the consultant does not spend time with the patient while the patient verbally relays their history. Time taken for social formalities and other important patient–physician interactions is also avoided.

The major disadvantages of digital still photography integrated in store-and-forward teledermatology include the lack of instantaneous feedback from the patient, the inability to examine any areas of the patient's body which were omitted from the initial set of images, and the lack of visual and auditory clues from the patient which may assist in making a diagnosis. In addition, the lack of instantaneous feedback from the patient may cause delays in diagnosis and treatment of the patient due to the time required for requesting additional information and receiving a response. The inability to receive additional views quickly of body areas that were not initially photographed, such as the oral cavity and tongue to check for candidiasis, can also lead to delays in diagnosis. This can be important in cases where the simultaneous observation of two areas of the body is helpful in the diagnosis.

Without the guidance of the consultant for positioning the camera relative to the patient, the photographer using store-and-forward teledermatology must be very well trained in consistently and properly positioning the patient and taking photographs which demonstrate the patient's lesions well. This requires thorough training in the use of the camera as well as a good understanding of the principles of medical photography. A detailed protocol for positioning the patient for photographs must also be provided for the photographer.

Despite high-bandwidth requirements, lower-resolution images and an extended length of time taken for consultation, real-time video links are still commonly employed for dermatological consultations. There are several attractive features of the technique. One feature is the ability to use additional accessories, such as close-up cameras that can transfer high-resolution still images and dermoscopes. Another useful characteristic of real-time telemedicine is the consultant's ability to seek additional information and views of the patient immediately by directing the patient and medical personnel at the other end.

Features of digital cameras in teledermatology

Magnification

Magnification is a mixed blessing in digital imaging. The reviewer can receive still pictures or video images from the patient's skin at various magnifications, allowing a clear, close-up view of the lesion. However, many dermatologists are not accustomed to viewing lesions at such high magnifications. Unfamiliarity with magnified views of lesions can lead to difficulties in diagnosis as well as a tendency to overdiagnose lesions. The key to using the magnification capabilities of digital imaging systems successfully is familiarity with diagnosing lesions from magnified images. This requires practice. Practice is also necessary for using specialized accessories such as digital dermoscopy cameras. Even the use of hand-held dermoscopes in face-to-face practice tends to lead to overdiagnosis in clinicians with an untrained eye.

Dermoscopy

Several manufacturers now offer dermoscopes that can be attached to an existing telemedicine system. The major manufacturers include American Medical Development and Welch Allyn.

Macro imaging

Macro imaging allows photography of lesions at very short distances from the camera. This is often not possible with standard lenses and flash settings. On digital and 35-mm film SLR cameras, a special macro lens is employed to allow focusing at short distances. The lens itself may have a built-in sensor to calculate the distance from the lens to the subject. Many fixed lens digital cameras also allow macro photography. This is usually a special mode where the flash is forced off and optics may or may not be internally altered to allow close-range photography. Once a fixed lens digital camera is in macro mode, images should not be taken at a distance exceeding the maximum range of the macro mode. The usable range of the macro mode is normally listed in the camera's instruction manual. If the flash is forced off while the camera is in macro mode, it is essential to have the subject well lit, otherwise the longer automatic exposure times required in low-light situations will produce blurry pictures. If the fixed lens camera has the capability, a supplementary external flash unit may be used.

White balance

White balance is extremely important in both still and video imaging. It allows the camera to compensate for the colour hues given to the patient's skin by the 'white' light sources used to illuminate the subject. Every light source has a different hue, which is designated by the 'temperature' of the light source. Table 4.1 lists the hues and temperatures of different light sources. The camera's white balance allows a digital camera to compensate for the colour temperature of the light source and therefore avoids inappropriate tinting of the resulting images.

43

Table 4.1. Colour temperature and apparent colour of various light sources

Light source	Colour temperature (degrees Kelvin)	Apparent colour
Sunless blue sky	11 000	Blue
Fluorescent light	7700–9000	Green
Bright sunlight or strobe	5000–6000	White
Flashbulb	4000	Yellow
Floodlamp	3000	Orange
Incandescent bulb	2500	Orange/red
Candlelight	1000–2000	Red

See http://cybaea.com/photo/color-correction.html (last checked 26 July 2001).

Photographic technique in digital imaging: controlling image quality

The basic guidelines discussed below are applicable to both standard film photography and digital imaging. Most of the published material relating to photography of patients is based on conventional photography using 35-mm film. However, the basic principles are similar for digital imaging. Perhaps the greatest benefit from using digital imaging, apart from the convenient storage format, is the ability to see the photograph immediately after it has been taken. This can be done by viewing the captured image on the liquid crystal display (LCD) of the digital camera or by transferring the image to a PC with a high-resolution monitor. This has the advantage that the photographer can evaluate multiple variables such as composition, positioning and lighting and make any necessary adjustments to ensure good-quality images.

Serial imaging

Perhaps the single most important aspect of clinical photography involves achieving a consistent image of the patient on multiple occasions. Whether the images are intended for use in comparing treatment outcomes of the same patient over time, or recording multiple patients with the same pathology, it is crucial that consistent photographic technique is employed in order to allow objective comparisons. The nature of dermatological diseases is that they can often have very different appearances over time regardless of treatment interventions. Therefore, the disease course may play an important role in deciding which images are to be captured for digital recording. For instance, if one were to evaluate a patient with new-onset psoriasis who presented with plaques limited to the elbows, it might be sufficient to photograph those lesions and follow the areas over time to evaluate the skin's response to treatment. However, since it is well established that psoriatic plaques can develop over time at multiple sites, it may be beneficial to photograph several areas of uninvolved skin at the initial presentation and compare these images with future ones. This is particularly valuable in evaluating a patient's response to treatment in clinical trials. Knowing the natural history of the disease being examined is paramount in choosing the areas of the body to photograph. It is also important to record disease duration, onset, previous treatments, secondary lesions and co-morbidities, since they may influence the pictures captured.

Once the areas of the body to be photographed have been chosen, it becomes necessary to decide how to photograph the patient in order to achieve the highest quality image and to produce consistent images over time. The following section is devoted to an analysis of the factors that are important when taking high-quality photographs. The practice of these methods can consistently lead to pictures taken at or near publication quality. Of course, not every practitioner of digital photography will need to address each of the issues in every session. However, paying attention to the principles of good photographic technique can result in excellent images time after time. Moreover, how many times have you said to yourself, 'I wish I had a good photograph of this patient before treatment was initiated'? Careful adherence to the basic principles of photography can lead to future benefits.

Backgrounds

The choice of the background material is one of the most important elements in both conventional and digital photography. The background material is used to block out extraneous information that distracts the viewer's attention from the lesion being imaged. It also provides sufficient contrast to allow evaluation of the lesion being imaged. The selection of the background material must be done in conjunction with selection of the lighting system, which is discussed below.[2]

There are four types of background. These are white (and off-whites), black, grey and coloured. Regardless of which type is chosen, it is generally accepted that the background material should have a dull or matt finish in order to absorb reflected light. It should also be free of distracting seams, debris or visible imperfections. White backgrounds offer certain advantages in the digital imaging of clinical lesions. For example, they tend to be readily available outside the studio – a bed sheet can be used when imaging in an emergency room or medical ward. In addition, white backgrounds provide good contrast for most skin types and lesions. For journal publications, white backgrounds tend to reproduce adequately.

However, there are two factors that must be carefully controlled when photographing a subject against a white background. The first is the undesirable shadows cast by the subject onto the background. These tend to be more prominent in images with backgrounds of lighter colours, and especially troublesome with a white background. The second problem is flare production. Flare is the bright washout resulting from patches of intense light in the image. Flare tends to occur if a white background is overilluminated, whereas shadows tend to be more of a problem if the background is underilluminated. Both factors can be controlled with proper lighting and positioning of the subject.[3]

An additional consideration is whether the image generated will be used in a slide presentation to be shown in a darkened room. For instance, some viewers may become distracted if presented with a series of slides with text on a dark background, followed by a clinical slide with a white background. This can be distracting and uncomfortable to an audience whose eyes have adjusted to the dark. Because of these disadvantages, white backgrounds tend to be used less commonly in dermatological photography.

Black backgrounds offer several advantages over white backgrounds in standard and digital photography. Black backgrounds tend to give the subject the most dramatic presentation when photographed appropriately. In addition, due to the absorptive nature of the colour black, there is rarely a problem with shadowing or flare production. Black is also a non-distracting colour which can provide superior contrast and detail of the outline of the subject or lesion. However, it is often difficult to find a homogeneous solid black background in practice. Also, the lighting of a black background has to be carefully adjusted to ensure that the edges of the subject are not lost in the background.[4] Therefore, black backgrounds tend to rely more heavily on accessory lighting to produce high-quality images.

After discussing the distracting nature of white backgrounds during dark auditorium presentations, one would think that a black background would be ideal. Although it is true that a dark colour such as black is the least distracting background, digital projectors rarely yield a 'true' solid black projection. This is primarily due to the contrast limitations of digital projectors. Moreover, many scientific journals are unable to reproduce a solid black background in print. Most journals produce black backgrounds that appear as dark grey and sometimes lack homogeneity.

For these reasons, many photographers consider grey backgrounds to be a good compromise. One reason is that shades of grey provide a good background for photographing both light- and dark-skinned patients. Although images generated against these backgrounds will tend to be less dramatic than those created against black backgrounds, flare and shadow production are more easily controlled compared to photography against white backgrounds. In addition, grey backgrounds tend to have less influence on the colour tone of the subject being photographed than coloured backgrounds. Although grey backgrounds do provide a good compromise between solid white or black backgrounds, care must be taken to ensure proper lighting and exposure of the image, especially if serial images are to be followed over time.[3]

Despite the suitability of grey, coloured backgrounds such as pale blues and greens are probably used more in dermatology than any other background. This is probably because these backgrounds, usually in the form of surgical towels or disposable drapes, are readily available for image capture at the bedside. Moreover, these backgrounds are complementary to the skin tone of the patient. If used properly, coloured backgrounds can provide satisfactory isolation and contrast for the subject. They also have the added benefit of providing a visually pleasing appearance when projected on a screen in a dark auditorium. The major drawback of coloured backgrounds is that they may impart a false hue to the subject. This is especially apparent when the background occupies a disproportionately large area compared to the size of the subject being photographed (Fig. 4.1). However, if care is taken to frame the shot so that the subject occupies the majority of the photograph, this effect can be minimized. Ideally, the photographer should choose a dull or matt, seamless light blue or green background. This must be coupled with judicious lighting to

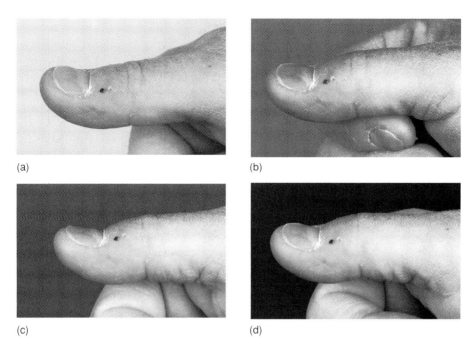

Fig. 4.1. Images taken with various background colours. The nuances of colour from the background influence the subtle colour in the thumb: (a) white background; (b) grey background; (c) blue background; (d) black background.

minimize shadowing and flare, while positioning the patient to minimize the ratio of background to subject appearing in the frame.[5]

Apart from hospital linen and surgical towels, background materials come in many different forms and colours. Photographic suppliers offer fixed or portable background materials in various sizes, as well as disposable background materials. The disposable background material is useful for photographing subjects with infectious or draining lesions.

Subject positioning

After the choice of background material and lighting, patient positioning is the next most important consideration in dermatology imaging. Clearly, the disease process being photographed will influence patient positioning. Several factors should be considered when deciding how best to capture a representative image of the lesions in question. These factors include the size, shape, colour, edge configuration and distribution of the lesions.[2] In addition, the intended use of the photograph also plays an important part in considering how the patient is to be positioned. For example, if the photograph will be used to evaluate disease progression over time, a significant effort should be made to ensure that subsequent images are obtained in the same manner as those taken before. To do this, one must take care to record not only the appropriate camera settings and lighting setup used in the original shoot, but also the precise position of the patient relative to the camera (including the distance and angle from the camera). Slight changes in either the distance from the camera or the angle of the shot can significantly influence the resulting photographs and therefore perceived patient responses to intervention. Incidentally, this is one area where digital imaging may offer a significant advantage over standard photography. The advantage lies in the fact that a digital image can be manipulated by the user through cropping or magnification/reduction so as to produce a more consistent series of images for evaluation. In many cases, this process can compensate for slight variations in photographic technique over time.

To assist in standardizing the distance between the lens and the subject, the photographer may choose to use a distance guide attached to the camera. These guides are commercially available and generally attach to the tripod mounting hole under the camera body. The guide consists of a fixed or adjustable length arm which projects forward. Some models even have a small ruler at the end of the guide. Although they provide a reliable method of maintaining a consistent distance between the camera and the subject, as well as a linear element which can be used to help adjust the axis of the shot, care must be taken to avoid contamination of the end of the guide. It may be best to disinfect the distal end of the guide between patients. Another way to help keep a consistent distance from the subject without the use of a physical guide is to choose a manual focus setting which focuses the lens at a known distance. After recording the position of the manual focus ring for that distance, subsequent images can be taken by setting the manual focus ring to the known position, and focusing on the subject by moving closer or further from the patient until the subject is in focus through the viewfinder.

When considering the composition of the photograph, it is important to include some identifiable frame of reference within the picture so that the location of the lesions on the body can be ascertained easily by the observer. For example, if a close-up picture of a small (<2 cm) lesion located on the thigh is taken to emphasize its surface characteristics, rapid evaluation by the observer can be hindered if its location is not readily identifiable (Fig. 4.2). An image which includes the lateral edges of the thigh will assist in the recognition of the distribution and location of the lesions. In some instances, a macro image including such landmarks may be sufficient for both studying the details of the lesion as well as identification of the distribution of the lesions. This can eliminate the need for 'scout' images. If such an identifying landmark cannot be included in a macro photograph, it is best to include a scout image, as discussed below. In addition to assisting in the identification of the distribution lesions, landmarks may allow the size of the lesion to be judged. However, the best scale of reference to give the viewer an idea of the size of a lesion is the inclusion of a ruler in the photograph. Different options for rulers are described in a section below.

To document the size and shape of a particular lesion accurately, one should ensure that the lens of the camera is parallel to the plane of the lesion. In addition, the camera should be on axis with the lesion, and not at an angle to it. Altering any of these angles

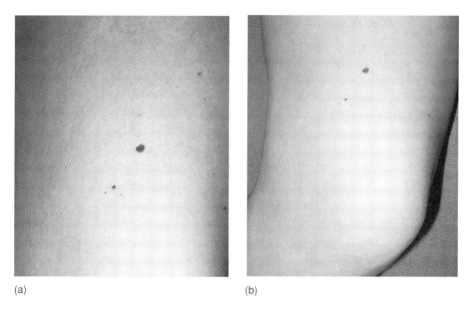

(a)   (b)

Fig. 4.2. Although the lesion is easy to detect in (a), it is difficult to determine its anatomical location because there are no reference points. However, the viewer can be assisted in finding the location of the lesion by including landmarks such as the knee shown in (b).

can result in a distorted image of the lesion in question. The drawback of using a direct axis when shooting an image is that this vantage provides little information about the texture or edge configuration of the lesion if the elevations and depressions are very fine.[6] However, additional images can be obtained off the axis to emphasize the height of the lesion (Fig. 4.3(a)–(c)). The fine texture as well as the elevations and depressions of a lesion can also be emphasized by increasing the incident angle of the lighting relative to the subject (Fig 4.3(d)). When possible, it is preferable to demonstrate such surface details by adjusting the lighting so that it is no more than 10–20 degrees off the axis. This allows proper representations of the elevations or depressions on the surface of the subject by casting subtle shadows and bright areas. However, if accessory lighting is not used, it may be acceptable to angle the camera slightly in order to bring out the surface details. Note that this technique will distort the image and should only be used with an accompanying on-axis view of the lesion.

It is important to remember that the overall colour of the lesion being imaged can be influenced by the choice of background material, as discussed above. If coloured backgrounds are employed, ensuring that the background occupies a relatively small area of the frame and is relatively out of focus compared to the lesion in question will reduce its influence on the colour of the subject.

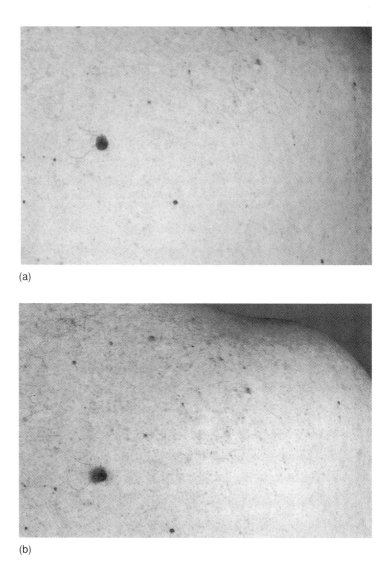

(a)

(b)

Fig. 4.3. The perceived depth of a lesion (a) can be enhanced by taking additional images off axis (b).

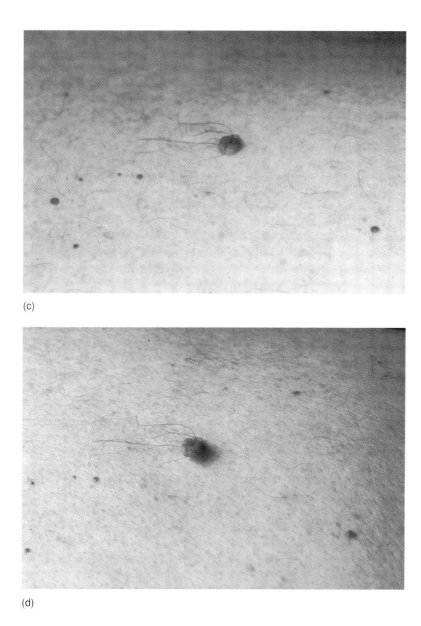

(c)

(d)

Fig. 4.3 – continued. The perceived depth of a lesion (c) can also be enhanced by increasing the angle of the incident light (d).

Scout images

It is often helpful to demonstrate the location of the lesion in question by providing an image taken at a distance from the subject. This image is called a scout image. It need not be very detailed since its purpose is to give the viewer an idea about the distribution of the lesion or lesions. The scout image can be taken by moving far away from the subject or by using a lens such as a 50-mm lens. When possible, the area covered in the scout image should not include more than 50% of the height of the patient. This allows the location or distribution of most small lesions to be identified. After taking the scout image, subsequent medium distance and macro photographs of the lesions in question can be taken to show the details of the lesions. This may require changing the lens on the camera to one suited for macro photography. Adjustment of the lighting may also be necessary between photographs taken at various distances.

Effective scales of reference

The most effective and accurate scale of reference for medical photography is a ruler. The ruler helps the viewer to appreciate the size of a lesion being imaged. The ruler should be placed next to the lesion being photographed and on the same plane. When choosing a ruler to use in medical photographs, there are several considerations to keep in mind. First, you need to select the correct size of ruler for the photograph. Ideally, the ruler should be as long as the lesion itself or slightly larger.[3] Rulers should be marked in metric units with centimetres marked with longer lines and millimetre increments marked with short lines.

The best materials for rulers are those with dimensional stability. For this reason, it is best to avoid paper or tape rulers. Also, the ruler should be rigid in order to avoid flexing. Flexing may lead to portions of the ruler being out of focus in the final image. This is especially likely for images that are taken with camera settings that provide little depth of focus. To ensure that both the lesion and the ruler are in focus, it is necessary to place the ruler on the same plane as the lesion. Because the ruler is marked with a series of straight lines, it is easy to see if it is out of focus. It is best to place the ruler at the bottom of the frame so that it does not distract from the image. It is also important to select a ruler that lacks distracting text, such as advertising matter, which can take the viewer's attention away from the subject. Distracting colours or highly reflective surfaces on rulers may also produce poor images of the subject.

Good rulers to use are brushed stainless steel machinist rulers. These produce a dark grey, non-reflective image with light lines. Another excellent ruler commonly used in legal medical photography and forensic work is the ABFO #2 scale (Fig. 4.4). This ruler consists of an L-shaped piece of plastic angled at 90 degrees. The 90-degree marking can help identify distortion at the periphery of an image due to a smaller or lower quality camera lens. Also, the scale has a greyscale marking which can be used to standardize the image if it is subsequently manipulated using software to compensate for small variations in exposure or lighting intensity.

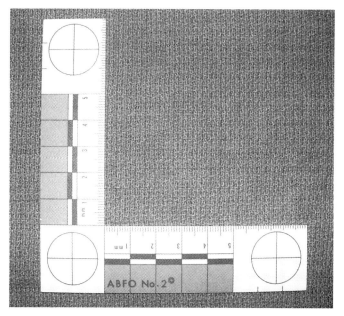

Fig. 4.4. The ABFO #2 Scale.

Lighting

Effective lighting is an essential part of good medical photography. There are many considerations when choosing lighting units for a studio as well as flash units for a particular camera. Both the ambient lighting and the studio flash units have an effect on the quality of the image. The most dramatic effects of lighting can best be seen by photographing a subject without using a built-in camera flash or a hot shoe-mounted flash.

A detailed discussion on the practice of light placement is beyond the scope of this chapter. Moreover, most practitioners who utilize digital imaging for convenience are unlikely to have elaborate lighting setups available to them. However, a few important points will be considered here. First, if one does have access to accessory lighting, use of these lights can significantly improve the quality of the images captured. In general, a frontal light source is beneficial for differentiating colour in a lesion, but often this is at the expense of texture detail. Similarly, side lighting or spot lighting significantly improves texture detail but diminishes colour detail and edge configuration. Thus a combination of both frontal and side lighting often yields the best results. With regard to lighting and background selection, it is important to focus external lights depending on the shade of the background. When shooting a patient against a light-coloured background, aim the lights so that they converge behind the patient on the background. With dark backgrounds, dramatic results can be obtained by focusing external lights behind the subject. In general, it is best to avoid any type of extreme lighting on the lesion, as this can introduce distortion with little gain in image resolution.[2]

Several companies make lenses which can be adapted to include both a ring flash and a point light source flash. Both types of flash have useful capabilities in capturing digital images. The ring flash provides even illumination and is used for imaging lesions that are in cavities, because the ring flash will penetrate the cavity. The point light source flash provides directional lighting and is useful in showing more edge detail or raised surfaces areas.

Tungsten lights versus electronic strobes

Many tungsten lighting kits are available for digital photography. Examples include kits by Lowel, Smith-Victor, Calumet and Arri. These units are relatively cheap. The disadvantages of tungsten lights are the heat produced, which can adversely affect the patient, especially in smaller office settings, and the high electrical current required to operate them. If both digital and conventional photography are being considered, then electronic strobes are the best choice. These allow the use of daylight-balanced film for conventional photography as well as digital photography. Electronic strobes are recommended due to their daylight colour temperature, low power utilization and relatively low heat generated. There are many manufacturers of electronic studio strobes including Novatron, Norman and Speedotron. In addition to studio strobes, smaller battery-powered units such as Vivitar, Metz, Nikon and Canon are available for digital photography.

Macro mode imaging

Images taken at various distances from the subject can prove useful to the consultant. An image taken from a distance for an overview of the patient can provide information about the patient's health as a whole. It may even show signs of disease processes, which may be a significant aid in the diagnosis of a specific lesion or in the treatment plan for the patient.

Imaging system optimization: trial and error?

When designing a digital imaging system for use in teledermatology, a team approach is required. The team members must include the physicians, nursing staff, technical support personnel, the director of telemedicine services, and the staff who will be performing digital photography or video filming and data entry at the patient's end of the system.

Many suppliers offer pre-configured teledermatology systems. Examples include systems designed and serviced by Polycom and V-Tel. The advantage of choosing such equipment lies in the customer support offered. This is attractive for health care providers who do not want to invest resources in installation and troubleshooting. A difficulty often encountered with piecemeal constructed telemedicine systems is the tendency for the manufacturer of each component to blame a problem on a different component of the system that is not manufactured by them.

The disadvantage of purchasing a pre-configured system is the loss of autonomy in choosing components to fit your needs and budget. Options and accessories may be quite limited or may be more expensive than comparable products from different manufacturers. Maintenance and support contracts for these systems can also be expensive.

Despite the problems of troubleshooting a custom-built system, the flexibility of choosing components best suited to your facilities and needs is valuable. This allows easy upgrading of individual components as required. It may also allow the ability to take advantage of technologies that are already available such as high-bandwidth lines and existing computer systems.

References

1   Loane MA, Bloomer SE, Corbett R, et al. A comparison of real-time and store-and-forward teledermatology: a cost–benefit study. *British Journal of Dermatology* 2000;**143**:1241–1247.
2   Williams R, ed. *Medical Photography Study Guide*, 4th edn. London: MTP Press, 1984:8–10, 14–17, 94–96.
3   McGaven MD, Thompson SW, eds. *Specimen Dissection and Photography*, 1st edn. Springfield: Charles C. Thomas, 1988:44–45, 54, 75–83.
4   Blaker AA, ed. *Handbook for Scientific Photography*, 2nd edn. San Francisco: W.H. Freeman, 1977: 43–44.
5   Tardy ME, ed. *Principles of Photography in Facial Plastic Surgery*, 1st edn. New York: Thieme Medical Publishers, 1992:12–15.
6   Hansell P, ed. *A Guide to Medical Photography*, 1st edn. Baltimore: University Park Press, 1979:15–20.

Section 2: Current Experience – Diagnosis and Patient Management

5

A Survey of Teledermatology in the USA

Bill Grigsby and Nancy A. Brown

Introduction

In the USA, dermatology has consistently been one of the most active clinical specialties for teleconsultation, both in terms of the overall levels of activity and the number of telemedicine networks doing it. We have examined teledermatology activity in the context of overall clinical activity in the telemedicine sector. The present study represents a recent survey of teledermatology providers in four of the more active networks in the USA in 1999–2000. The data were obtained from a series of annual surveys commissioned by the Association of Telehealth Service Providers[1-3] and conducted by staff at the Telemedicine Research Center (Portland, OR). The surveys focused on the telemedicine 'programme' or 'network' as the relevant unit of analysis. A network generally consists of one or a few resource-rich healthcare facilities (often large hospitals or academic medical centers) providing services in multiple clinical specialties to a larger number of resource-poor sites serving geographically or institutionally isolated populations (e.g. in the latter case, prisons).

The surveys were conducted via questionnaires distributed by mail, supplemented with Web-based and faxed versions. Dillman's[4] 'Total Design Method' was used. Response rates are difficult to calculate, because a good deal of duplication and redundancy was built into the sampling frame. To account for staff turnover, surveys were sent to multiple individuals within the same network, who were often geographically dispersed. Table 5.1 shows the observed response rates and adjusted response rates, which attempt to account for the duplication. The adjusted response rate compares the sample size to the number of *known* networks from the sampling frame (an effort was made to make telephone contact to confirm the existence of networks). There are obviously networks that exist that are not within the sampling frame, and networks within it that were not confirmed and listed among the *known* programmes.

Table 5.1. Survey sample size and response rates[3]

Year	Sample size	Response rate (%)	Adjusted response rate (%)*
1996	96	49	73
1997	141	31	90
1998	132	30	73

*The adjusted response rate attempted to compensate for the duplication built in to the sampling frame (see text).

Survey results 1996–1999

The results of the surveys show that five clinical specialties (Table 5.2) were the most active, both in terms of teleconsultations and numbers of networks: mental health, cardiology, dermatology, neurology and orthopaedics. They had become sufficiently widespread that their activity did not depend on the fortunes of individual networks.

A focus on the programme level from the 1999 survey reveals more about the use of teledermatology (for a complete list of programmes active in 1999, see Appendix 5.1). While there were no 'typical' programmes, a few generalizations seem warranted. First, most networks depended on one to three dermatologists to provide teleconsultation to remote sites – only three of 44 responding programmes from the 1999 survey reported more than three participating specialists. Second there was a great deal of variation in activity among the programmes. For 1998, nine programmes reported 10 or fewer teleconsultations; 11 reported 11–50; six reported 51–100; and 11 reported over 100. Fifteen networks listed dermatology as their most active specialty (second only to mental health, reported by 33 programmes as their most active specialty).

The most common service offered by networks providing teledermatology services was referral for specialist consultation (initial diagnosis or second opinion) (Table 5.3). Ongoing management and follow-up were also reported by nearly every responding programme. The most common means of delivering these services was through remote 'clinics' – blocks of time during which patients from specific sites were scheduled for a store-and-forward or an interactive consultation. Twenty-three programmes reported using remote specialist clinics to deliver care in dermatology. Generally clinics are convenient for patients, staff and providers, and can potentially reduce telecommunications charges through consolidation of the teleconsultations.

The data also show that a mixture of technologies was used to deliver care. In 1999, 21 networks responding to the Association of Telemedicine Service Providers' (ATSP) survey were exclusively using interactive video to provide care, accounting for 52% of activity. Five store-and-forward programmes accounted for 12% of activity. Four were using 'audiographic' technology (non-video interactive, allowing remote sharing of still images with an audio connection) and accounted for 3% of total consultations. Thirteen programmes were using a combination of the above three technologies, and accounted for the remaining 33% of activity.

Table 5.2. Activity for the most active specialties: 1996–99[1-3]

	No. of programmes				Total teleconsultations reported			
	1996	1997	1998	1999	1996	1997	1998	1999*
Mental health	25	43	57	55	2886	7404	11 974	3972
Cardiology	27	48	32	32	2282	6839	3469	955
Dermatology	28	40	38	36	1958	2345	3278	1387
Orthopaedics	18	29	24	25	1083	2306	4554	2912
Neurology	15	23	17	16	555	699	801	353

*Includes only first quarter statistics (1 January to 31 March).

Table 5.3. Services reported by 43 of the 44 programmes[3]

Service	Number reporting
Specialist referral/second opinion	32
Ongoing management of patient	22
Follow-up	13
Patient case review	4
Medication management	2
Patient screening	2
Total no of programmes responding	**43**

The latest survey showed that the 'mixed' category was increasing. This may be because asynchronous teledermatology is generally considered more effective when supplemented by some form of interactive communication with the patient or referring provider. However, the use of audiographic or store-and-forward technology to transfer information can potentially reduce telecommunications charges, and the store-and-forward technique provides greater flexibility for the specialists (who seem to be in short supply). Ten of the 15 networks reporting dermatology as their most active specialty were using multiple media to deliver care.

The survey questions did not identify the telecommunications services used for dermatology specifically. As far as the overall telemedicine activity was concerned, the three most commonly reported services were ISDN (128–512 kbit/s, reported by 45%), T-1 and fractional T-1 lines (384–1540 kbit/s, reported by 40%), and standard telephone lines (up to 33 kbit/s, reported by 24%). A variety of peripheral devices were used for telemedicine generally, including digital cameras (54), dermoscopes (29) and general examination cameras (12), although their specific use for dermatology was not reported.

Teledermatology has become an important component of many telemedicine networks, and its activity levels have increased, as have those for the telemedicine sector in general (Table 5.4). However, overall levels of growth tend to mask the uneven distribution of activity across states, across organizations and across clinical specialties. Prison telemedicine accounted for almost 30% of activity in 1998. The point is that remote access to specialists, dermatologists included, varies greatly from one area, one state or from one network to the next.

Table 5.4. Growth in number of programmes and telemedicine activity from 1993 to 1999

	1993[5]	1994[6]	1995[7]	1996[1]	1997[2]	1998[3]	1999[3]
Number of programmes identified	10	24	49	86	132	157	179
Number of teleconsultations	1750*	2110	6138	21 732	41 740	52 223	74 828†
Mean teleconsultations/ programme‡	175	88	125	253	316	428	608
Total number of facilities					747	1345	1521
Mean no. of facilities/programme					8.3	10.3	11.1

*The data from 1993 to 1995 focused exclusively on video-mediated interactive consultations.
†Based on projections for first quarter 1999.
‡Averages are based on the number of respondents, not the number of identified programmes.

It is also difficult to assess the extent to which growth in telemedicine depends on federal funding. Fifty-six out of 132 networks reported receiving some funding from the Federal Government in 1999.[3] Another indicator of the relative immaturity of the field is that 49% of the programmes relied on multiple sources of funding (25% relied on three or more).

Regardless of the success of any single application, the fortunes of telemedicine programmes are to some extent subject to larger forces within the healthcare industry. Survey results point to a lack of reimbursement for specialists as the most important barrier to the continued growth of telemedicine. However, the complexity involved in bringing together diverse organizations and individuals under one organizational umbrella (including many physicians with little affiliation to the consulting facilities) suggests great difficulty in developing an incentive structure conducive to the participation of the relevant parties – rural facilities, rural physicians, professional staff, patients, specialists, tertiary hospitals, even the parent organization. The role of the government, and the ability of the Internet to address the technical barriers and operate within the tightly regulated environment of health care will be critical to continued growth in the field.

Results of the year 2000 teledermatology survey

In December 2000, four telemedicine networks were surveyed via email about their teledermatology activity in 1999 and the first quarter of 2000 (these survey results are unpublished). We attempted to contact the six most active teledermatology programmes, but two did not respond. All of the networks were large, relative to average network size. The four networks were the University of California–Davis (UCD) (35 sites), the University of Missouri (MU) (23 sites), the University of Arizona (UA) (13 sites) and Mountaineer Doctor Television (MDTV) at West Virginia University (16 sites). The remote sites consist of a mixture of smaller hospitals, outpatient clinics and mental health clinics. All had been recipients of major federal grants, which were instrumental in the development of their networks.

Table 5.5 shows the teledermatology activity reported over the last 5 years, with total consultations in all specialties for 1998 provided for comparison. Dermatology was either the most active or the second most active specialty for all four of these programmes (where teledermatology was second, mental health was the primary activity). While dermatology comprised a substantial proportion of total teleconsultations, all four programmes were fairly robust in terms of specialty coverage.

How are teleconsultations generated?

Each of the networks relied on patient referrals from rural practitioners to bring patients into the telemedicine network. Their teledermatology initiatives were designed to address poor specialty coverage in rural areas (with the exception of a small number of correctional facilities at UCD and UA, and a military base hospital at MU). Three of

Table 5.5. Dermatology activity for the networks surveyed, 1996–2000. The total number of teleconsultations (all specialties) in 1988 is also shown for comparison

Network	Years active	No. of teleconsultations					Total teleconsultations
		1996[1]	1997[2]	1998[3]	1999	2000	1998
Missouri University (MU)	6	27	83	217	209	75*	694 (31%)
University of California–Davis (UCD)	5		19	201	256	556	1032 (19%)
University of Arizona (UA)	4		no resp.	201	240	60*	572 (35%)
MDTV (West Virginia University)	8	166	475	397	506	398†	680 (58%)
Total				1016 (34%)			**2978**

*Activity for the first quarter of 2000.

the four networks reported that they had adequate resources to meet the demand for teledermatology consultations. However, MDTV had reached maximum capacity with one dermatologist, who averaged 43 teleconsultations per month. UCD reported that its two clinic sites were consistently filled, with a total of 25 patients per week.

The number of physicians referring patients for teledermatology consultation varied from one network to the next. MU and UCD estimated that 35–50 providers referred patients, MDTV reported 13 providers who referred patients, and UA up to 100. We were unable to collect information on variation within these groups of physicians with respect to referrals. Two of the networks reported that referrals were increasing over time, while MDTV reported a decrease in the number of referrals. One could speculate that, with a smaller pool of physicians seeing more skin cases, the primary providers were gaining competence with the straightforward cases, and referring only the more complex ones. An interesting research question is whether the opportunity costs of learning from dermatologists during teleconsultation (i.e. seeing other patients in their practices) outweighed the benefits. In many cases the referring provider did not present the patient for teleconsultation.

What services are offered?

In general the networks were providing patients with remote access to a specialist for diagnosis or treatment. Each of the networks surveyed organized some of its teledermatology as remote 'clinics'. The clinic setting offered several advantages for the physicians and the network staff. Perhaps the most important was the convenience for specialists – who are arguably the most important component in a telemedicine network. Scheduling patients during pre-arranged blocks of time is more efficient, allows them to see more patients, and permits them to work telemedicine into their schedules in a predictable way.

The clinic setting streamlined scheduling for the network as well. It is important to remember that most programmes offer a variety of services within multiple specialties.

Scheduling patients on a one-on-one basis and coordinating those schedules between two sites would greatly increase the setup time and potentially the telecommunications costs per patient. In fact, the 1999 data show that all but one of the most active programmes reported using clinics. UA reported the least use of the clinic setting, however, because their method of working was store-and-forward, so that some of the advantages of clinic organization do not apply.

Two of the networks reported using telemedicine to facilitate the review of patients between providers. This can be especially helpful in the case of store-and-forward or audiographic teledermatology. It not only allows the physicians an opportunity to interact professionally, but in terms of telemedicine protocols, it provides a critical link in ensuring that the information from the teleconsultation is transferred to the patient's primary physician. This is useful in terms of increasing the likelihood of patient satisfaction with the process, and of managing risk associated with remote delivery of patient information and healthcare services.

What sorts of technical arrangements are used?

Three of the four programmes used interactive video exclusively to deliver care. One reported supplementing this with images captured by a digital camera (which presumably could transmit still images). All three seemed satisfied with the medium, and reported that the physicians preferred the interactivity. UA reported that 97% of its teleconsultation was done via store-and-forward technology, which the respondent characterized as 'easier and less time consuming'. The UCD respondent believed that store-and-forward telemedicine would probably be effective as well, and also reported that it was in the process of developing this capability. There was some reservation on the part of a few clinicians about whether store-and-forward telemedicine offered acceptable diagnostic quality (presumably because of the lack of interactivity with the patient).

Only one programme reported any extensive use of the Internet. MU stated that they were developing a 'virtual private network' instead. The programme director mentioned several advantages of using Internet protocols – easier maintenance, troubleshooting and upgrading, greater compatibility with PC-based systems in clinics, and more convenient scheduling because any site can communicate with any other site. This sort of network architecture has implications not only for cost, but also for ease of operation, especially within networks where facilities serve multiple roles (i.e. as a requestor and provider of services). UCD occasionally used the Internet to communicate about scheduling, and MDTV to receive or transmit distance educational material. All seemed to be looking for opportunities to expand in this area.

Sustainability

None of the survey questions directly addressed the issue of sustainability. However, a few responses addressed the issue indirectly. All of the networks reported that they were receiving reimbursement for teleconsultations, although it is not clear who was being reimbursed: presumably the specialist. Sustaining teledermatology may require more compelling incentives for the rural participants, both the organizations and the individuals concerned, who in most cases represent gateways for patients to enter the system. Rural providers play an important role in the sustainability of any telemedicine programme. They do not necessarily have to become involved in the teleconsultation process itself, although the more reasons they have to participate, the better. Incentives for providers to participate might include: learning from dermatologists or other specialists; working from office PCs; possessing clear information about telemedicine protocols (as opposed to clinical protocols – the procedures and responsibilities of each party); ability to access patient records electronically within the network; potential for remote back-up coverage in a local emergency room (where physicians perform this role); and availability of continuing medical education opportunities. Efforts to recruit providers to an area, as well as to retain them, will be easier if connectivity is perceived as an advantage. Physicians comfortable with the idea of integrating telecommunications technologies into their practice may be more likely to consider such opportunities.

From the specialist's point of view, reimbursement is crucial to sustainability. All four programmes reported some level of reimbursement. Two of the networks reported that they were near to full capacity in terms of utilization. Supply of dermatology expertise can be a limiting factor, and addressing it may have more to do with competition within regional markets than anything else. In this respect, larger healthcare networks may enjoy a comparative advantage in terms of programme expansion; for instance, UCD participated in a network affiliated to Blue Cross of California, an important insurance payor in a state with a population of more than 30 million people. Teleconsultations are also generally reimbursed by the Medi-Cal system as mandated by the state Telemedicine Development Act of 1996.

From an organizational point of view, it seems that much of the expertise in terms of providing care from the specialist's end was concentrated among a handful of dermatologists. Organizations would do well to find some mechanism of documentation that would ensure continuity in the event of staff turnover, as well as reduce the burden of training for current staff should new specialists enter the network.

Lessons learned

The four programmes surveyed represent an impressive accumulation of knowledge about how to provide teledermatology (over 15 years of collective experience). Two of the survey items were devoted to collecting a list of lessons learned. With respect to planning and design, MDTV emphasized the importance of having clinical need to drive the process. Physicians should be involved from the beginning, and a thorough understanding of their needs and technical competence is critical. Both MDTV and MU mentioned the importance of specialist–primary provider relationships. There needs to be a high level of trust and confidence. It is unlikely that, without information technology support, rural facilities would be able to integrate this service into their delivery system.

MU emphasized the importance of equipment choice and purchase. The process should be thorough and should involve product demonstrations. In addition, those entering the field should contact other teledermatology programmes and should take advantage of any existing technical guidelines for remote delivery of dermatology (such as the Telehealth Technology Guidelines at http://telehealth.hrsa.gov/ pubs/tech/techhome.htm [last checked 3 November 2001]).

From an operational perspective, MU stressed the importance of teledermatology emulating the face-to-face clinic setting as far as possible – in terms of delivery, medical records, scheduling and billing. Three of the four programmes mentioned the importance of the role of personnel at the patient site. UCD considered the site coordinator to be a critical factor in the success of the programme, both from an organizational standpoint (e.g. scheduling and patient consent), and also to ensure that the consultations run smoothly for the specialists. The camera operators and technicians are also extremely important – this was emphasized by the two dermatologists with whom we spoke, as well as the network administrators. They must be well trained, preferably in a process that involves the dermatologists with whom they will be working. This becomes more important with asynchronous working.

In addition, while organizing teledermatology delivery in a clinic setting was not mentioned with respect to lessons learned, it may be that because it is so much a part of the operation of real-time teledermatology that it was taken for granted.

Conclusion

There seems to be little doubt that technology has great potential for bridging coverage gaps. There are limiting factors, however, such as competition between healthcare systems, interstate licensure, liability concerns, or a host of individual attributes (e.g. physician attitudes about technology, willingness to modify established practice patterns, or to refer to 'closer' surgeons if need be). There is a shortage of specialists, whether for in-person or remote consultation. One of the dermatologists we interviewed said that he was confident that he could fill as many remote clinics as he could offer.

The sample of four relatively successful programmes (in terms of utilization) is probably not representative of the 30 or more programmes delivering teledermatology services. It is likely that the participants in the four programmes, especially the specialists, represent 'early adopters' of a new technique. Thus their reasons for practising teledermatology may not be relevant to the majority of specialists. Most will be concerned about the business aspect of the application, and with the opportunity costs of providing services remotely. This means that planning and design are critical components in the success of telemedicine initiatives, and places a premium on involvement of the relevant stakeholders. All four programmes were also based at academic medical centres, which presumably offered advantages in terms of infrastructure, personnel, funding and specialist availability.

Participation at the remote sites is another important component of any telemedicine network. Sites must have good reasons to devote space, staff and resources to telemedicine. 'Improving patient care' may be a necessary but insufficient benefit of teledermatology. All programmes listed the skill and expertise of remote site staff as important to the enterprise, as well as the cultivation of a sound working relationship between site coordinators, camera operators, and referring and consulting physicians. In some cases the individuals participating in the telemedicine network may be only marginally affiliated with the organizations.

It could also be that the growth and relative success of teledermatology is partly due to the suitability of dermatology to the medium. It appears to be ideal for remote diagnosis, permitting relatively short patient visits and productive clinics where many patients are seen.

It does not seem that lack of demand – often cited as a reason why rural telemedicine has not grown faster – has held back the development of teledermatology. This does not imply that investment in equipment is warranted solely for delivering services in a single clinical specialty. That is a situation requiring careful planning and evaluation, or a generous source of financial support. In most cases (and for all four surveyed networks) teledermatology is part of a larger package of expertise and services available through a telemedicine network. Operational changes needed to take advantage of remote delivery of care in one specialty can be transferred to other specialties as well.

Where demand for specific services within a given rural area can be aggregated at some larger network level, and combined with other services for which a clinical need has been identified and for which a delivery infrastructure exists, telemedicine is worth considering. Given sufficient commitment from individuals and organizations, teledermatology seems well placed to become a prominent part of networks offering multi-specialty telemedicine services.

Acknowledgements

We thank the staff of the four programmes surveyed in December 2000. Their willingness to provide additional information on their programmes is much appreciated. They include: Elizabeth A Krupinski PhD, Research Associate Professor, and Mary Dolliver, Programme Coordinator, at the University of Arizona; Kathy Chorba, Operations Lead, Robin Alexander MD, and Patricia Tyee, Clinic Coordinator, at the University of California–Davis; Joe Tracey, Director of Telehealth, and Ron Swinfard MD, at the University of Missouri; and Chris Budig, MDTV Programme Manager, at West Virginia University.

References

1   Grigsby B. *1997 Report of US Telemedicine Activity.* Portland, OR: Association of Telemedicine Service Providers, 1997.
2   Grigsby B, Brown N. *1998 Report on US Telemedicine Activity.* Portland, OR: Association of Telemedicine Service Providers, 1998.
3   Grigsby B, Brown N. *1999 Report on US Telemedicine Activity.* Portland, OR: Association of Telehealth Service Providers, 2000.
4   Dillman D. *Mail and Telephone Surveys: The Total Design Method.* New York: Wiley and Sons, 1978.
5   Allen A. Top ten North American programs. *Telemedicine Newsletter* 1994;**1**(4):1,3–4.
6   Allen A, Allen D. Telemedicine programs: 2nd annual review reveals doubling of programs in a year. *Telemedicine Today* 1995;**3**(2):1,10–16.
7   Allen A, Scarbrough M. 3rd annual program review. *Telemedicine Today* 1996;**4**(4):10–17, 34–48.

Appendix 5.1

US telemedicine networks reporting activity in dermatology, 1998–1999[3]

Name of programme	State	Technologies used	No. of providers	Services offered (see key below)	Teleconsultations 1998	Teleconsultations 1999 *
UAMS Rural Hosp. Telehealth Prog	AR	IATV/audiogr.	1	1,3,4,6	22	1
Arizona Telemedicine Program	AZ	IATV/S&F	3	1,3,6,8,20	201	56
Northern Sierra Regional TM Sys.	CA	Interactive video		1,3	7	5
University of California–Davis	CA	Interactive video	1	1,2,3,4,6	201	68
Telemedicine Services Program	CA	Interactive video	2	1,3,4,5,7	106	21
High Plains Rural Health Network	CO	Interactive video	1	1	4	0
Denver Health Telemedicine	CO	Audiographic	1	1,3	20	6
Americares Free Clinic of Norwalk	CT	Interactive video	1	1		
Walter Reed Army MC TM	DC	Store-and-forward	7	1	327	120
Georgetown–Nairobi Project	DC	IATV/S&F/audiogr.	1	1,3,4	0	0
Univ. of Miami Teledermatology	FL	Store-and-forward	1	1	22	
Georgia Statewide Telemedicine	GA	IATV/S&F/audiogr.	3	1,2,3,4,6	42	115
National Lab. for Study of Rural TM	IA	Interactive video	2	1,3,4,6,8	71	21
MRTC (Mercy)	IA	Interactive video	2	6	51	10
Clarian Health Partners	IN	Store-and-forward		20		
Kentucky TeleCare	KY	IATV/audiogr.	1	1,6	24	6
S. Cameron Memorial Telemedicine	LA	Interactive video	1	4	1	1
Louisiana Telemedicine Program	LA			1,6		
Allina Health System TM	MN	Store-and-forward	1	1	37	6
Univ. of Minnesota Telemedicine	MN	Interactive video	2	6,3	109	58
Univ. of Missouri Telemedicine	MO	Interactive video	3	1,3,6,20	217	105
Eastern Montana TM Network	MT	Interactive video	2	1	15	
East Carolina Univ. Telemedicine	NC	IATV/S&F	3	6,1,4	274	94
New Hanover Regional MC	NC	Store-and-forward	2	1	10	1
St Alexius TeleCare Network	ND	Interactive video	1	1,6,3	39	22
Dakota Telemedicine System	ND	Interactive video	1	6	50	11
Mid-Nebraska TM Network	NE	Interactive video	2	3,5,6		

Programme	State	Technology		Services offered		
Nevada Telemedicine Project	NV	Interactive video	1		10	6
Ohio State Univ. Telemedicine	OH	IATV/audiogr.	8	1,3,4,6,18	251	120
Crozer-Keystone Health System TM	PA	IATV/S&F/audiogr.	2	3,6,12	78	39
Avera McKennan TeleHealth Network	SD	Audiographic	1	1	7	3
Univ. of Tennessee TM Network	TN	Interactive video	1	6	18	10
Texas Tech Univ. Telemedicine	TX	Interactive video	2	1,4	61	15
Utah Telehealth Network	UT	Audiographic	2	5,6,3	84	45
Rural Utah Telemedicine Associates	UT	IATV/S&F	2	1,3	0	1
MCV Campus Telemedicine	VA	Audiographic	1	1,6		
Univ. of Virginia Telemed.	VA	IATV/S&F/audiogr.	3	3,6	97	30
Univ. of Wash. Telehealth	WA	IATV/S&F/audiogr.	3	1,2,3,4,5	58	11
Inland NW TeleHEALTH	WA	Interactive video	2	6	4	5
Virginia Mason Med. Ctr. TM	WA	IATV/S&F	3	1,18,20		
Marshfield Clinic Telehealth	WI	Interactive video	1	1,3,4,6.	100	86
MDTV (West VA University)	WV	Interactive video	4	1,6	397	257
MDTV–Charleston Med. Ctr.	WV	Interactive video	1	6,1,3,4	225	30
Wyoming Integrated Telehealth	WY	IATV/S&F/audiogr.	1	1,5,3	38	2
Total: 44 programmes	**30**	**IATV: 21** **S&F: 5** **Audiographic: 4** **Mixed: 13**	**83 (41)****		**3278 (37)****	**1387** **(33)****

*Activity for the first quarter in 1999.

**Numbers in parentheses denote the number of responding programmes reporting activity.

Key to services offered:

1 specialist referrals/2nd opinions
2 emergency room/triage
3 ongoing management of patient condition
4 medical/surgical follow-up
5 diagnostic examination
6 specialist clinics
7 physiological monitoring
8 medication management
12 nursing home/asst living
18 patient screening
20 patient case review

6

Real-time Teledermatology in Norway

Gisli Ingvarsson and Dagfinn Moseng

Introduction

The major referral centre in northern Norway, the University Hospital of Tromsø (UHT), has been involved in a variety of telemedicine activities since the late 1980s. Because of the considerable geographical distances in this northernmost region, communication is a costly and challenging problem. A pilot project,[1] started in 1989, included monthly teledermatology sessions between the UHT Department of Dermatology and a specially trained general practitioner (GP) in a studio in Kirkenes, some 800 km away (Fig. 6.1). Four years later (in 1993) a dermatological outpatient clinic was established at Kirkenes Hospital supported by weekly afternoon teledermatology sessions. Phototherapy is the mainstay of dermatological practice in

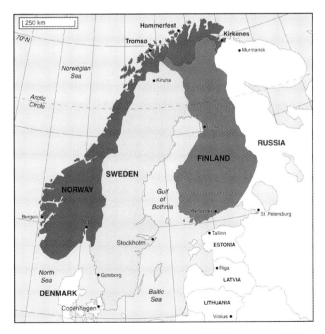

Fig. 6.1. Teledermatology sessions are held between the Department of Dermatology at the University Hospital of Tromsø and a specially trained GP in a studio in Kirkenes, some 800 km away.

these areas of the Northern Hemisphere. Teledermatology resulted in a welcome reduction in travelling for both the specialists and the patients involved. Indeed, this was partly because the assisting GP could function as a 'bare foot' dermatologist after a while. Subsequently in 1996 a phototherapy unit was established in Hammerfest, another town 500 km away from the UHT; this was also backed up by teledermatology services (Fig. 6.1). Between 8 and 15 patients are seen at afternoon sessions twice a week. Routine teledermatology practice has become firmly established.

The healthcare system in Norway is primarily publicly funded, with the government paying for most services. Averaged over a patient's lifetime, approximately 95% of all healthcare expenses are paid for by the government. Patient access to the healthcare system is fair in most parts of the country. The northernmost parts, however, comprise a vast area that is sparsely populated (less than 1 person per km^2), and the terrain is difficult to cross in wintertime, which is the prevailing season for 8 months of the year. It is therefore worthwhile to facilitate telecommunication whenever possible.

The aim of the central government is to give all the inhabitants of Norway equal access to medical services irrespective of their geographical location. In 1996, Norway became the first country to implement an official telemedicine fee schedule, making telemedicine services reimbursable by the national health insurer. Without this measure, delivery of these services would come to a halt.

In Tromsø the National Centre of Telemedicine (NCT), run by the UHT, is the interface between the specialist and the GP. The NCT chooses and supports all telemedicine equipment. No telemedicine sessions are held without a technician being available.

Methods

The videoconferencing system

To use videoconferencing, the parties need a studio at both ends. The equipment used until 1999 was a Philips Titan codec, with 384 kbit/s bandwidth, which complied with the H.320 standard. The video resolution was 352 pixels × 288 lines with up to 30 frames per second. Still-images had a better resolution of 720 pixels × 576 lines, which is important at times. The video screen was 69 cm. For close-up views of particular lesions we had a Sony 3CCD camera mounted on a mechanical arm. It was possible to reach most parts of the body easily with this. Illumination used to be from a mobile lamp, but recently a camera fitted with a light source has been acquired (Figs 6.2–6.4). Since 2000 we have been using a Tandberg Vision 6000 system with larger, 84-cm monitors and a 100-Hz refresh rate. The communication speed is 384 kbit/s from Kirkenes and 512 kbit/s from Hammerfest. In reality we have not upgraded the quality of video transmission despite the new monitors. More bandwidth is of course desirable.

The dermatologist acts alone and makes notes using a dictating machine, which are subsequently typed up in the hospital by a secretary. A copy is sent to the relevant GP. At the other end, the GP and the patient share the studio with a nurse who takes care of

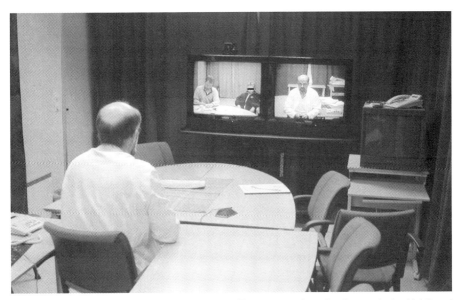

Fig. 6.2. The videoconferencing studio in Tromsø. The screens show the dermatologist (right) and the GP (left).

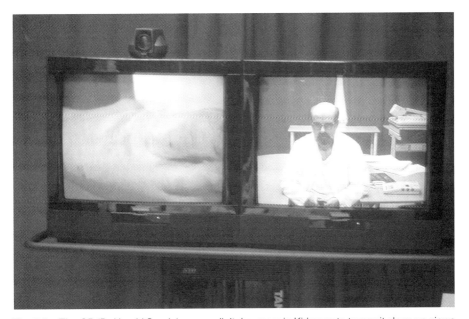

Fig. 6.3. The GP (Dr Harald Sunde) uses a digital camera in Kirkenes to transmit close-up views of the dermatology problem.

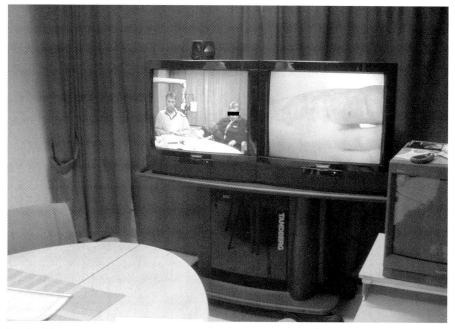

Fig. 6.4. The digital camera and its supporting arm can be seen on the left-hand screen.

the patient both before and after the consultation when necessary. The consultations are held in hospitals where phototherapy, bathing and surgical facilities are available. This amounts to quite a sizable system around each patient. Dermatology at hospital level is never about pencil and paper.

Videoconferencing has a tendency to create 'tunnel vision' and interacting with the patient as in a surgery consultation is impossible. Nevertheless, the traditional surgery consultation is really the point of reference when delivering these services. The specialists usually try to imitate surgery settings at videoconferences, mainly because it gives them a sense of control over a situation that is quite the contrary. A sensitive GP at the other end can usually cooperate and make the illusion work flawlessly for the specialist involved.

Patient selection

Teledermatology is based on a strict referral system. GPs and specialists can refer directly to the nearest studio where the specially trained GP selects patients that are suitable for videoconferences. This GP has some years' experience in general practice in addition to a few weeks in an outpatient dermatology service. 'Suitable' is a rather broad term and only a few guidelines exist. In practice, moles,[2,3] genital lesions, impaired hearing or poor communication skills are the exclusion criteria. Others, are qualitative, such as unidentified tumours, eruptions on dark skin, and cases where there are discrete lesions or none visible. These may include lesions in the scalp, hair loss, itch, chronic urticaria and very old and debilitated patients.

Discussion

Workload

About 700–800 patients are seen annually by telemedicine in the studio. In comparison, the annual outpatient workload at the UHT department of dermatology is about 19 000 consultations.[4]

Funding

Videoconferencing is rather expensive, and is time- and resource-consuming. Five specialists share this practice in a rotation. This means that each has the responsibility for one or two sessions per month. On the one hand, the specialists work in their spare time for a modest fee. The GPs involved, on the other hand, work on a regular basis at their normal salary.

Teledermatology is a good business for the national health insurer. The doctors are 'cheap' and reliable. We have estimated that the average fee for the dermatologist involved is US$30 per patient (about 300NKR). The travel expenses in northern Norway are high by almost any standard. The airfare from Kirkenes to Tromsø is at least $260. As technology advances and telecommunication costs become lower, the cost–benefit ratio will continue to improve.[5–7] That is, of course, when teleconsultations are viewed in isolation from the huge resources that it takes to implement these services. The National Centre of Telemedicine represents a heavy investment in staff and equipment. The sessions are run in a non-profit-making manner, giving no room for accumulation of capital for further investment in personnel and instruments. These services are provided purely as political goodwill and as such are very sensitive to the ever-changing tides of public funding.

Patient satisfaction

Doctors tend to believe that their patients would prefer to meet them in person. This may be so in cases of grave illness and when agonizing pain needs relief, but normally patients seek attention for less serious reasons. Symptoms usually appear gradually and the patient has already adjusted to them but needs the doctor's skill to alleviate anxiety or for symptomatic relief. In these cases, medical opinion is valuable, but not priceless. A chronic rash, a mole or an itching spot will all in due course need some kind of professional attention, but not at any cost. A patient will not travel hundreds of miles for a specialist opinion if their local doctor refuses to support their request for referral, because the skin lesion will probably be benign anyhow. But if the patient can see a specialist at their GP's surgery simultaneously, they are bound to be impressed. Videoconferences were rated highly by patients in Kirkenes when they were asked to compare them to ordinary consultations with a specialist.[8,9] Only 10% preferred direct contact with the specialist to videoconferencing. In a normal setting, 90% patient satisfaction would be welcomed by most physicians. When this study was evaluated, the specialists involved found this somewhat odd, but in the discussion they pointed out that the role of an attentive and supportive GP made up for the qualitative disappointment that a flat screen communication predictably delivers.

Diagnostic evaluation

Comparing diagnostic accuracy between videoconferencing and on-site specialist evaluation, the diagnostic agreement was almost 90% and the total disagreement was about 2%.[8] The total and partial disagreement was not serious enough to have a significant effect on patient management in the short term.[2,3] In a study from Northern Ireland, the diagnostic agreement was less than we found, perhaps because more doctors were involved and the number of patients was higher.[10] Long-term consequences of diagnostic inaccuracy are always a problem but are not particularly alarming in the context of videoconferencing. The most likely occurrence is delayed diagnosis of a skin tumour, as occurred in one of our cases. An elderly man was referred because of a chronic lip infection. Later, a biopsy taken after traditional clinical examination revealed squamous cell carcinoma. In a subsequent review, an independent expert concluded that diagnostic delay was due to the telemedicine process.

Recent studies comparing videoconferencing to still-image evaluation give rather similar results for inter-investigator agreement.[11] That may indicate that specialists trained at the same institution tend to concur in a given situation. Whether specialists from different institutions or different continents disagree more is not a significant issue in the context of teledermatology in northern Norway, because we are comparing the practice of local specialists.

Initially, patch testing was not part of the teledermatology service. We had serious doubts about the quality of such specialized evaluations. Despite this, we are now conducting patch testing remotely, as a screening procedure. This is made possible by means of a digital camera capable of transferring high-resolution still images to the consulting dermatologist's monitor and standardized, easy-to-use patch test material. A selection of patients is referred for further testing in a more appropriate setting.

Standardization

Do we need standard procedures for videoconferencing? In ordinary consultations standard procedures include:

1. the patient is invited to the office

2. introduction/recognition takes place

3. both parties observe each other

4. a history is taken

5. inspection, palpation, percussion and auscultation are performed

6. a conclusion or diagnosis is reached

7. management is planned.

In videoconferencing the sequence is similar. However, each component is truncated and the specialist must rely on the GP. The specialist does not control the consultation. Even when a conclusion has been reached or a diagnosis has been made, the GP may have the last word, at least to the patient – this is a problem in practice, but the legal responsibility of the parties involved must be considered carefully. Our GP makes his own separate notes. Some of our colleagues, not themselves experienced in videoconferencing, challenge our integrity and consider our practice unworthy of the reputation of the specialty. They compare videoconferencing to the casual, fragmented corridor consultations that are frequent amongst hospital colleagues. We see it as a service to a neglected population lacking regular specialist care. As the patient is under the supervision of a GP, we feel confident that videoconferencing is effective and, when appropriate, is more than satisfactory for both the patient and specialist. It is important that patients are properly selected for teledermatology consultations. We need to formulate guidelines to reduce the possibility of error.

The GP's guidelines for the selection of appropriate patients have been listed above. When in doubt, the specialist involved should ask for a conventional consultation. Nevertheless, there are a number of inappropriate referrals to the telemedicine clinic, and we depend on the GP's support to see such consultations through. The GP must therefore think carefully when referring a patient whose condition is inappropriate for viewing on a TV monitor. Many of these patients will end up travelling to the dermatology outpatient clinic.

Ideally a conventional clinic visit should be arranged every time the GP fails to select a patient according to our guidelines. In practice we do not operate strictly to such standards. We are placing our confidence in the GP involved and the primary healthcare system. Dismissing the problem because it cannot be assessed on a monitor, and not giving the patient a chance to be seen by videoconference, is not an option medicolegally.[12] Standardization in strictly technical terms is of course a very important issue, which is dealt with elsewhere in this book.

Maybe you do not like to see the esteemed doctor–patient relationship dwindle in the misty dots on the screen. Maybe you fear for the reputation of your specialty. Maybe you fear losing the specialist's traditional paternalistic control over the situation, rather than accepting the noble gain of being present as a humble advisor on dermatological issues. None of these attitudes should prevent the implementation of telemedicine in situations where it is appropriate.

General management and funding

Decreasing public spending on health care is the main goal of the Norwegian administration. Organization and funding are of great concern for the future viability of teledermatology services. The cost of establishing videoconferencing as we practise it is too high for private medicine.

In sparsely populated areas a public insurer is the only investor who will benefit from telemedicine. However, this service is possible because equipment and facilities are supplied by the referral hospital. The local healthcare budget funds most of the technical and medical support. The novelty of telemedicine is its main appeal when arguing for further investment. In due course we can expect the referral hospital to lose interest as decreasing resources demand further cuts. The public purse helps to pay the telemedicine GP's salary. Other possible dangers are that the specialists may find telemedicine consultations uneconomic or the local GPs may be unable to find the time required for telemedicine on a regular basis.

In bigger communities, the need for telemedicine might not look as pressing. However, store-and-forward telemedicine can be conducted on the Internet, which is easy for the patient to access and use. This will be open to private enterprise and less dependent on public revenue. Private medical companies may be able to make extra income by offering telemedical services and/or using the Internet as a shop window for special treatments, reaching patients far away, who would otherwise be inaccessible.

User satisfaction

A teledermatology clinic with 10–15 patients is a strenuous job for the specialist and requires maximum concentration. In our system we do not allow scheduled breaks between consultations because the appointments are tightly scheduled. The bandwidth (384 kbit/s) is inadequate for a relaxed ergonomic posture.

For the specialists, the main gain from videoconferencing is the reduction of a cumbersome travel schedule that takes them away from their main work at the hospital. Administration and funding are matters for the institutions' managers. This may be frustrating for the specialists at times. Lay people, technicians or administrators have set the standards at the lowest possible level, despite the specialists' objections. An example is the reduction in bandwidth from 2 Mbit/s to less than 384 kbit/s, the upper transmission rate at the moment. This resulted in staccato movements on screen and audiovisual disharmony. It took many years before there was any reaction to the specialists' complaints, and this came about solely because the telephone company had reduced their prices. High-resolution still images allowed us to continue our teledermatology service during this period.

When criticizing public health agencies, we see many examples of resources meant to improve the quality of care for the individual patient being diverted into projects that are otherwise difficult to finance. Teledermatology is a real administrative dilemma: delivery of health care is not separated financially from experimental development, and though important is not essential. The GP is easier to please as telemedicine gives more regular and direct access to a specialist. Skin problems are particularly challenging in general practice and the teledermatology sessions have played an important educational role for the GPs involved. As a result, more problems can be dealt with locally. However, teledermatology has resulted in a steady rise in referrals as the population becomes accustomed to a whole new field of medical services not available to them before. This tendency for increased referrals may now be levelling out.

Patients seem to be the main beneficiaries of teledermatology. They avoid travel with consequent savings in money and time, they benefit from a local skin clinic, and they experience a lower threshold for referral to a specialist dermatologist. We believe these are reasons for the high levels of patient satisfaction reported by many authors.[3,8,9,13] In our setting having their 'own' local clinic seems particularly important.

The road ahead

Whether bumpy or smooth, there will always be dead ends and short cuts on the road ahead. Telemedicine is a bridge in terms of this metaphor. Although the technology is 'sufficient', it is more of a thread in the wind than the Golden Gate Bridge in San Francisco. It is frail in structure and the travellers are both brave and insecure. The technical fabric is full of loose ends that need tying up; the financial support is unreliable, and the handful of regular users have little more than a vision to live up to, the vision of an endless variety of medical communication via the Internet. While the Internet is still in its infancy, so telemedicine is basically an idea that is taking on a form that cannot yet be fully grasped. Our solution has been to imitate conventional medical practice as accurately as possible and nurture it via the same institutions and legislation that came into being centuries ago. By doing so we hope to shape the future of telemedicine in the traditional mould. Only when future technology has reconstructed our institutions and legislation follows suit, will we experience the true blossoming of telemedical services.

References

1   Jøsendal O, Fosse G, Andersen KA, Stenvold SE, Falk ES. Fjerndiagnostisering av Hudsykdommer. [Distance diagnosis of skin diseases.] *Tidsskrift for den Norske Laeforening* 1991;**111**:20–22 [English summary].

2   Oakley AMM, Astwood DR, Loane M, Duffill MB, Rademaker M, Wootton R. Diagnostic accuracy of teledermatology: results of a preliminary study in New Zealand. *New Zealand Medical Journal* 1997;**110**:51–53.

3   Gilmour E, Campell SA, Loane MA, et al. Comparison of teleconsultations and face-to-face consultations: preliminary results of a United Kingdom multicentre teledermatology study. *British Journal of Dermatology* 1998;**139**:81–87.

4   Allen A. Teledermatology survey 1998. *Telemedicine Today* 1998;**3**(2):12–15.

5   Oakley AMM, Kerr P, Duffill MB, et al. Patient cost–benefit analysis of realtime teledermatology – a comparison of data from Northern Ireland and New Zealand. *Journal of Telemedicine and Telecare* 2000;**6**:97–101.

6   Bergmo TS. A cost-minimization analysis of realtime teledermatology service in northern Norway. *Journal of Telemedicine and Telecare* 2000;**6**:1–5.

7   Wootton R, Bloomer SE, Corbett R, et al. Multicentre randomised control trial comparing realtime teledermatology with conventional outpatient dermatological care: societal cost-benefit analysis. *British Medical Journal* 2000;**320**:1252–1256.

8   Nordal E, Moseng D. Lecture at the Nordic Congress of Dermatology, Bergen, June 1998, abstract 55.

9   Moseng D. Teledermatology –.the north Norwegian experience. *Tidsskrift for den Norske Laeforening* 2000;**120**:1893–1895 [English summary].

10   Loane MA, Corbett R, Bloomer SE, et al. Diagnostic accuracy and clinical management by realtime teledermatology. Results from the Northern Ireland arms of the UK Multicentre teledermatology trial. *Journal of Telemedicine and Telecare* 1998;**4**:95–100.

11   Moseng D, Ingvarsson G. Lecture given at the Norwegian Congress of Telemedicine 1999, Tromsø, October 1999.

12   Stanberry B. Telemedicine: barriers and opportunities in the 21st century. *Journal of Internal Medicine* 2000;**247**:615–628.

13   Loane MA, Bloomer SE, Corbett R, et al. Patient satisfaction with realtime teledermatology in Northern Ireland. *Journal of Telemedicine and Telecare* 1998;**4**:36–40.

7

Telemedicine at East Carolina University – Dermatology and the Prison

Vivian L. West and David C. Balch

Introduction

North Carolina (NC) is divided into three major regions. The eastern region, in which Greenville and East Carolina University (ECU) are located, encompasses 38 000 km^2 and is mainly rural. Approximately 17% of the region lives below the federal poverty level, compared to 14% in the USA as a whole and 13% in North Carolina.[1] The unemployment rate is 6%, compared to 4% in the USA and 3% in North Carolina. In 1995, North Carolina ranked 38th among the 50 states (1 = the best, 50 = the worst) for health outcomes, with the eastern region the worst of the three regions.

The eastern region is characterized by small rural towns with limited healthcare facilities. There is a shortage of primary-care providers, with a ratio of 1800 people per primary care physician, compared to a ratio of 960 : 1 for the USA as a whole. The highest concentration of physicians in eastern North Carolina is in Greenville, an urban community in the middle of the region. There are both medical and nursing schools at ECU that focus on training primary-care providers, with an emphasis on retaining practitioners for rural health care.

In 1992, administrators at the Central Prison, the maximum-security prison in Raleigh, North Carolina, wanted to reduce the costs of providing health care to the inmates. They believed that this could be done by avoiding transporting inmates from prison to surrounding healthcare clinics for medical consultations. The Center for Health Sciences Communication at the ECU had a staff who provided live video for educational purposes at the hospital and the schools of medicine and nursing. The Telemedicine Center evolved from this department, responding to the prison's need, to become the first telemedicine programme in North Carolina. This chapter describes the telemedicine programme at ECU and its dermatology services to the North Carolina prison system.

Telemedicine at East Carolina University

Clinical specialists and allied healthcare professionals at the medical centre provide teleconsultations, both interactively and by store-and-forward methods. The telemedicine network connects ten rural hospitals and clinics, one maximum-security prison and two smaller state prisons. There are also links to a health department, two home health agencies, two elementary schools, two high schools, two mental health centres with 12 clinics, a physician's office, a high-risk obstetrics management clinic and the North Carolina School for the Deaf (Fig. 7.1). The services include: consultations in 32 different medical specialties, diabetic nutrition and medication management, physical rehabilitation, speech pathology, pharmacy services, home health care, medical social worker services, obesity and nutrition clinics, and several nurse practitioner services. Over 6000 consultations have been provided since the telemedicine programme began in 1992. Three specialty groups account for over 60% of the consultations: dermatology (38%), adult cardiology (13%) and adult psychiatry (11%).

The telemedicine programme includes health education to the eastern region of NC. For distance learning, a microwave network provides full duplex connections to 42 sites with three discrete channels of audio, video and data. The ECU network is part of the North Carolina Information Highway, an ATM (asynchronous transfer mode) network that connects 400 data sites and 131 video sites, including schools, libraries, state and federal government agencies, criminal justice and economic development networks. This network also includes partnering relationships between the schools and the four major telephone carriers using a variety of wireless, satellite, microwave, cable and telephony modalities running on the ATM backbone network. The Telemedicine Center offers continuing education for primary care practitioners in rural facilities who participate in weekly grand rounds transmitted from the ECU. They can

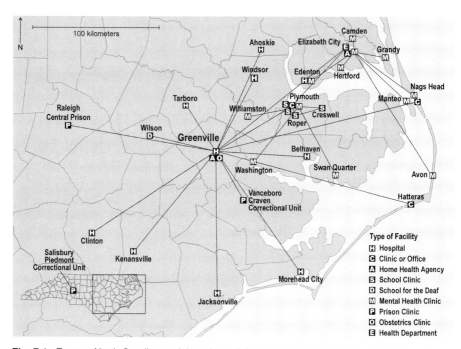

Fig. 7.1. Eastern North Carolina and the telemedicine network from East Carolina University.

also receive statewide educational programmes from the four medical universities in NC. In addition, the Telemedicine Center runs a training centre in which over 300 medical professionals from 25 different countries have participated in education and training on advanced telemedicine techniques.

The Telemedicine Center employs various telecommunications technologies in its network, including microwave, T1, ATM, videophones and ISDN. This permits each site to use the most cost-effective technique. The Telemedicine Center links the distant sites where specialty services for a patient are needed to a specialist who provides the care (Fig. 7.2). Engineers and support staff use algorithms to assist in decision making for rapid communications connections. In future, a nurse will probably become an additional contributor to activities at the bridge, providing a human interface with the sites to solve the problems not solved by an algorithm.

The Telemedicine Center has an active research programme. In May 2000 ECU became the first medical centre in the USA to use the Intuitive da Vinci Surgical Robot surgical tools. Dr Randolph Chitwood replaced a mitral valve in a 57-year-old woman during cardiovascular surgery using the robotic arm (Fig. 7.3). The Telemedicine Center is currently developing a 3D vision system for use in virtual training. The 3D vision system has additional potential uses, including application in dermatology. The images that a dermatologist sees wearing the 3D vision system are visualized in the same way the presenter at the distant site sees the lesions. Dermatological lesions become more realistic, because they have depth and clarity (Fig. 7.4).

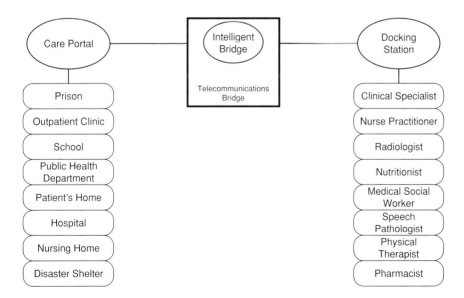

Fig. 7.2. Distributed Medical Intelligence system of care at East Carolina University.

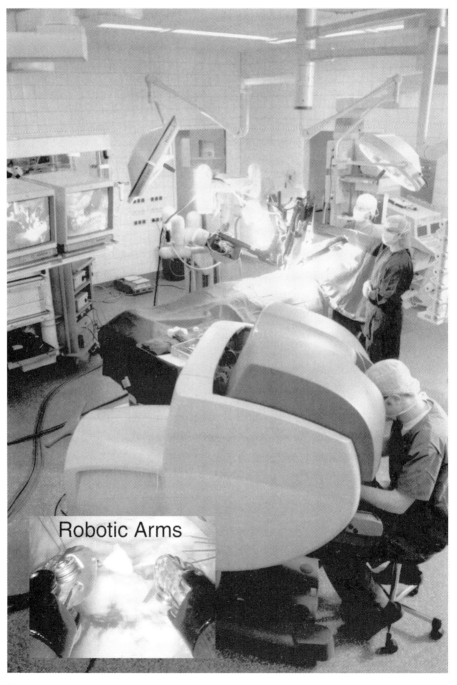

Fig. 7.3. The Intuitive de Vinci Surgical Robot in use during cardiovascular surgery. Insert at bottom left shows the surgical arms that are being operated by the surgeon who is sitting at the controls of the system. (Photo credit: Intuitive Surgical, Inc.)

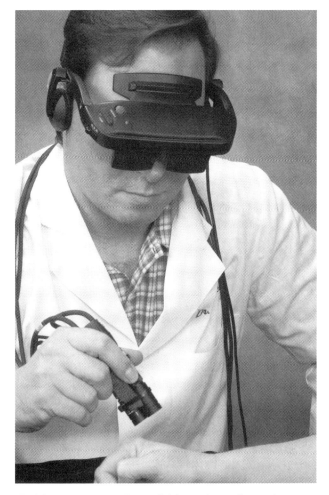

Fig. 7.4. The 3D-vision system worn by a clinician using a dermatology camera to transmit images to the dermatologist. The dermatologist in the remote site wears similar headgear.

Telemedicine to the prison

The North Carolina Department of Correction maintains 82 correction facilities throughout the state. The Central Prison, located near Raleigh, is a maximum-security facility and the point of entry into the prison system for male offenders sentenced to more than 20 years. (Women are housed in two smaller facilities outside Raleigh.) The prison occupies 29 acres, and includes an acute care hospital and two mental health wings with beds for 224 inmates, an operating suite, laboratories and a pharmacy. Physicians are contracted to provide services to the acute care hospital at the Central Prison, with specialty services obtained primarily through the University of North Carolina clinics in Chapel Hill, 48 km west of the prison.

For the 81 correctional facilities outside the Central Prison, the Department of Correction contracts with local physicians from the communities around the facilities. These are often retired primary care physicians. For care that cannot be provided locally, inmates are referred to the Central Prison. North Carolina is a large state, approximately 127 000 km^2 in area. Transporting prisoners is therefore often time consuming. In many cases a round-trip cannot be made in the same day, necessitating an overnight stay and the use of two guards.

The Telemedicine Center, located 140 km east of the prison, has provided specialty consultations to the Central Prison since 1992. In 2000, the Telemedicine Center began providing medical consultation services to two more prisons: Craven Correctional Institution in Vanceboro (40 km south of Greenville) and Piedmont Correctional Institution (330 km west of Greenville). The Department of Correction noted in a memorandum to the Telemedicine Center that renewal and expansion of the contract were the result of documented benefits and cost savings from telemedicine, and particularly the costs avoided in the areas of security, escape, transportation, private physician fees, reduction in litigation over lack of specialty medical care, and the increase in public safety resulting from not having to transport sick prisoners outside the prison environment. The majority of our references to the prison programme are from experiences with the Central Prison.

Physicians from the ECU School of Medicine provide the consultations using both interactive video and store-and-forward methods. Equipment used at the correctional facilities and its installation, equipment maintenance, operations support personnel, troubleshooting, and on-site service and training are provided by the ECU. In 1992 a videoconferencing unit (PictureTel 4000) was installed at the Central Prison. In 1997 we upgraded it (to a model 4000E) to increase its performance to 30 frames per second and increase the resolution of the graphics. In 2000, a VitelNet Medvizer system was installed. This had some initial teething problems, but after six months it replaced the PictureTel unit. The VitelNet system uses IP (Internet protocol) connections at 768 kbit/s, instead of ISDN at 384 kbit/s. It can operate in store-and-forward mode, as well as doing videoconferencing (Fig. 7.5).

Over the years we have used three generations of dermatology peripherals in the prison telemedicine programme. In 1992, a Welch Allyn camera was installed. This was awkward to hold, making it difficult to focus the camera when the presenter was trying to show a lesion to the dermatologist. In 1995 it was replaced by an Andries Tek macro camera. The Andries Tek camera had better resolution, but was too small to manipulate easily. It was also difficult to identify the top of the camera, so that images were often upside down unless the dermatologist questioned the presentation. In 1999, an AMD (American Medical Development) dermatology camera was installed that has zoom capabilities and a close-up lens with a built-in ring light. The camera has a freeze frame feature, so that movement can be eliminated, resulting in a higher resolution of the image. It also uses a polarizing filter, which removes surface light reflection and permits skin visualization to the capillaries.

Medical records at the ECU are stored electronically, while the Department of Correction uses paper records at its correctional facilities. At the Central Prison, a physician's assistant and a licensed practical nurse are responsible for consultation

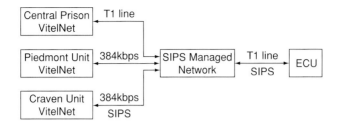

Fig. 7.5. Network configuration from the prisons to the Telemedicine Center at East Carolina University.

preparation, presentation of the patients and distribution of the specialists' recommendations for follow-up by the prison medical staff. In 2000, the electronic record system was implemented at the three prisons.

As is common in other correctional facilities around the USA, the Department of Correction has difficulty in filling its vacancies for physicians and nurses. Lower salaries and less desirable working conditions contribute to the inability of the correctional institutions to attract and keep qualified clinicians. Therefore, as clinicians are hired for the various specialty positions in the prisons, the needs for specialists through telemedicine change. In 1999 and 2000, only four specialty services were provided.

Dermatology at the prison

Dermatology has consistently been the most requested specialty over more than eight years of telemedicine to the prison, with neurology and pulmonology second and third (Table 7.1). There has been a significant change in the method for providing dermatology consultations. At first, interactive consultations were requested on a regular basis. In 1998, store-and-forward consultations accounted for 87 of the 234 consultations (37%). By mid-1999, however, the store-and-forward consultations began to outnumber the interactive ones. In 2000, 213 of the 225 consultations (95%) were provided using store-and-forward methods.

Interviews with dermatologists show that they agree that still photographs are satisfactory for diagnosing many dermatological conditions, and that they prefer store-and-forward consultations for dermatology. In the prison system, 846 of all dermatology consultations (72%) were for black patients, compared to 61% for patients seen outside the prison system. The inability to see lesions on dark-skinned patients is a common problem in dermatology.[2,3]

The specialists rotate their responsibilities for telemedicine. Consultations to the prison are booked at least two days in advance, and occur during normal business

Table 7.1. Most frequent specialty consultations to the prison: August 1992 to December 2000

Year	Annual consultations (no.)	Dermatology (%)	Neurology (%)	Pulmonology (%)	Other* (%)
1992	25	28	12	4.0	56
1993	197	46	18	3.6	32
1994	117	37	26	2.6	35
1995	144	47	16	2.8	34
1996	326	53	8.6	4.6	34
1997	299	56	7.4	12	25
1998	356	66	2.6	9.6	22
1999	370	79	0	3.8	18
2000	240	94	0	0.4	5.8
Total	**2074**	**63**	**7**	**6**	**25**

*Other includes: allergy, cardiology, endocrinology, gastrology, general surgery, haematology, oncology, infectious disease, internal medicine, nephrology, ophthalmology, rheumatology, urology and vascular surgery.

hours. Teledermatology clinics are scheduled several weeks in advance. A computerized scheduling system has been developed for booking all telemedicine consultations. This allows an appropriate date and time to be identified quickly.

The image of the lesion is critical for diagnosis in dermatology. Video pictures are not as sharp as static images. Real-time video pictures at the H.320 standard (as used in videoconferencing) have a resolution of 352×288 lines, while images on photographic film provide a resolution equivalent to about 2000×2000 lines. Digital still images have improved to be near the resolution obtained with conventional clinical photography. Studies have shown that substituting good quality digital images for conventional clinical photographs is satisfactory in most cases.[4-6] One study demonstrated that the diagnostic accuracy and confidence were not compromised when lower-resolution digital images were used, and concluded that experienced dermatologists could interpret digital images of 720×500 pixels correctly in most clinical settings.[7]

The most common diagnoses in patients in the prison system are eczema, dermatitis and acne, and these account for almost half of all diagnoses. Infections (viral, bacterial and fungal), tumours, inflammations and pruritic complaints are other common conditions. This is similar to the types of conditions seen by telemedicine at our non-prison facilities.

There are approximately 1861 prisoners housed at the three correctional facilities, with 942 male prisoners at the Central Prison, and 73 women and 919 men at the Craven and Piedmont Correctional Institutions. Of these, 27% are white, 72% are black and 4% are Indian, Asian/Oriental or Spanish/Mexican. The age groups with the highest numbers are 25–39 years, although in the black male population the largest group is 20–24 years of age. The patients for whom dermatology consultations are provided are representative of the overall prison population, with the mean age of dermatology patients slightly higher than the mean age of all patients from the prison.

Compared to the dermatology patients who receive consultations at the rural telemedicine sites, there are fewer white patients and more black patients in the three prisons. A comparison of the patient demographics is shown in Table 7.2.

In 1993, interviews were conducted with 11 physicians at the ECU who were providing consultations to the Central Prison. Three of the 11 were dermatologists. As a result of their observations various changes were made, correcting such things as room glare and lighting. A darker background was employed to soften the glare, a small floor lamp was used for direct lighting to facilitate close-up examinations, and a camera with a polarizing lens was used to lessen skin surface shine.

Table 7.2. Demographics of patients (August 1992 to June 2000) at the prison, compared with patients from the non-prison, rural locations in the ECU Telemedicine Programme

	Non-prison telemedicine		Prison telemedicine	
	All patients (n = 4145)	Dermatology only (n = 1562)	All patients (n = 2048)	Dermatology only (n = 1184)
Age (years)				
Mean (SD)	38.7 (24.4)	37.0 (22.7)	34.4 (10.5)	40.0 (10.4)
Range	1–97	1–97	19–80	20–80
Race (%)				
White	43	37	21	26
Black	51	61	74	72
Other	6	2	5	3
Sex (%)				
Male	41	37	100	100
Female	59	63	0	0

In 1999, the physicians who were still consulting via telemedicine – which included the three original dermatologists – were again interviewed to determine how their perceptions of consultations at the prison had changed. They continued to question the patients' motives for some consultations, stating that patients occasionally try to manipulate the examination, might sometimes use a visit as an escape from daily routine and often exhibit some degree of hostility. There was agreement that the patients seem happier with consultations via telemedicine compared to prisoners who are brought to their clinics in person. One physician suggested that this was because the telemedicine patients have the opportunity to discuss their personal healthcare concerns with a physician without a guard standing close by.

The biggest change in dermatology consultations to the prison, however, has been the presenter. In 1993, a physician at the prison acted as the presenter; this was thought to inhibit the consulting physician, who felt that conversations tended to be from physician to physician rather than between physician and patient. Over the last four years a physician's assistant (PA) and a licensed practical nurse (LPN) have presented the patients. The skills of the PA include administering potassium hydroxide and scabies preparations, two procedures that are lacking in other settings and often cited by dermatologists as drawbacks for using telemedicine.

The organizational skills of the PA and LPN have contributed to the efficiency of the telemedicine visits. The PA obtains a complete history and performs a physical examination prior to every consultation, interactive or store-and-forward, permitting the dermatologist to read information about the patient's condition prior to the consultation. These extra steps were noted in the dermatologists' comments about improvements in the consultation process.

According to discussions with the PA at the Central Prison, the patients have never questioned the use of telemedicine for consultations, most being very interested in the technology and 'seeing myself on TV'. This is consistent with a previous study that investigated satisfaction with telemedicine in the Federal Prison system. Although inmates can file grievances about the various aspects of their treatment as prisoners, this comprehensive study showed that few grievances are filed about health and medical care.[8]

From the perspective of the care providers who are responsible for implementing the consultant's recommendations, using telemedicine enhances the care to the patient. Orders are received immediately, so that laboratory tests or prescriptions can be filled while the patient is still in the prison clinic. Unlike consultations provided when the patients are taken off-site for care, the visit is well documented and there are no questions about future care for the patient.

Costs for prison services

Telemedicine contracts with prisons have proved to be profitable.[8,9] These contracts tend to be either flat rates based on a per year/per inmate charge, or a maintenance fee with a fee-for-service for each consultation. The Telemedicine Center charges a monthly maintenance fee for the equipment. A flat rate charge is made for each consultation. The telecommunication charges are paid by ECU, but installation and maintenance of the lines is the responsibility of the Department of Correction.

Once the equipment has been installed, little maintenance is required. Experienced engineering staff can quickly troubleshoot, and with the assistance of the staff in the prison most of the technical problems have been solved without travelling to the prison. This makes the model cost-effective from the standpoint of the provider.

More important, however, is that the correctional facilities realize cost-savings. It has been estimated that the cost of providing health care in a prison represents at least 20% of its operating budget.[9] Numerous factors are responsible for the high cost of providing health care to prisoners outside the facility: healthcare personnel time in preparing for an outside visit, transportation, the use of one or two escorts, any precautions taken to protect the public from harm when an inmate is transported outside prison walls and overnight stays when prisoners are transported a long distance. Telemedicine, particularly when prison staff maximize use of the system, produces significant taxpayer savings.

Challenges and potential solutions

In providing telemedicine for dermatology patients in prisons, there are several challenges, the first being the cost. The expense of providing healthcare services in any prison system like that in North Carolina can be very high. The litigious nature of inmates in the USA, together with constitutional law that requires prison officials to provide health care to prisoners, encourages administrators of prison systems to seek cheaper solutions for health care. Although telemedicine from the Central Prison is a cost-effective solution for the prisoners housed there, it is an expensive solution when inmates from smaller facilities are transported to the Central Prison for telemedicine, particularly when they must spend the night because of the travel distance. The addition of two telemedicine systems, one on the eastern side of North Carolina and one on the western side, are attempts to reduce the travel time and costs associated with travel. Dermatology at these remote sites can be provided most efficiently from inexpensive telemedicine systems using store-and-forward applications. Dermatologists frequently comment about the success of store-and-forward for their specialty; here a low-cost solution is perhaps the best solution.

Just as telemedicine is a promise for better access to care in rural locations, telemedicine is a promise for improved access to care at remote prisons. The success of any telemedicine programme regardless of location, however, depends on the motivation of the people who are responsible for implementing it. The decision to provide telemedicine in the Craven and Piedmont facilities was made by state administrators, and was not a solution generated by the local administrators. Without the initiative driven by the two prisons where telemedicine was to be employed, it has taken longer to see the cost savings from these sites. There will be no improvement in access to care at these remote locations unless there is a concerted effort to use the system as originally intended, and this requires that the local administrators actively support telemedicine.

Another challenge for telemedicine to a prison is the possibility of lawsuits. When the Central Prison telemedicine consultations began in 1993, one of the biggest concerns of the consultants was the fear of being sued by patients at the prison, as lawsuits by prisoners are common in the USA. A solution that was satisfactory to the consultants was to record each consultation and archive the tape, so that it could be used if future litigation was to occur. This was acceptable to the Department of Correction and was incorporated into standard practice. To date, there have been no lawsuits involving telemedicine at the prison. Furthermore, in Louisiana telemedicine has been mandated by the courts to answer disputes over lack of care in prisons.

An added concern expressed not only by dermatologists, but also by most physicians participating in telemedicine, is the confidentiality of the visit. The physician cannot control the environment and ensure that only authorized individuals are present with the patient. During interactive consultations, specialized hardware is used at each end of the link, which minimizes the possibility of interception of signals and provides secure connections. When store-and-forward telemedicine is performed, the medical records are encrypted.

The presenter's skills and organizational management play a large part in the efficiency of any interactive consultation, as previously discussed. It is important to have appropriately trained and motivated personnel to assist throughout interactive consultations, and well-trained support staff to process store-and-forward consultations. In the USA the educational level of a presenter is an unresolved issue. Some telemedicine experts think that non-licensed staff can become good presenters. From our experience at the ECU Telemedicine Center, professional staff have been quick to learn the skills needed for presenting patients. With additional training and experience, and with changes in practice laws, professional nurses and physicians' assistants could provide many of the laboratory tests that dermatologists perform in their offices to assist them in diagnosis. As evidenced by the skills of the PA at the prison, this has not only improved the care to patients, but has also resulted in greater satisfaction of the dermatologists who rely on the presenter to conduct a satisfactory examination of the patients.

Finally, scheduling has presented problems in the prison telemedicine programme. Over half of the cancelled appointments for teleconsultations have been from the Central Prison. Most of them occurred because patients have simply not shown up for their appointments, although prisoners being paroled or moved to another correctional facility are also frequent reasons for cancellation. With interactive visits, the dermatologists schedule blocks of time during the week to conduct consultations. When the patient is not ready to be seen or does not arrive, not only is this time lost for the consultant, but the time is also not reimbursable. If the consultation is provided using store-and-forward technology, lost or down time no longer occurs. We have found that combining interactive with store-and-forward work improves the efficiency of the dermatology clinics, because the dermatologist can view store-and-forward images while waiting for patients.

Conclusion

In 1994, a report commissioned by the General Accounting Office of the USA identified four problems in the Federal prison system:

1. special medical care needs

2. quality assurance programmes to detect problems and develop corrective action

3. qualified healthcare providers

4. cost-effective alternatives to meet medical care needs.[10]

These problems are not unique to the Federal prison system; they are probably common to all correctional facilities in the USA. Telemedicine could be a solution for problems such as these. The most frequent use for telemedicine is specialty care, providing high quality care with qualified healthcare providers. Telemedicine is also expected to be a cost-effective alternative to current models of care, although it is difficult to determine cost-effectiveness accurately because of the complex financial environment.[11]

In general, delivery of health care using telemedicine is still relatively new and there are many unanswered questions. Teledermatology has progressed several years ahead of many of the other telemedicine specialties, and its successes and shortcomings can now be seen. For dermatology in a prison setting, future expansion of these services should be encouraged.

References

1   East Carolina University, Center for Health Services Research and Development. *Eastern North Carolina Health Care Atlas: A Resource for Healthier Communities.* Greenville, NC: East Carolina University, 1997.
2   Tachakra S. Colour perception in telemedicine. *Journal of Telemedicine and Telecare* 1999;**5**:211–219.
3   Vidmar DA. Plea for standardization in teledermatology: a worm's eye view. *Telemedicine Journal* 1997;**3**:173–178.
4   Perednia DA, Gaines JA, Butruille TW. Comparison of the clinical informativeness of photographs and digital imaging media with multiple-choice receiver operating characteristic analysis. *Archives of Dermatology* 1995;**131**:292–297.
5   Bittorf A, Fartasch M, Schuler G, Diepgen TL. Resolution requirement for digital images in dermatology. *Journal of the American Academy of Dermatology* 1997;**37**:195–198.
6   Whited JD, Mills BJ, Hall RP, Drugge RJ, Grichnik JM, Simel DL. A pilot trial of digital imaging in skin cancer. *Journal of Telemedicine and Telecare* 1998;**4**:108–112.
7   Vidmar DA, Cruess D, Hsieh P, et al. The effect of decreasing digital image resolution on teledermatology diagnosis. *Telemedicine Journal* 1999;**5**:375–383.
8   McDonald DC, Hassol A, Carlson K, McCullough J, Fournier E, Yap J. *Telemedicine can Reduce Correctional Health Care Costs: An Evaluation of a Prison Telemedicine Network.* Washington, DC: National Institute of Justice, 1999.
9   Zincone LH, Doty E, Balch DC. Financial analysis of telemedicine in a prison system. *Telemedicine Journal* 1997;**3**:247–255.
10 US General Accounting Office. *Bureau of Prisons Health Care: Inmates' Access to Health Care is Limited by Lack of Clinical Staff.* HEHS-94-36. Bethesda, MD: Government Printing Office, 1994.
11 Emery S, Whitener BL. *The Issue is not Geography: Health Care Markets and the Diffusion of Telemedicine.* Chapel Hill, NC: North Carolina Rural Health Research Program, 1997.

8

Teledermatology in the US Military

Hon S. Pak

Introduction

In the early 1990s, the US military began to evaluate telemedicine. The goal was to make specialty care available, while also attempting to reduce healthcare expenditure and the costs related to medical evacuations. During the initial trials of telemedicine, dermatology cases made up a significant proportion of the consultations, and thus began the military's interest in teledermatology. Several military facilities began to experiment with teledermatology systems. Much of the early work was based at the Walter Reed Army Medical Center (WRAMC), the National Naval Medical Center/Uniformed Services University of the Health Sciences and the Tripler Army Medical Center.

The WRAMC used telemedicine to support US armed forces deployed in peacekeeping, humanitarian aid and disaster relief missions. Gomez et al[1] described 240 WRAMC telemedicine consultations held from February 1993 to February 1996. The consultations originated from Haiti, Somalia, Macedonia, Croatia, Ivory Coast, Egypt, Panama, Germany, Kuwait and elsewhere. The clinical histories and images were transmitted via modem to the WRAMC using combinations of commercial telephone lines and/or satellite communications (e.g. INMARSAT B). Videorecordings were transmitted at the relatively slow data transmission rate of 56 kbit/s. The quality of many of these consultations was considered to be poor. Dermatology accounted for 29% of the telemedicine consultations, most of which included diagnostic-quality, high-resolution still images. Walters[2] reviewed 114 telemedicine cases that were received at the WRAMC from February 1993 to March 1995, of which 39% were dermatological. He reported that the most common reason for the consultation was to obtain recommendations for additional therapy, and in only 17% was there a request for confirmation of diagnosis or treatment. In several cases the consultant initially viewed live video images but requested supplementary still images because of their generally better quality overall.

With the telemedicine experience from Bosnia and other deployments, the WRAMC developed a rudimentary store-and-forward consultation system using a point-to-point connection between Fort Myer, Virginia and the Walter Reed Army Medical Center. The images were transmitted via a T1 line while the clinical history was sent by fax. The printed images and the clinical history were then hand-delivered to a dermatologist at the WRAMC. The dermatologist wrote the diagnosis and treatment plan on a sheet which was then faxed back to the referring physician. An

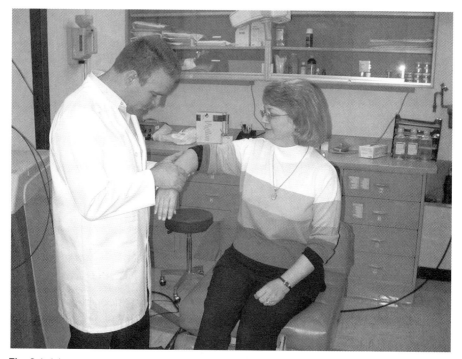

Fig. 8.1. (a)

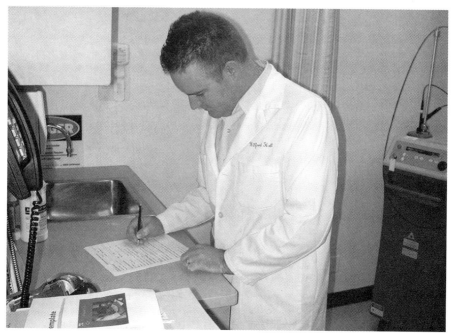

Fig. 8.1. (b)

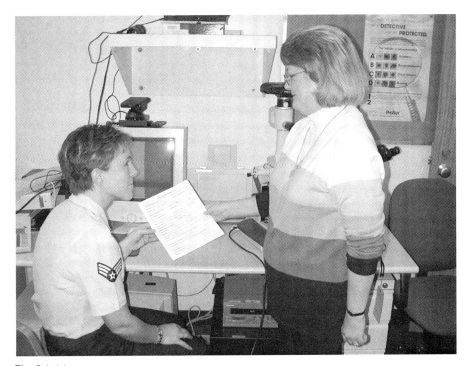

Fig. 8.1. (c)

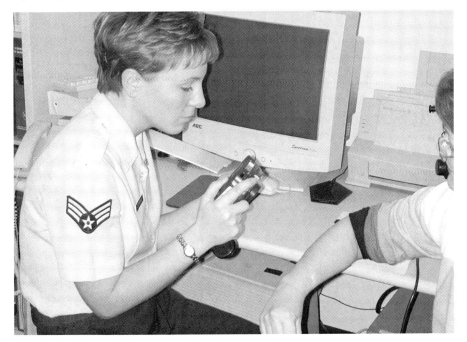

Fig. 8.1. (d)

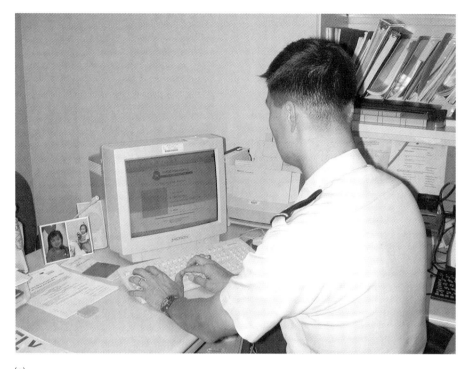

(e)

Fig. 8.1. Consultation flow. (a) Step 1: a referring physician examines a patient and decides whether a dermatology consultation is required. (b) Step 2: the referring physician completes a template-based consultation form and gives it to the patient. (c) Step 3: the patient takes the completed form to a consultation manager. (d) Step 4: the consultation manager takes the appropriate images and transcribes the information from the form into the teledermatology system. Images are sent to the server along with the patient's clinical information. (e) Step 5: a dermatology consultant logs in twice a day to answer any new referrals. The recommendations of the consultant are automatically sent to the referring physician.

economic analysis of this early system showed that although generally well received, it was not cost-effective because it was so labour-intensive.

A telemedicine demonstration project began in 1993 between Tripler Army Medical Center (TAMC) in Hawaii and Kwajalein Island in the South Pacific to improve the clinical support of remote locations and reduce the cost of transporting patients to Honolulu or Manila for consultation, which amounted to US$1million per year. Using real-time audio and still images transmitted over satellite links and local telephone lines, this system was considered to be slow but satisfactory. Norton et al[3,4] summarized Tripler's initial telemedicine experience but did not report a reduction in off-island travel to specialty care.

The National Naval Medical Center in co-operation with the Departments of Military and Emergency Medicine and Dermatology at the Uniformed Services University of the Health Sciences (Bethesda, Maryland) took part in 89 teledermatology consultations from April 1996 to January 1998. These consultations originated from a wide variety of sources, ranging from aircraft carriers with videoconferencing capabilities to submarines and large amphibious ships, which had digital cameras and email. More than 95% of cases were received by email. The incoming case files were received by a server at the National Naval Medical Center. The consultant then manually transferred the history and image files to a PC, reviewed them and sent a reply via email. Although somewhat labour intensive, this approach allowed rapid responses, usually within 12 hours, regardless of the location of the consultant.[5]

Current state of military teledermatology

Following the cost-effectiveness analysis, a web-based store-and-forward consulting system was developed at the WRAMC. This was felt to be more cost effective as it used the Internet and commercially available digital cameras. The system was written using 'Allaire's Cold Fusion v. 3.11', 'Dream Weaver' and Microsoft's 'SQL Server Database v. 6.5'. With minimum training, any military site with Internet access using a web browser could submit requests for consultations (Fig. 8.1). It had 40-bit built-in encryption as well as a user password for security. We instituted a digital imaging algorithm for teledermatology and incorporated a standard template for entering clinical information, to improve the likelihood of making the correct diagnosis (Figs 8.2–8.4). We eliminated unnecessary manual steps to decrease cost and response time. To use this system the following were required: Internet access, a PC, a web browser, a digital camera with at least 1024×768 pixel resolution with 24-bit colour, and a trained person to take appropriate images.

With the overall reduction in military strength, there has been a significant shortage of military dermatologists. The web-based consulting system has proved simple and inexpensive and has been widely accepted throughout the military in Europe and elsewhere. Over 1200 consultations have been handled using the WRAMC system (Table 8.1).

A different teledermatology system was developed in the military Tricare Region 10, based in Northern California. They initially used a software package called 'Visitran' to answer consultations, but it was replaced by a package ('RAVLIN 10') with improved encryption and data security. About 100 cases have been dealt with using the Tricare Region 10 teledermatology system.

In addition to using the WRAMC teledermatology system, videoconferencing has been used in the Great Plains region for teledermatology. This is partly because videoconferencing is used to support all specialties, not just dermatology.

Tripler received congressional funding through the AKAMAI project (Theatre Telemedicine Prototype Project) and developed a sophisticated store-and-forward telemedicine system that allows dermatology consultations as well as other special-

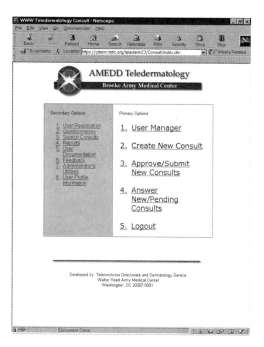

Fig. 8.2. Screen shot: teledermatology home page/log-in page.

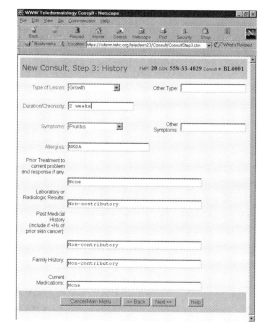

Fig. 8.3. Screen shot: template of clinical history.

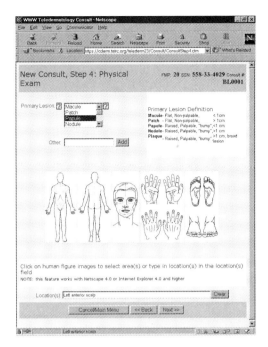

Fig. 8.4. Screen shot: template of physical findings.

Table 8.1. Number of web-based, store-and-forward teledermatology cases in the US military: September 2000

Region	Sites (no.)	Cases (no.)
North Atlantic	30	670
Great Plains	8	73
Europe	16	114
Southeastern	25	382
Total	**79**	**1239**

ties, such as orthopaedics. The system allows capture of workload, tracking of consultations and also interfaces with the military's medical database system, CHCS, which is used for ordering laboratory tests, radiology and prescriptions and also stores the results. Unfortunately, due to recent funding changes, the future of the project is uncertain. Currently, there is some discussion about combining the WRAMC web-based teledermatology system and the Tripler system.

Several years ago, the Army Medical Command gathered military telemedicine experts in various specialties to discuss the telemedicine support which will be needed in the future. During this meeting, there was general consensus that teledermatology support via store-and-forward methods or videoconferencing should be available in Echelon II level facilities (large field hospitals) or higher, to allow rapid diagnosis and minimize unnecessary evacuations of soldiers. At present tele-dermatology support for army operations is provided by the Special Medical Augmentation Response Teams located at all major military medical centres. These teams have satellite communication equipment that can supply medical expertise to the units they are supporting. In the navy, most of the larger ships are capable of store-and-forward teledermatology via email.

Military teledermatology studies

In addition to the studies mentioned above, Pak et al[6] reported the initial findings with the WRAMC web-based teledermatology system. The first 100 teledermatology cases resulted in a 50% reduction in face-to-face referrals, while requiring one-third of the dermatologists' time compared to face-to-face evaluations. We also observed that biopsy rates were higher with teledermatology.

There have been several published studies about the effectiveness of teledermatology as a diagnostic tool. However, much of the data relates to live two-way videoconferencing consultations and very little to store-and-forward consultations. Moreover, most published studies have compared diagnoses from two different dermatologists (i.e. interpretation is complicated by interobserver variation). There is little information about interdermatologist diagnostic variability. Pak et al conducted a study of intraobserver diagnostic correlation in teledermatology. In this study the diagnostic concordance was compared between a teledermatologist and the same dermatologist seeing the same patient face to face. A secondary goal was to measure diagnostic certainty: 404 participants were randomly selected from patients who had routine appointments at a tertiary medical centre. Teledermatology and face-to-face diagnoses were in complete agreement in 70% of cases (95% confidence level: 65–75%), 20% were in partial agreement, and in 10% there was disagreement. The diagnostic certainty level between the two groups differed significantly (teledermatology 7, face-to-face 9), and this difference was found in every category of disease ($P = 0.0065$) (Table 8.2). There was a 10% higher recommendation rate for biopsies by the teledermatologist (unpublished data).

Table 8.2. The levels of agreement differed significantly ($P = 0.03$) between categories of disease

Category of disease	Complete		Partial		Disagreement		Total
	No.	%	No.	%	No.	%	No.
Infectious	26	84	4	13	1	3	31
Premalignant/malignant	45	83	5	9	4	8	54
Acneiform eruption	23	82	4	14	1	4	28
Pigmented lesion	26	76	6	18	2	6	34
Benign tumour	57	70	17	21	7	9	81
Eczematous rash	29	66	13	30	2	4	44
Papulosquamous rash	62	59	28	27	15	14	105
Other	15	56	6	22	6	22	27

The diagnostic agreement rate was similar to previously published studies using interobserver comparisons and we therefore concluded that teledermatology appears to be an effective method of delivering dermatology care in the appropriate setting.

In reviewing the literature, there appear to be an adequate number of teledermatology studies indicating its clinical efficacy. What is lacking is an outcomes study to determine if patients do as well with teledermatology as with traditional face-to-face management. I believe that in order for teledermatology to become incorporated into routine military healthcare practice, a study must show that teledermatology is equal to or better than the traditional face-to-face medical system in terms of cost-effectiveness and the patient's ultimate outcome (as measured by a quality of life index and objective improvement or resolution of the patient's skin condition).

Diffusion of teledermatology

Despite the military experience in teledermatology, there are many issues that inhibit its widespread adoption. The main problem is that there is no centralized telemedicine organization. Telemedicine operations usually come under the control and direction of each local Tricare region, which has resulted in many disparate systems. Furthermore, each region competes for funds annually from the same limited allocation for telemedicine. All new telemedicine research projects are now reviewed centrally to reduce duplication of effort. However, this has not resulted in a unified military telemedicine system. One of the main reasons is that each service (army, air force and navy) has a slightly different medical mission with different capabilities. Moreover, each service and healthcare facility is organized differently and has different communications infrastructure. For example, some sites have a local area network (LAN), and others have a dial-up telephone connection to the Internet. Given this variability, building a system that meets all requirements with the flexibility to serve all customers is not straightforward.

Lessons learned

The lessons learned from the military experience of teledermatology include:

▷ Store-and-forward telemedicine appears to be preferable to real-time videoconsultations for teledermatology. Store-and-forward teledermatology is easier to use, it is easier to co-ordinate and it appears to be more cost effective.

▷ To be successful, the project should be led by a convincing clinician.

▷ The system must be user-friendly.

▷ The system must not interfere with normal patient flow or it will not be used much.

▶ Training is essential and should be continuing, no matter how user-friendly the system may be.

▶ Proponents of teledermatology should not oversell technology and nothing should be promised that cannot be delivered.

▶ Equipment breakdowns should be expected. The system must be reliable, preferably being available more than 95% of the time.

▶ Prior to implementing teledermatology, a business plan is required for each site. Developing such plans requires adequate resources.

▶ The number of likely consultations should be determined, and where the patients are going to be referred from.

▶ Participants should be prepared to modify and adjust the programme.

Unique features of the military

In implementing teledermatology, the military is somewhat ahead of civilian practice in the USA for several reasons, which include:

▶ lack of interstate licensure restrictions

▶ little dependence on third-party reimbursement (insurance and Medicare)

▶ medicolegal issues may not apply to the same degree in the military.

Telemedicine is becoming a necessity to support military missions during peace and in wartime. Since there is a shortage of military dermatologists, teledermatology may be a solution for the troops, their families and retired military personnel.

Future of military teledermatology

In the future, it appears likely that teledermatology will become incorporated into the daily delivery of health care instead of being a novel tool. I envisage that in the near future, telemedicine will be an integral part of a universal military electronic patient record. This new system will incorporate smartcard technology to allow soldiers in the battlefield to be identified, tracked, diagnosed, treated and evacuated expeditiously. Information on every patient/soldier will be immediately available. Furthermore, as has occurred in teleradiology, digital images in dermatology will become standardized and will conform to DICOM standards to allow integration and interfacing with other systems.

Teledermatology represents a change in the way that health care is delivered as it shifts more responsibility to the referring primary-care physicians while educating them to improve their management of patients with skin conditions. Military teledermatology will allow more efficient utilization of dwindling medical resources.

References

1 Gomez E, Poropatich R, Karinch MA, et al. Tertiary telemedicine support during global military humanitarian missions. *Telemedicine Journal* 1996;**2:**201–220.

2 Walters TJ. Deployment telemedicine: the Walter Reed Army Medical Center experience. *Military Medicine* 1996;**161:**531–536.

3 Norton SA, Burdick AE, Phillips CM, et al. Teledermatology and underserved populations. *Archives of Dermatology* 1997;**133:**197–200.

4 Norton SA, Floro C, Bice SD, et al. Telemedicine in Micronesia. *Telemedicine Journal* 1996;**2:**225–231.

5 Vidmar DA. The history of teledermatology in the Department of Defense. *Dermatologic Clinics* 1999;**17:**113–124.

6 Pak HS, Welch M, Poropatich R. Web-based teledermatology consult system: preliminary results from the first 100 cases. *Studies in Health Technology and Informatics* 1999;**64:**179–184.

9

International Teleconsultations in Dermatology

Joseph C. Kvedar and Eric R. Menn

Introduction

A woman in an isolated region of Northern Indonesia develops a widespread blistering rash in her third trimester of pregnancy. Her providers manage the illness, using their best knowledge, with antibiotics and topical steroids. Because of concern for the mother and her fetus, an email message is sent to dermatologists at USA centres of excellence. The message includes a brief history and several images (Fig. 9.1). At one of the centres, the history and images are presented at a departmental teaching conference at which several world experts are present. Return email messages are sent back to the doctor in Indonesia; the majority of which suggest that the patient has been misdiagnosed and has an illness that will threaten both her life and the life of her fetus. Confident in his own diagnosis and treatment plan, the Indonesian provider does not alter his approach to his patient's care. He sends a second email message a few weeks later noting the improvement of the patient on his original regimen.

This vignette, a true story, illustrates much of what is right and wrong with international teledermatology. While international consultation in dermatology has great promise, there has been only limited experience so far. Various factors account for this apparent contradiction. First, the primary beneficiaries from such a service are mostly unaware of its existence; second, a clear reproducible revenue model is lacking. Issues of standardization of technology, infrastructure and business process remain to be resolved. Finally, cultural and language barriers may inhibit its adoption by providers and patients.

This chapter explores the use of teleconsultation across national boundaries as a method of care delivery. There is almost no literature on this topic from which to extract objective data. The Department of Dermatology at Harvard Medical School has been providing international teleconsultations for the last six years. During this time we have directly experienced both the opportunities and limitations noted above.

History of remote consultation

Teleconsultation permits a profound realignment of medical practice patterns. Care has always been performed in face-to-face encounters in which a possessor of specialized knowledge brings that expertise to the care or healing of another individual. It was only with the development of telecommunications that a concept

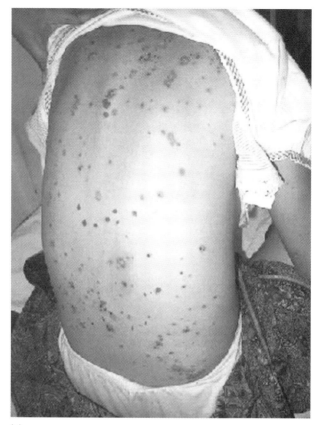

(a)

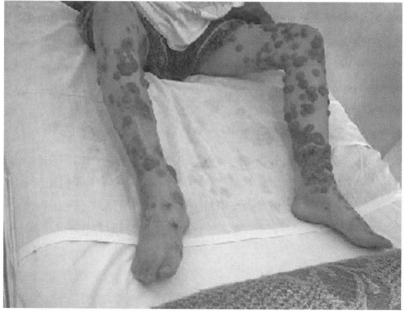

(b)

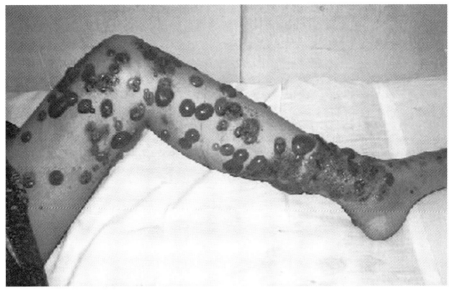

(c)

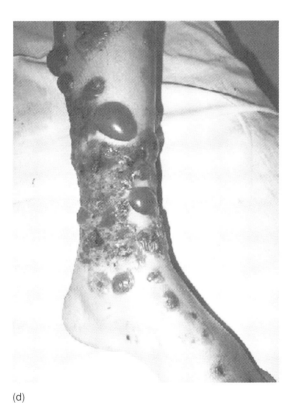

(d)

Fig. 9.1. Low-resolution JPEG images of a patient from Indonesia with an acute blistering eruption of pregnancy. (a) Patient's back: file size of 33 kByte allowed easy transmission as an email attachment, while preserving adequate colour and spatial resolution. (b) Legs (file size, 27 kByte). (c) Left leg (file size 26 kByte).(d) Left lower extremity (file size 27 kByte).

such as remote care could be considered. Telecommunications have now evolved to allow both real-time and store-and-forward interactions.

The first experiments, both in the USA and other parts of the world, centred on the delivery of health care to rural populations who traditionally have suffered from a lack of access to specialist expertise.[1] This geographical maldistribution of health care has long been recognized as a serious issue.[2] For example, in the USA, the New England states with a population of 13 400 000 had almost 50 000 physicians, while the Mountain states, comprising a much greater geographical area, had only 36 000 physicians serving a similar population. This issue is not confined to the USA.

The delivery of health care to these remote populations via teleconsultation has been studied extensively,[3,4] and shown, for the most part, to be preferable to the former paucity of care. Teleconsultation, however, represents a major change in the delivery of care. Reliance by providers in a remote setting on the expertise of a caregiver who may be hundreds or even thousands of miles away demands a significant leap of faith. Teleconsultation also upsets traditional healthcare financial models.

Over time, albeit slowly, recognition has arisen that in those instances in which care cannot be provided at the local level, teleconsultation is not only feasible and desirable, but can also be life saving. Further, it has been demonstrated repeatedly that care delivered at a distance compares favourably with opinions rendered in a face-to-face setting. This has been demonstrated in many specialties including neurology, cardiology, trauma and especially dermatology.[5-9]

Physicians, particularly those from academic medical centres, have always participated in the training of colleagues from other countries. As a result of this exchange of expertise, a global network of physicians has developed who make referrals to, and seek expert advice from, each other. As advanced telecommunications have evolved, and teleconsultation has been proved at the local level, it was inevitable that these discussions would take place on an international level.

Demand for services

Demand for international teleconsultation is driven by a variety of factors. These include the perceived burden of disease and need, the record and distribution of local healthcare providers, awareness of telemedicine services and any value they might bring, and finally the price sensitivity of the local population. Emerging international markets for teleconsultation generally share the characteristics of having a relatively high level of industrialization, education and technology infrastructure. Further, there is often either a distrust of local healthcare workers, or a perception by the population that the quality of care is poor.

The technology required for teleconsultation is less of a problem than it once was. The equipment required for teledermatology includes a digital camera capable of capturing high-resolution images, a PC on which to store the images and access to an Internet service provider for transmitting the images to a specialist via email or a website. The Internet has provided a standardized, inexpensive way to connect individuals around the world.

The most fertile ground for international teleconsultation is a country or region where a certain degree of affluence exists, together with some level of suspicion of local providers and some penetration of standard technologies, such as the Internet. There are millions of people around the world who fit this description. Why is it, then, that the volume of international teleconsultations in dermatology is so small?

Cultural barriers

Teleconsultation is best seen as a way of connecting healthcare providers. Thus if telemedicine is being considered, the local provider must be involved in making recommendations and carrying them out. In situations where the local population is interested in importing another culture's health care, the local providers are usually not. This is because teleconsultation is a disruptive force that may be perceived as threatening by local physicians. This mistrust on the part of local providers has severely limited the penetration of teleconsultation in many countries. Those who have successfully overcome this barrier have done so by partnering with local personnel and reassuring the local providers that care will remain local; that teleconsultation is a tool for them as much as it is for consumers. One of the largest commercial providers of international teleconsultations is WorldCare, Inc. (http://www.worldcare.com [last checked 28 July 2001]). In brokering over 10 000 consultations over the last six years, the experience of WorldCare is that teleconsultants recommend a change in the diagnosis and/or management about half of the time, but that care remains local in more than 90% of cases (H. Sharif, personal communication). Thus, experience shows that local providers can benefit from the advice of experts, but that care remains local in the majority of cases.

Consumer and provider awareness

The majority of the world's population still conceives of health care as an activity that is constrained by time and geography. The ability to break down barriers of time and place via teleconsultation will not be perceived as possible by the average person without some concerted effort to educate them. Because most teleconsultation services are priced as an alternative to travelling abroad for care, they are often more expensive than care by a local physician. Therefore, they are perceived as solutions for grave illnesses. Dermatological illness does not usually rise to the level of concern that would drive a consumer to seek care from a second provider, let alone an expert from another country. For teledermatology to achieve a meaningful workload, there must be a focused effort to educate consumers and providers. That education effort needs to explain the increase in quality of care that teleconsultation can provide.

Teledermatology at Partners Healthcare

The introductory vignette in this chapter discussed a specific teledermatology consultation that arose in Indonesia. Since its inception, Partners Healthcare affiliates including the Massachusetts General Hospital and Brigham and Women's Hospital have investigated teledermatology from both a research and an operational perspective. Protocols have been developed for obtaining the patient history, capturing images, transmitting that information to the specialist and handling the specialist's response. Teledermatology is offered as part of a more comprehensive teleconsultation service. Several hundred teledermatology consultations are performed every year. Almost all are store-and-forward, although an occasional interactive video consultation is also performed. Anecdotally we have noted that dermatology is rarely the specific impetus for a consultation. The case mix for our teleconsultation service is shown in Figure 9.2. While dermatological conditions are perceived by sufferers as important to their well-being, they are rarely of such urgency that remote care is needed or requested. When referring practitioners request dermatological consultations, it is usually to help with cases representing diagnostic dilemmas or therapeutic challenges. Diagnoses have included cutaneous T-cell lymphoma, morphoea, vitiligo, chondrodermatitis nodularis helicis and others. A pattern has emerged in handling these international teleconsultations that is not unique to dermatology. Often the specialist consultants ask questions of the referring practitioner in return. This usually takes the place of the questions that would be asked of the patient in the office in a live visit. A common consultation response is:

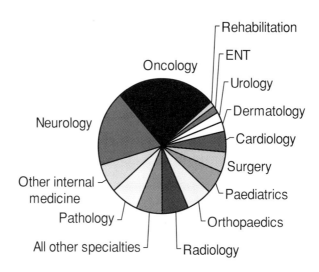

Fig. 9.2. Distribution of the international teleconsultations for the year 2000 (Partners HealthCare System).

You have presented a patient with X history and Y additional data. If A, B and C have been done and are negative or normal, then I would suggest the following diagnosis and treatment. If A, B and C have not been done, I would recommend doing them and would be happy to review the case again in the context of the additional data.

Telemedicine process

When possible, the preferred method of case handling is via the Internet.[10] Referring physicians assemble case materials, including digital images where possible. These can be transmitted to a server using standard web techniques. An automated email message is sent to the consulting dermatologist to inform him/her that a case is in need of comment. Consultants can review cases and offer their opinion through a secure, password-protected website. The process of case handling is that a coordinator reviews materials, assigns each case to a specialist, tracks case progress and turnaround and reviews the consultation for quality assurance. As Internet access improves around the world and physician adoption of the Internet increases, it is expected that more and more cases will be handled online.

Next steps

Growth in demand for teledermatology will depend on the resolution of a number of issues. The need for mass consumer education regarding the availability of the service has already been mentioned. A major difficulty is the identification of a financial model for the delivery of teledermatology internationally. Many of those who could most benefit from the service cannot afford it. The technology is certainly in place in most of the industrialized world, as evidenced by the rapid growth of the Internet. In due course it is to be expected that the same level of access will be possible in the most remote parts of the world. It has been shown clearly that teledermatology is feasible whether the transmission medium is ordinary telephony, ISDN, wireless or satellite communications. As the cost of the required technology is likely to continue to fall, it will represent a smaller and smaller component of the price of teleconsultations in future. International standards for image capture and clinical data will facilitate collaboration between colleagues in different academic centres.

Perhaps the most important factor in its growth will be a demonstration that teleconsultation positively affects the quality of care in a meaningful way. In the introductory vignette, although a remote physician sought expert consultation, he chose to ignore the advice from the USA and the patient recovered nonetheless. The diagnostic acumen of academic centres is not in dispute. However whether this diagnostic acumen will positively affect the quality of care in a measurable way remains to be tested rigorously. The demand for an international teledermatology service may grow without this proof, but the demand will not be sustainable without it.

The future of international teledermatology

Dermatology as a subject for international teleconsultation may never achieve the workload of specialties concerned with more critical illnesses such as cardiology, neurology and oncology. However, teledermatology will remain an important, cost-effective method of diagnosis and treatment across widely separated clinics and tertiary care hospitals. The growth of the Internet into a robust, reliable communications medium will inevitably foster international teledermatology because of the removal of space and time as barriers to care and consultation. The globalization of dermatology will be encouraged by the dissemination of information and education to all healthcare providers. As standards of care, and technological and practice protocols emerge, the standard of care delivery around the world will be increased.

Conclusions

It has been demonstrated repeatedly that the quality of care possible by teledermatology is, in most cases, equal to that of a face-to-face consultation. Barriers to teledermatology are primarily cultural, and market based. Culturally, patients are often unaware of the availability of teledermatology, or indeed any variety of teleconsultation. Many of the physicians who are aware of teleconsultation fear it because of a perceived diminution of their role in care delivery, and threats to practice patterns that they have developed over their working life.

Market forces mitigate against the rapid deployment of teledermatology because no revenue model exists for the delivery of the service outside of national health schemes, for whom domestic care is the over-riding priority. Doctors providing the casual consultations that take place today could be completely overwhelmed by the demands of a global population whose desperate healthcare needs are not being met at any level. One area in which teleconsultation is likely to have a profound impact lies in the distribution of knowledge to the physicians, healthcare providers and patients who avail themselves of the rapidly expanding body of expertise that is available over the Internet. Online consulting is not without risk however, because of the difficulty of ensuring that the information obtained is reliable. It may be the case that centres of medical excellence should play a more prominent role in acting as repositories of high-quality information.

References

1   Field MJ, ed. *Telemedicine: A Guide to Assessing Telecommunications in Health Care*. Washington: Institute of Medicine, National Academy Press, 1996:34–54.
2   Randolph L, ed. *Physician Characteristics and Distribution in the US 1997–1998*. Chicago: American Medical Association, 1998.
3   Nesbitt TS, Ellis JC, Kuenneth CA. A proposed model for telemedicine to supplement the physician workforce in the USA. *Journal of Telemedicine and Telecare* 1999;**5**(suppl. 2):20–26.
4   Wootton R. Telemedicine and isolated communities: a UK perspective. *Journal of Telemedicine and Telecare* 1999; **5**(suppl. 2):27–34.

5   Levine SR, Gorman M. Telestroke: the application of telemedicine for stroke. *Stroke* 1999;**30:**464–469.
6   Perednia DA, Allen A. Telemedicine technology and clinical applications. *Journal of the American Medical Association* 1995;**273:**483–488.
7   Balas EA, Jaffrey F, Kuperman GJ, et al. Electronic communication with patients: evaluation of distance medicine technology. *Journal of the American Medical Association* 1997;**278:**152–159.
8   Kvedar JC, Edwards RA, Menn ER, et al. The substitution of digital images for dermatologic physical examination. *Archives of Dermatology* 1997;**133:**161–167.
9   Lowitt MH, Kessler II, Kaufman LC, et al. Teledermatology and in-person examinations: a comparison of patient and physician perceptions and diagnostic agreement. *Archives of Dermatology* 1998;**134:**471–476.
10   Kvedar JC, Menn ER, Baradagunta S, Smulders-Meyer O, Gonzalez E. Teledermatology in a capitated delivery system using distributed information architecture: design and development. *Telemedicine Journal* 1999;**5:**357–366.

10

Telemedicine for Wound Healing

Eliot N. Mostow and Jennifer Geras

Introduction

Telemedicine has many potential benefits when applied to the care of wounds since almost by definition patients with chronic wounds tend to be limited in mobility. This often makes ordinary office visits (that might otherwise enhance the care and healing of their wound) somewhat difficult. Using telemedicine, the patient and caregiver are spared the cost and inconvenience of transportation and office visits.

This chapter describes telemedicine for wound care. There are two possible forms of telemedicine. The first is real-time telemedicine, usually videoconferencing (which needs sophisticated equipment and requires all participants to be available at a specified place and time). The second is asynchronous telemedicine, often called 'store-and-forward' (take a picture and transmit it via email or by attaching it to a web page). We are participants in a multidisciplinary wound-healing clinic (see http://www.agmc.org/wound.htm [last checked 29 July 2001]) and have developed a telemedicine programme, based on the store-and-forward approach.

Costs and benefits

Fiscal responsibility demands that costs and benefits are considered before spending money on a new medical technique. The desire is to maintain the same quality of care with decreased costs to doctors, patients and insurers. In the case of telemedicine for wound care, we were unable to find published information about the economics. We therefore investigated:

- whether there was a cost difference (for the patient or for the caregiver) between seeing a patient in our wound clinic compared to having a digital image sent to us for comment on subsequent care;

- whether there was a difference in outcome (i.e. healing rate) of patients seen in the wound clinic versus telemedicine.

While it would seem to be a simple matter to compare costs, there are many variables to consider. Relevant telemedicine work has been examined, mainly in dermatology.[1-3] One study addressed the use of telemedicine in nursing home care and demonstrated the ability to replace some on-site dermatology consultations for cost-efficiency.[4]

Another addressed the ability to follow pressure ulcers in patients with spinal cord injuries, an example of the benefit of telemedicine to patients with obvious transportation problems.[5]

The direct costs of wound care include office visits, procedures, diagnostic tests, hospitalizations and dressing supplies. One study showed that patients with chronic skin ulcers accounted for $150 million in direct patient costs[6] and cost was noted in a discussion on the 'burden' of diabetic foot ulcers by Reiber et al.[7] Olin et al indicated that the average total direct cost of treatment of venous stasis ulcers was $9685 per patient.[8] We were unable to generalize from the published studies to the patients seen at our clinic, who have a variety of wound types (e.g. pressure ulcers and diabetic foot ulcers). Indirect wound care costs such as pain, suffering and inconvenience to the patient's family should also be considered when analysing the advantages of telemedicine. The budget must include funds (and time) for recruitment and training of staff, selection and installation of equipment, and project coordination.[9]

Table 10.1 suggests that the costs for a provider using telemedicine for wound care will be reduced if there are lower costs for rent (computer space) and staff (who might even work off-site). There are also non-monetary outcomes that may be considered beneficial. These include decreased time to diagnosis, decreased length of waiting time for treatment initiation, improved education, reassurance and patient comfort secondary to the lack of need for transport to an outpatient facility and an unfamiliar setting.[10]

Our primary use of telemedicine has been as an adjunct to our wound clinic. So far, most patients seen with telemedicine have also been seen on some regular basis in our outpatient wound centre.

Table 10.1. Cost of wound care in a general clinical practice, a hospital-based wound clinic and a telemedicine programme

	General clinic	Wound clinic	Telemedicine
Rent	Fixed	Fixed	Lower
Facility fee	None	Yes	None
Dressing costs	Paid by patient or provider	Billable to insurance	Paid by patient or billable to insurance through nursing home or home-care agency
Staff costs	Usual	Usual	Variable (patient, nursing home or home-care agency)
Physician fee	Usual	Usual	Negotiated
Travel costs	Fixed	Fixed	None
Travel hardship	Fixed	Fixed	None
Quality of assessment	In person	In person	Restricted (2D images with delegated verbal description)
Materials required	Clinic supplies	Clinic supplies	Camera, email

Basic equipment

The equipment necessary for telemedicine includes:

- a computer and monitor to receive images
- an email account accessible via a modem or other connection
- a security mechanism to avoid patient information being retrieved by others inadvertently (e.g. Verisign. See http://www.verisign.com [last checked 29 July 2001])
- one or more digital cameras
- someone to monitor the email account and check for new images
- personnel to read information and respond via email or telephone
- personnel to evaluate the patient in person if telemedicine does not seem appropriate (e.g. the image is not adequate, the image suggests hospitalization, or some other intervention, such as debridement, is required).

Personnel

Setting up a programme has a significant training requirement. Personnel will be needed to train the nurses at the extended care facility in the skills necessary to operate a digital camera, use a computer and transmit the photographs.

There are many ways to staff a telemedicine programme. We use a nurse or nurse practitioner to ensure that all the appropriate information is available with the images and that the images themselves are of reasonable quality. A nurse practitioner or physician then reviews the information and responds with recommendations.

Having technical assistance available has been very helpful to deal with questions about equipment problems and camera operations. It has improved the overall quality of the images. A photographer takes pictures of the wound at the nursing home or in the patient's home. This has presented problems because these people do not work for us and they may not see telemedicine as an advantage over simply arranging for a patient to be transported to our clinic. Nonetheless some centres have produced high-quality photographs. In one case of pyoderma gangrenosum, the patient, who travelled often, took his own pictures. He sent us photographs of the closing wound on his thigh for us to provide guidance on the tapering doses of prednisone (Fig. 10.1).

Liability

The details of liability need to be addressed with each provider's and corporation's malpractice carrier and legal counsel as appropriate. Our local carrier has verified that we are covered, as we would be if we saw the patient in our office. We take great pains

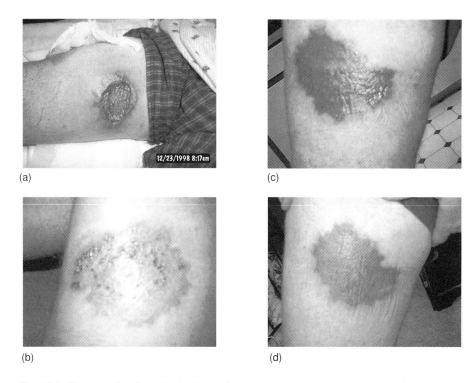

(a)

(c)

(b)

(d)

Fig. 10.1. Photographs of a patient with pyoderma gangrenosum sent to us to monitor progress. Treatment recommendations regarding tapering off the prednisone were carried out via email and occasional telephone conversations. (a) 23 December 1997: initial inpatient photograph. (b) 26 January 1998: patient's first attempt at photography; coaching helped later. (c) 4 February 1998: wound almost closed. (d) 12 February 1998: wound closed.

to make sure that we err on the side of direct patient contact if there is any question that a wound is not progressing as we expect.

Accuracy of diagnosis

With each image transmission, the nurse caring for the patient sends a basic wound description and past medical history, along with details of current treatment and the wound measurements. In our experience, diagnosis has been accurate using telemedicine when compared to assessment in person, based on pictures of reasonable quality. However, if the digital photograph is of poor quality, or the patient appears to have a diagnosis that requires emergency treatment, or if the wound needs debridement or some other diagnostic procedure, then more extensive plans for evaluation and treatment need to be arranged.

Roth et al found 87% agreement in diagnosis between digital and slide images.[11] Lesher et al found complete agreement in dermatological diagnosis using telemedicine versus on-site diagnosis 78% of the time, and partial agreement in diagnosis 21% of the time, and disagreement 1% of the time. They also found that telemedicine required a longer time for diagnosis in 90% of cases.[12] Gilmour et al showed that face-to-face consultations were more likely to result in an accurate diagnosis, but this may not necessarily apply to wound care.[13] Wirthlin et al found that diagnoses and treatment of wounds were comparable between viewing digital images and standard wound examination.[14]

Security

In order to prevent unauthorized access to medical records, we use a commercial service to encrypt the digital images and assessment information. The necessary software can be obtained via the Internet for a small annual fee. Each sender and recipient must obtain a digital certificate in order to read the encrypted information. We require patients and other healthcare facilities participating in the programme to obtain the encryption software. Other issues to consider include who is actually going to be receiving and viewing the images.[15]

Documentation

We have developed a basic wound assessment form for the information that is helpful in formulating a diagnosis and treatment plan. This form can be filled in and sent with each photograph transmission (Fig. 10.2).

Reimbursement

At the end of 1999, reimbursement for telemedicine was available only for certain cases and only for real-time telemedicine (i.e. not for the store-and-forward telemedicine described above). We have negotiated a fee structure with several nursing homes in our area. Three levels of telemedicine care are offered. The lowest level applies to an evaluation of a simple closing wound that requires no treatment change. The highest level applies to an initial patient evaluation, and to most reviews that require significant treatment changes. The reimbursement fees are $50, $100 and $150 for low, medium and high level telemedicine care respectively.

Performance evaluation

Performance evaluation should be part of any new programme, especially those with technology that may change rapidly.[16] Performance improvement for telemedicine

The Wound Center of Akron General – TeleWound™ Services
400 Wabash Avenue   Akron, Ohio 44307
330 / 376 – 4325 (HEAL)   -   e-mail: telewound@agmc.org

Initial Consult Request

Facility Name:	Assessment Date:	NH Wound Care Nurse / Primary Physician:
Resident Name:	Patient ID / SSN Number:	Allergies:

Wound Location:	PMH:

Wound Description:

Onset Date:
Wound Dimensions: cm x   cm x cm
Necrosis: ☐ Black ☐ Yellow ☐ Wet ☐ Dry
Debridement: Yes ☐ No
Debridement type:
Wound edges:
Wound bed:
Peri-wound area:
Exudate amount:
Exudate color:
Tunneling:
Undermining:
Edema:
Odor:
Pain:

Comments:

Tobacco Use: ☐ Yes   ☐ No   Pack Years: ____ years

INSERT PICTURE HERE

Current Treatment Order(s) Including Oral Meds Related to Wound Care:

Support Surfaces:	Nutritional Status / Specific Lab Results to Wound:

Page 1 of 3

Fig. 10.2. The template sent to participating sites for patient information. The template is sent by email or as a hard copy.

should address such issues as licensing and credentialing, data security and privacy, informed consent and peer review for evaluation of documentation. Our programme has evolved into a service tailored to each patient's individual needs and resources.

Barriers to utilization

We have found that telemedicine equipment should be both cost effective and easy to operate. Many extended-care facilities that we have approached to participate in our programme do not have basic computer equipment or Internet access. Furthermore, the cost of purchasing a digital camera has also been prohibitive. There has also been a lack of basic computer skills in nurses participating in the programme, as well as fear of new technology. Confusion and inability to use the equipment properly has increased the need for troubleshooting visits by our personnel.

Marketing telemedicine

Any marketing of a service must define the target population. While the patient is clearly one target, other important users of the service are the referring physicians, other wound-care specialists, nursing home medical directors and insurance companies. The target population needs to understand that telemedicine can provide high-quality care at lower cost, with reduced patient travel.[17] Patients who can benefit from telemedicine most are therefore those with hard to heal wounds living in extended-care facilities or those who are homebound. These patients would suffer financial and physical hardship if they needed to make a trip to an outpatient wound care centre. Our potential customers therefore include home health agencies and extended-care facilities.

These organizations were recruited through informational meetings and presentations at professional meetings. Brochures introducing the programme were also mailed to target clients throughout the local area. Distribution of brochures resulted in consultations from underserved rural and inner city areas.

We have not assessed patient satisfaction. Other studies have shown positive impressions that might be important to any insurer or organization concerned with quality care and capturing more 'market share'.[18,19] Lowitt et al observed a positive patient response in 97–100% of video examinations, although patients did show a preference for in-person examinations.[20]

Conclusion

To establish a successful telemedicine programme for wound care requires overcoming many obstacles, including reimbursement for store-and-forward telemedicine, rapidly changing technology and building a substantial clientele to ensure financial viability. In addition, a performance improvement programme should be put into place. Image resolution requirements should also be considered. Previous studies have used a variety of image resolutions (Wirthlin et al,[14] 756×504 pixels/inch; Gilmour et al,[13] 352 pixels, 288 lines; Roth et al,[11] 1000 pixels/inch; Vidmar,[3] 1524×1012 pixels). The appropriate resolution will depend on the needs of the programme as determined by its participants.

In our case, telemedicine is used as an additional service in a specialty wound-care clinic. We use it for patient follow-up in straightforward cases and for triage of questionable cases sent by the nursing home. Telemedicine has augmented our traditional medical practice and has made care available to otherwise unreachable patient populations.

Telemedicine activity has been much less than our initial expectations. We have found patients who have benefited from the service because of their geographical location and secondary inaccessibility to specialty consultation. For example, a young man visited our clinic with a chronic surgical wound. He lived approximately 400 km from our clinic in a medically underserved rural community. With weekly teleconsultation, the patient's wound healed in approximately four weeks without disrupting his work schedule or family life with journeys to our wound centre for re-evaluation.

We have found telemedicine to be most useful as an adjunct to ordinary clinic visits. The main barriers have been acceptance of new duties by nursing home staff and concerns about equipment costs by nursing home administrators. However we expect that telemedicine will become a standard form of medical care within the next few years.

References

1   Freeman K, Wynn-Jones J, Groves-Phillips S, Lewis L. Teleconsulting: a practical account of pitfalls, problems and promise. Experience from the TEAM project group. *Journal of Telemedicine and Telecare* 1996;**2**(suppl. 1):1–3.
2   Lewis P, McCann R, Hidalgo P, Gorman M. Use of store and forward technology for vascular nursing teleconsultation service. *Journal of Vascular Nursing* 1997; **15**:116–123.
3   Vidmar DA. The history of teledermatology in the department of defense. *Dermatologic Clinics* 1999;**17**:113–124.
4   Zelickson BD, Homan L. Teledermatology in the nursing home. *Archives of Dermatology* 1997;**133**:171–174.
5   Vesmarovich S, Walker S, Hauber R, Temkin A. Use of telerehabilitation to manage pressure ulcers in persons with spinal cord injuries. *Advances in Wound Care* 1999;**12**:264–269.
6   Huse DM, Oster G, Killen AR, Lacey MJ, Colditz GA. The economic costs of non-insulin dependent diabetes mellitus. *Journal of the American Medical Association* 1989;**262**:2708–2713.
7   Reiber GE, Lipsky BA, Gibbons GW. The burden of diabetic foot ulcers. *American Journal of Surgery* 1998;**176**(2A suppl.):5S–10S.
8   Olin JW, Beusterien KM, Childs MB, Seavey C, McHugh L, Griffiths RI. Medical costs of treating venous stasis ulcers: evidence from a retrospective cohort study. *Vascular Medicine* 1999;**4**:1–7.
9   Crowe BL. Cost-effectiveness analysis of telemedicine. *Journal of Telemedicine and Telecare* 1998;**4**(suppl. 1):14–17.
10 McIntosh E, Cairns J. A framework for the economic evaluation of telemedicine. *Journal of Telemedicine and Telecare* 1997;**3**:132–139.
11 Roth AC, Reid JC, Puckett CL, Concannon MJ. Digital images in the diagnosis of wound healing problems. *Plastic and Reconstructive Surgery* 1999;**103**:483–486.

12   Lesher JL Jr, Davis LS, Gourdin FW, English D, Thompson WO. Telemedicine evaluation of cutaneous diseases: a blinded comparative study. *Journal of the American Academy of Dermatology* 1998;**38:**27–31.

13   Gilmour E, Campbell SM, Loane MA, et al. Comparison of teleconsultations and face-to-face consultations: preliminary results of a United Kingdom multicentre teledermatology study. *British Journal of Dermatology* 1998;**139:**81–87.

14   Wirthlin DJ, Buradagunta S, Edwards RA, et al. Telemedicine in vascular surgery: Feasibility of digital imaging for remote management of wounds. *Journal of Vascular Surgery* 1998;**27:**1089–1100.

15   Eysenbach G, Diepgen TL. Patients looking for information on the internet and seeking teleadvice: motivation, expectations, and misconceptions as expressed in e-mails sent to physicians. *Archives of Dermatology* 1999;**135:**151–156.

16   Eliasson AH, Poropatich RK. Performance improvement in telemedicine: the essential elements. *Military Medicine* 1998;**163:**530–535.

17   Brunicardi BO. Financial analysis of savings from telemedicine in Ohio's prison system. *Telemedicine Journal* 1998;**4:**49–54.

18   Callahan EJ, Hilty DM, Nesbitt TS. Patient satisfaction with telemedicine consultation in primary care: comparison of ratings of medical and mental health applications. *Telemedicine Journal* 1998;**4:**363–369.

19   Huston JL, Burton DC. Patient satisfaction with multispecialty interactive teleconsultations. *Journal of Telemedicine and Telecare* 1997;**3:**205–208.

20   Lowitt MH, Kessler II, Kauffman CL, Hooper FJ, Siegel E, Burnett JW. Teledermatology and in-person examinations. *Archives of Dermatology* 1998;**134:**471–476.

11

Transcontinental Dermatology – Virtual Grand Rounds

Henry Foong Boon Bee

Introduction

'The art of knowing is the art of visual memory', said Walter Shelley.[1] We can never see too many patients, too many atlases or too many clinical photographs. While the traditional method of bedside teaching is still valuable, advances in global communication allow one to keep in touch with far-flung colleagues and share our patients' problems interactively, occasionally allowing one to solve difficult diagnostic and therapeutic cases. This activity facilitates both learning and teaching and may well be a model for future professional education. Over the past few years, I have consulted peers on many continents including North America, Australia, Asia and Europe. These colleagues have included experts with areas of special interest like paediatric dermatology, dermatopathology, dermatological surgery, collagen vascular disease, critical care dermatology, nail disease, laser surgery, oral medicine and contact dermatitis.

The Internet is quickly becoming a popular communications medium. In 1999 there were about 1.5 million Internet users in Malaysia and more than 15 000 new Internet accounts were being registered each month.[2] Modern technologies have expanded the possibilities for the Internet, turning it from a mainly text-based medium of communication into a global multimedia network. Most people are now familiar with the Internet via the telephone network though an Internet service provider (ISP). This system has proved useful for telemedicine.[3]

Virtual grand rounds

I am a solo practitioner in Ipoh, a Malaysian city with a population of about half a million. The nearest academic dermatology centre is in Kuala Lumpur, which is 200 km south of Ipoh. My ISP account allows me to transmit data and images to colleagues for dermatological discussion, a process we have termed 'virtual grand rounds' in dermatology. The Internet is widely available and low in cost. It has encouraged those interested in telemedicine to evaluate its usefulness.[4-6]

The concept of virtual grand rounds in dermatology was originally envisaged by myself and a colleague, David Elpern. We are both relatively isolated dermatologists and have shared cases for a few years via email. Gradually, it dawned on us that we could share cases with others, too, for teaching purposes, for consultation or just for interest.

The colleagues I most frequently consult using the Internet are dermatologists from Malaysia, Singapore and the USA. In the early days, we discussed cases by email, using a simple narrative process, but with the advent of digital cameras, we can now add images to the purely descriptive history. The ability to capture the images of skin lesions accurately and reliably with a good digital camera has added immensely to our discussions.[7] Digitized images of the histopathological findings will further enhance the value of this practice. The process that I employ in my daily practice is described below.

Patients are approached in the traditional way by taking a good history and performing a thorough physical examination. Laboratory investigations are available and utilized when appropriate. In addition, digital images of the patients' skin lesions can be captured with a digital camera (DC 265, Kodak). With regards to patient confidentiality, the patients are informed that their images may be transmitted electronically for discussion and consultation with other dermatologists.

The Kodak DC 265 digital camera has a 3× zoom lens (38–115 mm) allowing close-up pictures of subjects. The camera can record images up to a resolution of 1.6 million pixels, i.e. 1536×1024 pixels in high-resolution mode. The camera uses a removable memory card for storing the pictures.

For dermatology I use the digital camera in automatic white balance mode, automatic exposure mode, with automatic focus and automatic flash. The camera is set to record at the highest resolution. The images are stored in a compressed Joint Photographic Experts Group (JPEG) format and transferred to my computer using a universal serial cable (USB). On average, each case requires two or three images, each of about 200 kByte in size. Once transferred to my personal computer, the images can be saved on the hard disk and sent using any email program as an attachment. The recipient can then receive the email message and can open the attachment to view the images.

Case reports

Over the past three years I have discussed more than 300 cases with at least one colleague using email and digital images. Some recent cases that have been shared with colleagues are described below.

Case 1

A 22-year-old woman presented with an explosive onset of cystic acne upon returning home from Singapore. Her friends had described her face previously as 'spotless'. She had no constitutional symptoms. The lesions were tender and extensive, and disturbed her sleep. Examination showed multiple pustules, nodules, cysts and haemorrhagic papules on the face (Fig. 11.1). She was initially treated with isotretinoin 40 mg daily

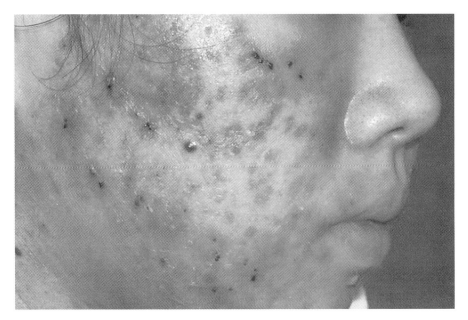

Fig. 11.1. Case 1: pyoderma faciale.

with little response. Her case was discussed in virtual grand rounds with images attached to email messages and there was general agreement that this was pyoderma faciale and that she would benefit from the addition of prednisolone (Box 11.1). Prednisolone 45 mg daily was prescribed and subsequently tapered off over the next six weeks. She experienced a complete resolution of the lesions over eight months of treatment with isotretinoin. As pyoderma faciale is a rare condition, the availability of case discussions through email helped me to treat her more confidently and appropriately.

Box 11.1. Excerpts of email messages relating to Case 1.

This unfortunate 22-year-old girl had severe acne for 2 weeks prior to seeing me. Her face was described as 'spotless' prior to that. Just 1 week upon returning to Malaysia from Singapore her face was swarmed by pustules and nodules. The lesion was tender and disturbs her sleep. I have initially given her oral Roaccutane and erythromycin 400 mg bd and intralesional triamcinolone for 2 weeks, but today on follow-up the lesions are not getting any better.

Her present treatment: Roaccutane 40 mg daily for another 2 weeks; prednisolone 15 mg tid for 1 week (and possibly tail to 15 mg bd on the second week); Isotrex gel and intralesional triamcinolone on nodular areas.

Appreciate your comments.

Case 2

An 8-year-old boy presented with fever and desquamation of the fingers. The fever began 10 days before the office visit, and a generalized maculopapular eruption became manifest two days later. A few days after that he developed desquamation of

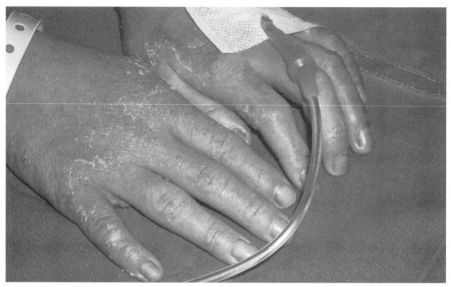

(a)

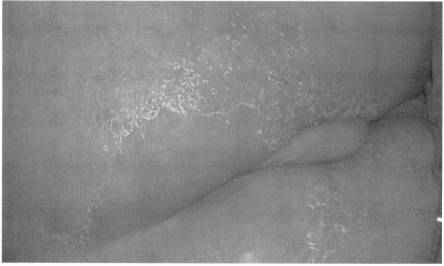

(b)

Fig. 11.2. Case 2: staphylococcal scalded skin syndrome affecting the fingers (a) and the perineal area (b).

the fingers and the perineal area. He had a past history of Kawasaki disease at the age of 2 years and was treated with intravenous immunoglobulins. He had a history of allergy to cephalexin. Physical examination revealed a temperature of 38°C with desquamation of the fingers.

A blood culture, antistreptolysin O titre and an echocardiogram were unremarkable. An email consultation with a complete description of the patient's history and physical findings was sent to a number of colleagues, together with the digital images (Fig. 11.2). There was general agreement among my peers that this was a variant of staphylococcal scalded skin syndrome, rather than a relapse of Kawasaki's disease. One of the colleagues was an academic paediatric dermatologist. The patient was started on fusidic acid 250 mg bd, which was associated with rapid resolution of fever and desquamation. In this instance, we were able to save the patient from an unnecessary and expensive course of intravenous immunoglobulins.

Case 3

Ms T. was an 18-year-old student who had had mildly tender purpuric indurated patches on the right arm for 4–5 years. The lesions had increased in size and number over the previous 2 years. She was otherwise well and had no constitutional symptoms.

Examination showed three purpuric lesions, 4–5 cm by 5–6 cm in diameter, with ill-defined margins on the extensor surface of the right arm. Her regional nodes were not enlarged. There were no other significant findings.

A skin biopsy taken from the lesion was initially interpreted as a variant of Kaposi's sarcoma. This biopsy was reported by a general pathologist and the diagnosis did not correlate with the clinical findings. The diagnosis of Kaposi's sarcoma led to uncertainty and caused the patient unnecessary anxiety. She was sent to Kuala Lumpur for further evaluation but I received no further definitive feedback. For further help, I sent a slide to another pathologist who had imaging facilities. He was of the opinion that this was a haemangioendothelioma and took digital photographs of the relevant sections (Fig. 11.3). These images were sent by email to a dermatopathologist who felt that Ms T.'s lesion was indeed a haemangioendothelioma. Electronic transmission of clinical photographs and histopathology sections was instrumental in making the correct diagnosis for this young woman.

Case 4

A 39-year-old-Chinese lady presented with a 3-month history of polyarthralgia, dry eyes, xerostomia and diffuse alopecia. In addition, she noticed stiffness of the metacarpophalangeal and proximal interphalangeal joints, elbows, wrists, shoulders, knees and ankles. She also complained of morning stiffness lasting for an hour every morning. Over the previous 3 weeks she had developed non-pruritic, tender discrete purpuras on the lower limbs. She had no history of Raynaud's phenomenon or butterfly rash and was not taking any long-term medications.

The physical examination showed extensive purpura on the dependent areas and lower limbs especially around the ankles. Some of the purpuric patches had

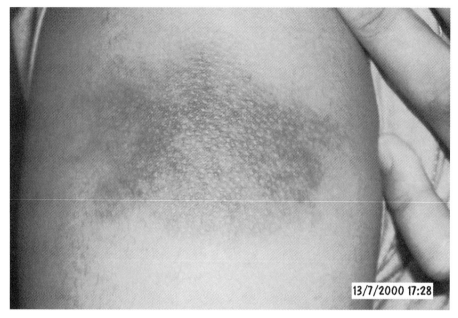

(a)

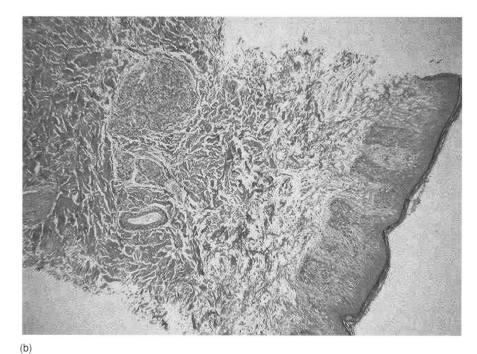

(b)

Fig. 11.3. Case 3: clinical (a) and histological (b) picture of haemangioendothelioma.

superimposed intact vesicles. There was no lymphadenopathy. Her joints were mildly tender on movement but there were no obvious swellings.

Initial investigations showed haemoglobin 12.6 g/dl, total white cells 3.6×10^9/l, platelets 363×10^9/l, ESR 65 mm/h with a positive rheumatoid factor but a negative antinuclear antibody. A skin biopsy was taken from the ankle and showed evidence of leukocytoclastic vasculitis. As Sjögren's syndrome is rare in Malaysia, her case was discussed by email with peers, one of whom was an expert in connective tissue disease. There was general agreement amongst the virtual grand rounds participants that this was Sjögren's syndrome rather than systemic lupus erythematosus. The patient was started on prednisolone and methotrexate, which resulted in a complete resolution of her lesions and symptoms.

Conclusion

The experiences reported here with teledermatology demonstrate that the ability to share cases over the Internet can be both a teaching and a learning experience. In the past we usually learned patient management from ward rounds and the teachers consisted of ward and clinic consultants. Now, we have the opportunity to learn from consultants and experts all over the world.

I believe that using the Internet for virtual grand rounds is similar to conventional grand rounds, in which a case is presented and feedback is obtained from various participants. In general, the views of various participants, some of whom are experts in their respective field, should significantly increase the chance of getting the right diagnosis. Therefore the Internet can serve as a modality to improve patient care. This seems to be a new paradigm for clinical practice, because a relatively isolated dermatologist can now consult with peers around the world. All that is required are an email facility, a digital camera and perhaps digital dermatopathology. Up-to-date antivirus software should be installed on the computer to protect against computer viruses, especially when images sent as attachments must be opened for viewing.

In the past when I faced difficult diagnostic and management problems, I usually wrote to an expert, but it could take several days to weeks before a reply was received. Now, using email, it is possible to obtain the reply within hours. This revolutionizes the consultative process and improves patient care and outcome tremendously. Digital-imaging consultations can result in reliable and accurate diagnostic outcomes when compared with traditional clinic-based consultations. This is a powerful tool that has the potential to transform the practice of dermatology.[8]

The Internet has created a powerful framework for communication between dermatologists and their patients. The ability to transmit high-definition images rapidly over the Internet will help dermatologists to see patients as efficiently as possible and can improve patient outcomes and reduce cost. This represents the beginning of a revolution in peer-group consultation.

Acknowledgements

I thank David Elpern MD for his encouragement, and all my colleagues and peers who have participated in the virtual grand grounds.

References

1 Shelley W, Shelley D, eds. *Advanced Dermatologic Diagnosis*. Philadelphia: Saunders, 1992.
2 Hizamnuddin Awang. The Internet, freedom of speech and Malaysian society. *Jaring Internet* 1999;**2**:19–20.
3 Della Mea V, Puglisi F, Forti S, et al. Expert pathology consultation though the Internet: melanoma versus benign melanocytic tumours. *Journal of Telemedicine and Telecare* 1997;**3**(suppl. 1):17–19.
4 Kirby B, Lyon CC, Harrison PV. Low-cost teledermatology using Internet image transmission. *Journal of Telemedicine and Telecare* 1998;**4**(suppl. 1):107.
5 Johnson DS, Goel RP, Birtwistle P, Hirst P. Transferrring medical images from the world wide web for emergency clinical management: a case report. *British Medical Journal* 1998;**316**:988–989.
6 Della Mea V. Internet electronic mail: a tool for low cost telemedicine. *Journal of Telemedicine and Telecare* 1999;**5**:84–89.
7 Ratner D, Thomas CO, Bickers D. The uses of digital photography in dermatology. *Journal of the American Academy of Dermatology* 1999;**41**:749–756.
8 Whited JD, Hall RP, Simel DL, et al. Reliability and accuracy of dermatologists' clinic-based and digital image consultations. *Journal of the American Academy of Dermatology* 1999;**41**:693–702.

12

The Florida Child Protection Team Telemedicine Program

J.M. Whitworth, Betsy Wood, Karen Morse, Howard Rogers and Michael Haney

Introduction

Child abuse and neglect is a common problem in the USA and internationally. However, it is difficult to determine the incidence and prevalence of child maltreatment around the world. History, culture, religious beliefs and law affect the way that countries define and respond to child abuse and neglect. Any discussion of child abuse and neglect or child protection services will therefore benefit from agreement about definitions. However, there is little agreement between countries on the reporting of child maltreatment and relatively few countries keep records that can be compared and used in legal and scientific inquiries across international boundaries. Virtually every country has different reporting definitions and criteria relating to how child abuse and neglect cases are identified and responded to. The legal and scientific literature tends to describe abusive or neglectful incidents, while policy-makers, researchers and practitioners describe the context in which the incidents occur before defining them as abusive or neglectful. This approach is defined as phenomenological. The weakness of this approach is one of tautology: behaviour becomes abusive when it is described as such. The challenge to any child protection system is to assess all the relevant information, which includes both the incident and context, and do so in a manner that protects the child.[1]

Even in the USA there are differences in definitions among the 50 states regarding terminology and interventions on behalf of abused and neglected children. Based on responses from the 1998 National Child Abuse and Neglect Data System (NCANDS), it is estimated that child protective service agencies investigated reports of alleged maltreatment on more than 2.8 million children in America in 1998. Of those children investigated, it was reported that 903 000 children were victims of abuse and neglect, which translates to a rate of 12.9 per 1000 children.[2] More than half (54%) of all victims suffered neglect, while almost a quarter (23%) suffered physical abuse; sexual abuse accounted for 12%. Psychological abuse and medical neglect accounted for 6% or fewer for each category. In addition, over 25% were reported to be victims of more than one maltreatment. The highest victimization rates were from birth to age 3 years.

The immediate and accurate assessment of alleged abuse or neglect is critical in enabling child protection staff to make valid and timely child safety and placement decisions. It is the primary mission of any child protection system to determine whether abuse or neglect has occurred and if there is an immediate threat to the child. It is then incumbent on that system to engage the necessary resources and take steps to ensure the safety of the alleged victim. When the child protection system fails, the result can be the serious injury or death of a vulnerable child. In Florida, Child Protection Teams (CPTs) are created under the authority of Florida Statutes 39.303 and are defined as medically directed, multidisciplinary teams of professionals available to assist in the immediate assessment of suspected abuse or neglect in children.

In 1998, 82 children died in Florida as a direct result of abuse or neglect. In addition, 39 deaths showed some indication of abuse or neglect. Seventy-six per cent of the 82 children who died were 5 years of age or younger.[3] Reports of abuse and neglect to the Florida Abuse Hotline Information System (FAHIS) increased from 122 115 in the fiscal year 1997–98 to 164 916 in the fiscal year 1999–2000, an increase of 35%. In 1999, the Florida Legislature placed additional responsibilities on the CPTs. All child abuse and neglect reports accepted by the FAHIS are required to be simultaneously transmitted to both the Department of Children and Family Services (the state agency responsible for investigating alleged child abuse and neglect reports) local service centre and the associated CPT. At the CPT, all reports must be reviewed by either a board-certified paediatrician; a licensed physician working under the direction of a board-certified paediatrician; an advanced registered nurse practitioner; a physician assistant or a registered nurse to determine whether a face-to-face medical evaluation is necessary.

The law further mandates that the Department of Children and Families refer to the CPTs reports of abuse or neglect involving the following circumstances:

▶ Injuries to the head, bruises to the neck or head, burns or fractures in a child of any age.

▶ Bruises anywhere on a child 5 years of age or under.

▶ Sexual abuse of a child in which vaginal or anal penetration is alleged or in which other unlawful sexual conduct has occurred.

▶ Any sexually transmitted disease in a prepubescent child.

▶ Reported malnutrition of a child and failure of a child to thrive.

▶ Reported medical, physical or emotional neglect of a child.

▶ Any family in which one or more children have been pronounced dead on arrival at a hospital or other healthcare facility, or have been injured and later died, as a result of suspected abuse, abandonment or neglect, when any sibling or other child remains in the home.

▶ Symptoms of serious emotional problems in a child when emotional or other abuse, abandonment or neglect is suspected.

These increased responsibilities have intensified the demands of working in the discipline of child abuse and neglect. The workload, combined with delivering services in a large and culturally diverse state such as Florida, coupled with an increase in the number of child abuse and neglect reports requiring medical evaluation, make recruitment and retention of medical experts in child abuse and neglect difficult. Even with increasing knowledge, child abuse and neglect continues to be a burden for many medical practitioners. Child abuse cases are time consuming, since they involve calling child protective services and dealing with local authorities, not to mention the probability of being called to testify in court at a later date. For these reasons and others, many medical staff consider child abuse and neglect work to be outside their scope of practice. Few areas of paediatrics generate as much emotion as child abuse and neglect.

As of 1 March 2000, Florida had 81 board-certified paediatricians or family practitioners and 24 advanced registered nurse practitioners (ARNPs) working for CPTs. Each year the recruitment and attrition rates for physicians and ARNPs remains approximately the same. The majority of these physicians and ARNPs are located in the more populous regions of the state, leaving large areas with limited access to child abuse and neglect expertise.

Telemedicine network

Child abuse or neglect is not only physically traumatizing but takes a severe emotional toll on the child and family. The shock and disbelief that occurs when these allegations are made can fragment and immobilize a family, and leave the child feeling abandoned, blamed or ostracized by those they love. The child may then be placed in the hands of a system that may require them to be separated from those they feel most attached to, at a time when they are most in need of physical and emotional support. They will then be transported to another location by child protection staff or law enforcement officers for an examination at the hands of someone they have never seen before, which will further compound an already traumatic event. Child protection teams are charged with the responsibility to medically examine and assess the child to see if abuse or neglect has occurred. The staff of the Children's Medical Services (CMS) Program have therefore investigated ways to make the assessment process less intrusive, more responsive and considerate of the needs of the child.

Florida is located in the extreme southeast corner of the USA. It has a population of approximately 15 million people, making it the fourth most populous state in the USA. Of this population, almost 26% (3 922 500) are children and adolescents less than 20 years of age (1999 Bureau of Census, population estimates). The CPT Program, composed predominantly of local, non-profit-making organizations, provides multidisciplinary assessment services in 25 different locations. Florida comprises 67 counties, so that many of these teams have large geographical areas to serve. Teams act as consultants to local providers and agencies who investigate allegations of abuse. However, access to team expertise for patients and local facilities is limited by the geography of some areas.

To meet the additional service needs mentioned earlier, the CMS implemented a real-time telemedicine pilot project, linking two 'hub' CPTs to local healthcare facilities such as hospital emergency rooms, county health departments and child advocacy centres. To our knowledge, this was the first time that real-time telemedicine has been used in this field. Five sites, including three 'remote' sites and two 'hub' sites participated in the pilot, which was a joint effort between the CMS, the State of Florida's Department of Management Services (DMS) and the University of Florida (UF). The pilot was established in a small number of sites in order to fine-tune the technology for this application as well as to assess what equipment and communications modality worked best in Florida. Currently, hub sites in Alachua and Duval Counties connect to remote sites in Marion, Suwannee, Citrus, Putnam and Lake as well as Clay, Polk and St John's Counties, respectively (Fig. 12.1).

The telemedicine network facilitates child abuse and neglect assessments between the hub sites and the remote sites. Hub sites are comprehensive medical facilities with a wide range of medical and multidisciplinary professional staff. Remote sites are smaller medical facilities in less urbanized areas with limited medical and non-medical expertise. Each hub site is responsible for providing expert levels of medical child abuse assessments to specific remote sites by using the communication infrastructure developed. To ensure around-the-clock coverage by medical experts, each remote site can be linked to the other hub site as well.

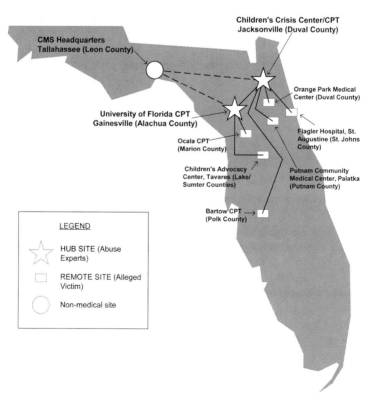

Fig. 12.1. Telemedicine network. There are hub sites in Alachua and Duval Counties. These are connected to peripheral sites in Marion, Suwannee, Citrus, Putnam and Lake, as well as Clay, Polk and St John's Counties, respectively.

The telemedicine unit selected included a rolling cart that allowed use in multiple locations. A personal computer was integrated into the cart (the codec operates independently of the personal computer) and was fitted with a video capture card and electronic medical record software for recording data and capturing digital still images. The equipment included:

➤ Tandberg Health Care System III (hub sites) and Tandberg Interns (remote sites). While these two models have different codecs which have different maximum bandwidth and differing numbers of video/audio inputs/outputs, they are fully interoperable.

➤ Leisegang colposcope model number 3DLSUL with LM2PR analogue camera.

➤ AMD colposcope with articulating arm model number 7800.

➤ AMD 2500 general examination camera, which uses a CCD sensor and 1× and 50× lenses which snap on.

A typical room setup is illustrated in Figure 12.2.

Regarding the infrastructure, the engineering team decided to build a parallel network to compare leased lines (using the SUNCOM backbone which is the State of Florida's telecommunications network) with ISDN lines (a non-SUNCOM offering). The other transport and/or equipment options were ruled out due to high expense, untested technology with perceived interoperability problems or poor video quality. Following advice from experienced telemedicine workers in Georgia and Vermont we chose to use a transmission speed of 384 kbit/s. This bandwidth can be provided by ISDN (three basic rate ISDN lines) or dedicated leased lines (one-quarter of a full T-1 line). The current hybrid network is shown in Figure 12.3.

Patient's reactions to telemedicine

A number of considerations must be addressed before the deployment of a telemedicine project that affects children, if there is to be any chance of success. Before implementation of our child abuse telemedicine programme, there were concerns about patient acceptance and comfort with the equipment used in the evaluation process, as well as the unknown factors governing parental acceptance and acceptability of the technology in a court setting. In evaluating the CPT Telemedicine Network, we do not request direct feedback from the children and families who are served using telemedicine technology. Because referrals for assessments are made through the child protection agency in Florida, families are not always happy about participating in the process. In many instances, they view a child protective investigation as intrusive and unwarranted. Therefore they often have an unfavourable view of the whole investigative process, of which the use of the technology is only a small part.

In our experience, children are intimidated by electronic equipment in completely different ways from adults. While adults often see electronic equipment as

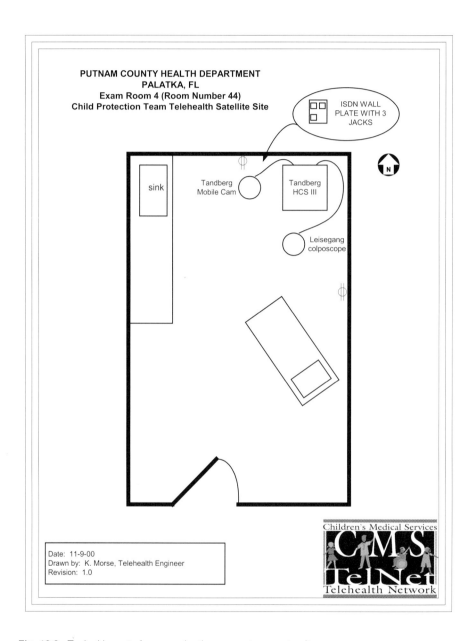

Fig. 12.2. Typical layout of an examination room at a remote site.

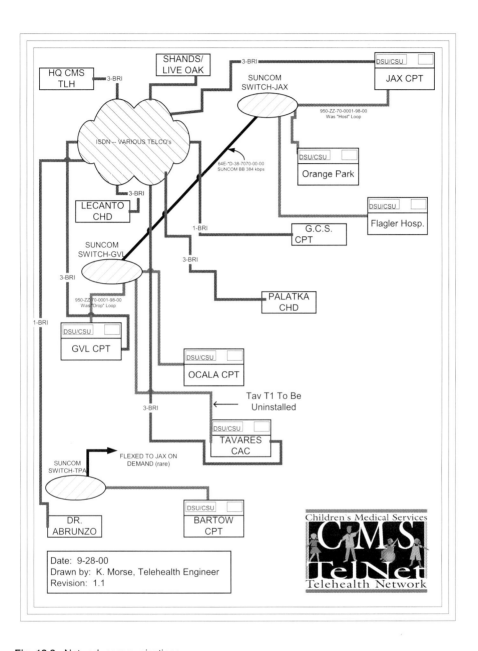

Fig. 12.3. Network communications.

a series of black boxes, which may be dangerous or invade their privacy, children think in much more basic terms – such as 'Does it hurt?' or 'Does it have a needle in it?' Verbal reassurances may suffice for adults, but children need to be shown or be able to touch the equipment and see it demonstrated on other people before they feel safe. They are often able to accept not knowing how it works as long as they are sure that it doesn't hurt. For these reasons, the orientation period before the examination is longer with children than for any 'hands-on' procedure. In our programme, the orientation period with the child is much longer than the examination itself and is essential to reduce fear of the unknown and assure a successful outcome.

Because of our concerns about the unknown stresses of being evaluated electronically at the already stressful time of a medical evaluation for abuse or neglect, we set out to field test our equipment in a group of children of various ages in the least stressful manner. Since our evaluation protocols preclude the presence of a parent at certain times during the evaluation, special attention was focused on the need to ensure that the equipment would not introduce a significant distraction to working with the child. Operating procedures were written based on the experience with young children and the examination equipment.

Information was gathered during interactions with children ranging in age from 3 months to 18 years. Twenty-six children were recruited from a continuity care (primary care) clinic population presenting for non-urgent assessments of various kinds, the majority being camp physical examinations. Children and parents were asked to volunteer to help evaluate new equipment. An attempt was made to select children with non-urgent complaints. Only the two hub sites were involved in this phase of the pilot, thus ensuring that the hub-site personnel became familiar not only with the reactions of adults and children to remote evaluations, but also with the equipment itself before it was deployed to the remote sites.

As stated earlier, the electronic equipment included video monitors, microphones, hand-held cameras, cameras in fixed mountings and a colposcope. While no child was fearful of the monitors or cameras, several required orientation to the peripheral devices, which were less familiar to them. It was clear from the beginning that young children interacted with the examiner as if they were in the room together: the equipment was transparent. Little familiarization with the equipment was necessary. As mobility and verbal skills increased, however, so did the need for specific orientation to the various technical 'gadgets'. This need for specific orientation increased with more complex equipment and with equipment for which the purpose was not obvious.

A trained registered nurse provided an orientation to the equipment and to the process of the examination. We found that children were usually intimidated when someone used any equipment without demonstration. Allowing children to touch the equipment and, where possible, participate in the examination by pushing the capture button appeared to alleviate their fear faster than simply describing the equipment's function verbally. Allowing the older children to use the equipment on the examiner was also very effective in alleviating any lingering mystery. It is also important to allow time for the nurse, who will be the examiner's virtual hands, to develop a rapport with the child to create an environment of trust and understanding. For this reason, every attempt was made to recruit project nurses with paediatric experience.

Infants are clearly oblivious to the electronics and relate well to the nurse at the peripheral site as long as the primary caretaker is close by. Older children conducted themselves as if a conversation with a monitor was no more unusual than having a conversation with a television set and did not seem to find a two-way conversation to be anything unusual. While seeing themselves may be initially distracting, they quickly became fascinated with seeing their image on the monitor. However, after a few minutes the children were able to concentrate on the image of the distant examiner and interact without difficulty. We therefore encouraged staff to turn the monitor on to self view, if time permitted, to allow the child time to react to their own picture before initiating the actual interaction. It was found that the children were able to relate to the peripheral equipment without difficulty if time was spent before the examination during which the child was allowed to touch the equipment and have a demonstration that it was neither painful nor otherwise intimidating. After appropriate orientation, there was no discernible difference between a live interaction and an electronic interaction.

Older children have voiced concerns that telemedicine images are, in fact, being broadcast on television stations or on a closed circuit. They must be assured that the connection is confidential and that their pictures can only be seen by a limited number of people. It is vital to make sure that all participants in the videoconference are identified to the patient and that no others are allowed into either site without the child's knowledge. Similarly older children want assurances regarding who will see any pictures taken, especially if intimate parts of the body are to be depicted. Occasionally children will express concern that the equipment can see things by X-ray vision or that the equipment may emit harmful rays during use. All such questions should be answered honestly. While it has not happened yet, it is not unreasonable to expect fairly sophisticated and advanced questions about the telemedicine equipment and network from children with advanced computer knowledge and skills. It is therefore suggested that either the nurse on site or the remote examiner be familiar enough with both the equipment and the network to answer this type of question honestly and intelligently. In addition, we believe that all telemedicine patients should provide informed consent to include all possible uses of the images.

Another issue that has been encountered, but which is not specific to the equipment, relates to the examiner. Older children and adolescents may object to an opposite-sex examiner for intimate examinations. There should therefore be a same-sex examiner available as a contingency. We require that the physician or nurse practitioner in the hub site wear a white coat with appropriate identification to lessen initial apprehension by the child. It is vital for the examiner to remember that the interviewing techniques and language used must be carefully matched to the child's age and level of functioning. Given that the establishment of trust is a core component to a successful telemedicine examination, the importance of communication between the examiner and child cannot be overemphasized.

The presence of a supportive and well-trained individual at the remote site is essential. This individual should be trained by the staff of the hub site regarding the needs of the telemedicine consultant and the specifics of the evaluation in which they will be participating, and more importantly, in the best methods of making children comfortable with essential procedures. Repeated staff practice with the equipment prior to an actual examination is strongly recommended and is a requirement of our programme.

The general procedure for a telemedicine evaluation is similar to a face-to-face encounter. In non-emergency situations, the connection between sites is established prior to the child and family being brought into the examination room. Introductions of hub and remote site personnel are made and the child and parent are asked questions pertaining to the child's past and present medical status. Once the medical history is obtained, and prior to the remote evaluation, the on-site nurse provides routine intake care. Measurement of height, weight, vital signs and examination of the head, eyes, ears, nose and mouth assists in putting the child at ease with the nurse. Evaluations of children alleged to be abused or neglected focus mainly on dermatological findings, such as bruises, abrasions, welts, scars and other marks secondary to child physical abuse. Remote evaluations of sexual abuse have been successfully performed on both males and females.

All participating healthcare providers (both physicians and advanced registered nurse practitioners) have consistently reported satisfaction with the quality of the interactions. However, there were several instances when a child could not be examined because the equipment was not working properly. Problems with the quality of the audio and issues with the communications lines topped the list of difficulties encountered. The initiation of weekly maintenance calls between the hub and remote sites have alleviated most of these problems.

From January 2000 through February 2001, a total of 75 children have been examined via the CPT Telemedicine Network. The majority of these evaluations were non-acute in nature, or scheduled evaluations. With time and experience, the examiners became much more comfortable with the process and equipment, which tended to help the children's comfort level. With experience, the examination time was reduced by 40% compared to the initial evaluations.

Dermatological findings

In the USA, more than 15 million children are injured each year, most unintentionally. About 750 000 of these injuries are intentional, however, and it falls to the medical practitioner to determine which they are and what children are at risk. The challenge to the examiner is to answer three basic questions:

1. What is the history?

2. What are the injuries?

3. Does the history explain the injuries?[4]

In addition to carefully documenting the physical examination, Florida protocols require the examiner to take photographs of the injuries, which become part of the medical and investigative file.

As reported by Krugman et al,[4] examiners must be alert to the following findings:

1. shape of the injury

2. pattern of injury

3. age of injury.

Children are prone to bruising from everyday events. These bruises tend to be on bony prominences on the extremities, forehead and chin. Bruises on the trunk, ears, genital area and back, however, are suggestive of abuse. Similarly, young children may burn themselves, usually on a hand, arm or leg. However, burns on both palms, both soles, the flexor surfaces of the thighs or the perineum are pathognomonic for abuse. Examiners should consider whether bruises or fractures in different stages of healing indicate intentionally inflicted injuries or abuse. For example, belt buckles, bites, electrical cords, rope, coat hangers and cigarettes, all leave distinct identifiable marks (Fig. 12.4).

Three different peripheral cameras have been used in the project to assess external and internal evidence of alleged child abuse. These cameras include the AMD general examination camera, the Leisegang colposcope and the Welch Allyn colposcope. Interviews with remote-site staff indicated that the lack of standardization in equipment across sites contributed to staff anxiety, which, in turn, inhibited usage in some remote sites. Each site had slightly different configurations, which either facilitated easy use of the equipment or presented challenges in getting the equipment activated in a user-friendly way. This was an unintended consequence of the way the

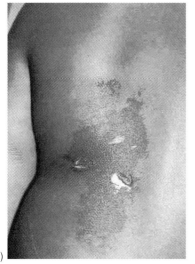

(a)

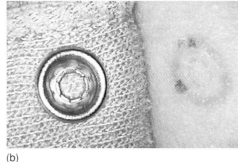

(b)

Fig. 12.4. Distinctive skin marks: (a) burn on the back; (b) bruising from a snap fastener.

pilot programme was designed. During the planning stages of the pilot programme, a decision was made to use different types of equipment and transmission lines. It appears that this strategy contributed to the confusion of field staff.

While the colposcope provides a clear image, which can be calibrated based on a fixed focal length for use in telemedicine at all the different magnification levels, the patient examination camera seems to have more flexibility. The AMD general examination camera has been most helpful in general physical abuse examinations. It is lightweight, very portable and can readily be moved over the child's skin by the nurse so that the examiner at the remote site can view the entire body, including intra-oral surfaces (Fig. 12.5). Still photographs can be captured and stored in an electronic medical record at any time during the examination by the hub-site examiner. The still images are normally captured and electronically stored at the hub site. The hub-site examiner has the option of controlling the remote cameras and therefore can capture the image prior to transmission – thereby receiving a still image captured at the remote end.

Dermatological findings that are significant for child abuse and neglect are easily seen and documented with the telemedicine equipment. The quality of the transmission allows distinction of marks such as those made by extension cords, telephone cords or looped belts. One can easily see details such as scabbing, scars or keloid, if present. There are varying degrees of magnification in each of the peripheral

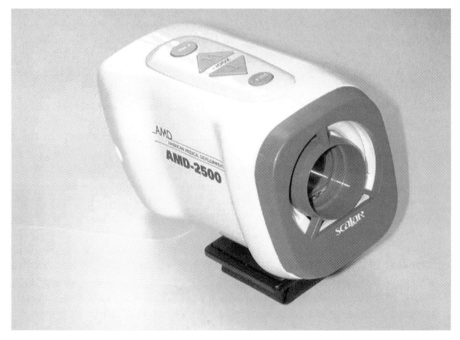

Fig. 12.5. The general examination camera can be moved over the child's skin easily by the nurse so that the examiner at the remote site can view the entire body, including intra-oral surfaces.

cameras that allows magnification to a size that individual hair and hair follicles can be seen (Fig. 12.6). The smallest lesion seen to date was approximately 2 cm, but marks less than 5 mm have been clearly discerned through the patient examination camera during tests. The other dermatological features that can be ascertained, in addition to loop marks, include the following: cigarette burns, iron burns, bruises, scratches, petechiae and slap marks. One can distinguish patterned injuries so that a pattern, if present, can be differentiated from a generalized reaction. Other dermatological findings that have been diagnosed via telemedicine include molluscum contagiosum, impetigo, herpes zoster and mongolian spots.

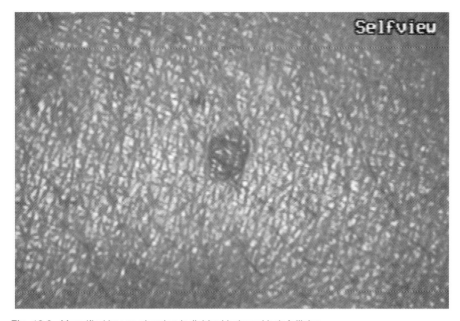

Fig. 12.6. Magnified image showing individual hair and hair follicles.

In terms of protocols, we require that all skin lesions be evaluated by capturing at least four views. This is to ensure that at least two images of each lesion will show adequate detail. Each includes the measurement standard and each series must include the colour standard (Fig. 12.7). A colour standard ensures standardization of hues on reproduction. In addition, a standard millimetre-measuring device is included in each photographic examination to reduce distortion in future enlargements of photographs. If a standard millimetre-measuring device is not available, one can use any standard object, such as a coin or a ruler to allow for additional measurements or comparisons. We have found that capturing short videoclips along with still photographs is useful. If still photographs are lost in transmission, the video can be used for reconstruction of still photographs, if needed.

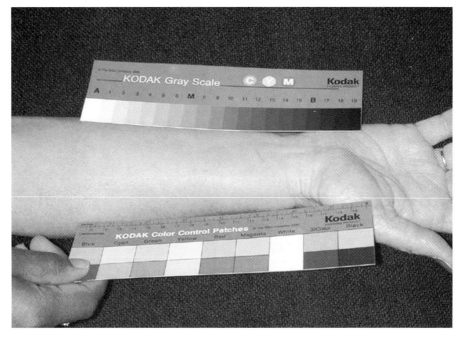

Fig. 12.7. Each series of pictures includes a colour standard.

We have experienced court challenges in two of our telemedicine cases so far, but were successful in defending the medical record as well as the images collected during the examinations. In one case, the digital images were challenged and in the other case the interview process was challenged. In both cases, the validity of the examination and interview via telemedicine equipment was upheld. The telemedicine consultant was considered the expert and provided testimony in the same manner as in on-site evaluations.

Conclusion

The goal of the CPT Telemedicine Network is threefold. The first is to offer medical and multidisciplinary expertise to more areas of the State of Florida. The second goal is to expedite the evaluation of children without having to transport them from remote areas. The third is to create a system of response that minimizes additional trauma to a child who is alleged to be abused or neglected. During the pilot stage of the programme, we have learned many lessons about what works best for this specialized telemedicine application. Clarity of the digital image through all of the peripheral cameras used in the network has been excellent, with clear pictures, observed and captured, of dermatological marks measuring less than 5 mm. With adequate explanation and given time to touch and even experiment with the peripheral devices, children are not intimidated by the technology. However, standardization of equipment and ease of use of the equipment must be continually pursued. As the project expands, the extension of child abuse and neglect expertise will be extended across Florida's many geographical and cultural barriers.

References

1   Bullock R, Little M, Millham S, Mount K, eds. *Child Protection: Messages from Research*. London: HMSO, 1995.

2   US Department of Health and Human Services. *Child Maltreatment 1998: Reports from the States to the National Child Abuse and Neglect Data System*. Washington, DC: US Government Printing Office, 2000.

3   Department of Children and Family Services, Office of Family Preservation, Quality Assurance. *Child Abuse and Neglect Deaths, Calendar Year 1998*. Department of Children and Family Services: Tallahassee, FL, 2000.

4   Krugman S, Wissow L, Krugman R. Facing facts: child abuse and pediatric practice. *Contemporary Pediatrics* 1998;**14:**131–144.

Section 3: Current Experience – Education

13

Online Dermatological Information for Patients*

Amanda Oakley

*Website addresses listed in this chapter were valid in June 2001.

Introduction

In the past, dermatological information has been the preserve of the specialist. In the main, the patient had very limited knowledge about the nature of their disease and its management options until the latter few years of the twentieth century. Information appropriate to the patient started to appear as health care became more consumer-focused. Conventional sources of information about dermatological topics are limited in number and quality. These include:

▶ Handouts prepared by an individual consultant for an outpatient clinic.

▶ Professionally produced brochures published by a college or by a pharmaceutical company.

▶ Home health encyclopaedias and short single-topic monographs on the more common topics such as acne, psoriasis or atopic dermatitis.

▶ Articles in magazines about cosmetic surgery, medical breakthroughs or an individual patient's battle with their disease or with authorities.

▶ Alternative medicine topics sold to those dissatisfied with mainstream medical practice.

Conventional health information can be out of date or misleading. It may offer a single viewpoint without supporting evidence. As experts may not review the content, misinformation can persist and propagate.

There are hundreds of published books on skin diseases, readily located on the online bookstore Amazon (http://www.amazon.com). In October 2000, Amazon listed 59 titles relating to psoriasis, 28 to eczema and 10 to urticaria, mostly aimed at a medical readership. The majority of 105 books about skin cancer, 100 about lupus and 156 about candida were aimed at the consumer. The listings included out-of-print self-help publications.

Some long-established home-help medical texts are also available online. The fourth printing of the 'Merck Manual of Medical Information Home Edition' (http://www.merck.com/pubs/mmanual_home/) includes a section on skin disorders.

Health information on compact disk

Technological solutions to reduce consumer ignorance have been slow to arrive. Although for the last decade or so many medical practitioners have had access to current literature on Medline through their local medical library or college/academic body, this has not been available to the public and until recently access was expensive.

An American Academy of Pediatrics publication, 'Patient Education on CD-ROM: Health Care Advice for Children, Teens, and their Parents' is sold by Amazon for US$433.75. One cannot imagine that many copies have been sold at that price. In 1997 a compact disk (CD) of consumer health information ('Everybody') was marketed in New Zealand but was not widely distributed among consumers. Contributors (mainly professional organizations and self-help groups) were not paid but production costs were high. The same information available on the Internet (http://www.everybody.co.nz/) has proved much more successful, with 42 000 page accesses in October 2000 (personal communication).

Health information on the Internet

The Internet has proved revolutionary in many sectors. A 1997 survey indicated that over 40% of the traffic of the Internet was due to searches for medical information.[1] The number of health-related sites is astonishing, with estimates ranging from the 17 000 medical listings on Yahoo to 100 000 sites including chat groups, online support groups and mailing lists.[2] The majority are American owned and operated.

Sources of information freely accessible on the Worldwide Web in June 2001 included websites owned by academic bodies and self-help groups, and commercial health portals.

Websites owned by academic bodies or professional societies

Websites owned by dermatological academic bodies, institutions and professional societies are generally inadequately funded and slow to produce content. The pages are usually peer reviewed, but are of variable quality and with unsophisticated navigation and formatting. Some of the most useful are:

▶ NZ DermNet, the website of the New Zealand Dermatological Society (http://www.dermnet.org.nz/). This site received 120 000 visitors in May 2001.

▶ SkinCarePhysicians.com, the consumer site of the American Academy of Dermatology (http://www.skincarephysicians.com).

▶ National Skin Center, Singapore's information on skin diseases (http://www.nsc.gov.sg/commskin/skin.html).

Other non-profit organizations

MedHelp International is a non-profit-making organization dependent on sponsorship, which offers a consumer health information library, question and answer forums, health news and a patient network (http://www.medhelp.org/).[3] Twenty-five thousand entries are listed by its search engine, which links to numerous sites with information on skin diseases. MedHelp claims to be the largest Consumer Health Network in the world, welcoming 5 million visitors to its website in October 2000.[4]

Commercial sites for medical professionals

Patients can often access review articles, textbook chapters, abstracts and news items at no charge. Such sites include:

▶ The comprehensive medical site Medscape (http://www.medscape.com/), which has links to CBS HealthWatch for consumers.

▶ The e-medicine World Medical Library, which includes consumer treatment guidelines for skin diseases (http://www.emedicine.com/derm/).

▶ MedlinePlus (http://www.medlineplus.gov/), which has been developed by the US National Library of Medicine to provide simple information for the public. It includes topics on skin, hair and nails, drug information, interactive tutorials, dictionaries, directories and links to other appropriate resources. MedlinePlus received 5 million page hits in late 2000.[5] But interpreting original clinical data is not easy for trained scientists and must be very difficult for most patients.

Dermatological sites created by private individuals

Several dermatologists or groups of dermatologists have set up health information sites. Useful sites include:

▶ The Skin Site, Michelle Soignée, Inc. (http://www.skinsite.com/), funded by product sales.

▶ DocDerm, Dr Rosen's private practice site (http://www.docderm.com/).

Patient support organizations

The websites of self-help groups are of variable size and quality. They depend on sponsorship and donations for survival. Apart from providing information about specific diseases, sites may include a calendar of events, news items, research findings, fundraising endeavours, directories of local resources, databases of affected individuals and links to other sites. Online support is provided as bulletin board forums, electronic mailing lists, newsgroups and live chat groups. Local organizations are benefiting from international collaboration. For example, the Mastocytosis Society is based in the USA, its web page is hosted in Australia, its email discussion list is moderated in the Netherlands and the chat line is based in Canada.[6] Online patient-helpers with a chronic disease can be valuable resources for other patients with the same condition and for health professionals.[7] Patients with breast cancer with computer support had significantly less depression, anxiety and distress than controls,[8] and one can expect this also to be true for those with skin diseases:

▶ Links to 24 American dermatological support groups (http://www.aad.org/patientadvocacy.html).

▶ Links to 36 British dermatological support groups (http://www.bad.org.uk/patients/patient_s/index.htm).

Private individuals have also set up disease-specific sites, such as:

▶ Mike's page – the Melanoma Resource Center (http://www.tustison.com/interests1.html).

Health maintenance organizations

American health maintenance organizations such as the Blue Cross and Blue Shield Association (http://www.bcbs.com/), Kaiser Permanente (http://www. kaiserpermanente.org/) and Aetna US Healthcare (http://www.aetnaushc.com/) are increasing their web presence but as yet have little consumer health information. Benefits to members may include preventative care, directories and interactive content such as personal health assessments, research about medications and diseases, discussion boards, answers to email questions and appointment scheduling.

Commercial health portals ('dot coms')

Commercial health portals, or 'megasites', derive funding from venture capital, advertising and product sales. Although of a general nature, they often include excellent articles about common skin conditions.

Websites of general consumer health portals with significant dermatological content include:

▶ http://www.healthcentral.com/

▶ http://www.drkoop.com/

▶ http://my.webmd.com/

▶ http://www.allhealth.com/

▶ http://www.healthanswers.com/

▶ http://health.discovery.com/

▶ http://thriveonline.oxygen.com/

▶ http://www.intelihealth.com/

These American health portals are comprehensive, providing more than simply diagnosis-specific content. Most web-enabled consumers only access health information online when they require it.[9] These health sites aim to build a relationship with their visitors so they will visit again, by providing health and wellness information to consumers, daily health news, discussion boards, newsletters and chat groups facilitated by health experts and interactive tools. Several offer health directories and reference centres; they are nearly always based in the USA.

Some sites offer more specific information – online private consultations (for a fee), or bulletin board 'agony aunt' responses to anonymous personal queries. The replies are of variable quality and not always factually correct, depending on the expertise of the 'consultant' (who is not always medically qualified).

WebMD has acquired Onhealth.com, which was the single most heavily used health site on the web in May 2000, with 5.2 million unique visitors.[10] The consumer section of WebMD.com lists more than 3000 documents about skin disease, including health news, disease topics and chats. The site aims to satisfy health performance and health research needs, e-commerce and community support. Some articles are written in-house and others are obtained externally from medical associations, government agencies, medical publishers, non-profit organizations and corporations.

Healthanswers.com also includes numerous pages about skin conditions as well as related health news, chat rooms and discussion forums, and more than 2000 audio and video broadcasts. Personalized content came from a variety of reputable partners. According to information on the website in November 2000, the average Healthanswers.com guest was a married female, aged 35–49 years with an average of two children and an annual household income of US$40 000. Two-thirds were the primary healthcare insurance provider for their family. In addition, more than one-third of the guests had college degrees. Fifty-four per cent of the site's traffic was from viewers of 35 years of age or older.

More than 150 top healthcare organizations contribute to Intelihealth.com, including Harvard Medical School and the National Institutes of Health. Intelihealth is a subsidiary of Aetna US Healthcare. It has developed extensive patient information, discussion boards and live forums on its own site.[11] Its material is distributed in print form as supplements to magazines and disease-specific newsletters, and electronically to many popular Internet sites. These include DiscoveryHealth Online, owned by Discovery Communications Inc. This online site is promoted on the Discovery Channel available to 75 million homes in the USA on network TV, cable TV and the Internet. Heathgrades.com provides databases on nationwide healthcare facilities and professionals on the Discovery site.

Thriveonline.oxygen.com is a subsidiary of Oxygen Media and is the key health site of America Online. Its skin section encourages interaction with a health expert (not a dermatologist) and has a number of dermatological message boards.

Although drkoop.com is one of the most heavily used health sites and has extensive affiliations and partnerships with other organizations, it has little content relevant to the patient with a skin problem. Interactive tools include entry into clinical trials. In October 2000, there were two drug trials relating to skin diseases (eczema and fungal infections).

A dermatological consumer site, myskinMD, was launched in June 2000, funded by venture capital and product sales. The parent company, Dermplace.com, boasted a network of over 3000 North American dermatologists to answer questions and provide information. Like many other web ventures, by January 2001 it had proved a commercial failure and closed.

Pharmaceutical industry sponsorship

Some professional sites such as NZ DermNet depend on funding by pharmaceutical company sponsorship and/or product advertising.[12] The commercial health portals also receive income from this source; for example, Ortho Dermatological sponsors a section about skin conditions on Allhealth.com.[13]

Some of the innumerable pharmaceutical company sites are named after the product, test or related skin condition. For example:

▸ http://www.nizoral.co.nz/ – Janssen Cilag's New Zealand-based site for Nizoral Shampoo

▸ http://www.truetest.com/ – Allerderm Laboratories' site about contact allergens (T.R.U.E. Tests)

▸ http://www.pimpleportal.com/ – Ortho Dermatological's acne site for teenagers.

It is sometimes difficult to identify pharmaceutical company ownership. Schering Corporation owns The Allergy Learning Lab (http://www.allergylearninglab.com). The only reference to the Corporation is on the 'Terms and Conditions' and 'Privacy Policy' pages. Schering manufactures an anti-allergy drug, loratidine.

Advertising issues

It has been said that 'while pharmaceutical companies are spending billions in off-line direct-to-consumer and health-related advertising, they have largely ignored the potential that the Internet affords for targeted marketing and customer relationship management'.[9] The biggest spender in 1999 was Schering-Plough for its antihistamine, Claratin (loratidine).[14]

The health megasites are investing heavily in infrastructure and advertising. Rather than developing their own material from scratch, they depend on aggressive acquisitions and partnerships with academic institutions. The commercial survival of the websites depends on buoyant advertising, sponsorship, cross-marketing deals in offline catalogues and on other websites, content syndication to other websites and hospital intranets and revenue-share opportunities. The scene is constantly changing. Several excellent sites surveyed in October 2000 while preparing this chapter had disappeared by June 2001.

Each site claims editorial independence despite the advertising. Complaints that Drkoop.com blurred the line between objective information and advertising resulted in a precipitous drop in the value of its shares.[15,16] This prompted the production of a 14-point set of ethical principles designed to ensure reliable health information and services. Major components of the Hi-Ethics principles include clear identification of advertisements and disclosure of paid sponsorships, giving consumers information about, and control over, how their personal data are used, and ensuring that health advice on the Internet is accurate and up to date.[17]

Online drug stores with information about skin conditions

Organizations primarily providing online information are merging with online and offline pharmacies to fund their ventures by e-commerce. For example, Healthcentral, which provides a vast resource of consumer health information and online product sales, acquired the Internet sites of Vitamins.com and Drug Emporium, Inc. to create the WebRx Health Superstore (http://www.webrx.com/). More recently Healthcentral has acquired online and offline assets from More.com and its subsidiary Comfort Living, Inc., a 13-year-old home and personal comfort products distributor. It has an affiliate agreement with the retail drugstore chain PharMor.[18]

E-commerce sites risk a conflict between editorial integrity and advertising, particularly if advertising is not clearly identified.

Internet health stores selling 'all-natural' products derive significant revenue from the sale of nutraceutical products and other items. Content about skin diseases is limited and non-evidence based. As an example, dermatologists will be surprised by the following statement read on Healthshop.com in October 2000: 'To maintain healthy skin, brush it daily with a vegetable-bristle brush, drink plenty of water, moisturize from the inside and out and get moderate sun exposure' (this website no longer exists). Vitacost.com acquired Healthshop.com in February 2001, and claims 'scientifically proven benefits' for its products.[19]

Domain site names

In June 2001, Whois.net lists 32 123 450 registered domains and a further 2054 846 on hold.[20] Many of these have no active website. A keyword search revealed 23 domain names relating to scabies, but only 'gotscabies.com' linked to useful information about the skin complaint (the National Pediculosis Association's 'headlice.org' site). Some companies have registered multiple disease-related domains. The online pharmacy PlanetRx.com owned 'www.acne.com' and others, but went into liquidation in March 2001. BetterHealthUSA.com, a division of the toxic food testing facility Immuno Laboratories, owns at least four dermatological domains; visitors to these sites are directed to have blood tests to determine the dietary cause of their yeast infection, urticaria, dermatitis or 'skin rashes'.[21]

Search facilities

According to a 1999 Consumer Survey by Jupiter,[19] more than 50% of online users turn to general search and directory sites to begin their health-related information visits. Information about skin diseases is not easily accessed using search engines or hierarchical medical directories. For example, in June 2001 Yahoo had 43 categories of skin diseases and nothing on hundreds of other conditions that patients may wish to investigate. Lawrence and Giles found that no engine indexes more than 16% of the web.[22] This is improved to 42% by using a metasearch engine, but newer sites with fewer links to them can easily be missed.[23]

Wu and Li compared seven search engines using consumer health topics.[24] Bykowski et al checked the first 100 listings for cutaneous laser surgery by each of three search engines. Only three sites were found by all three. Forty sites were evaluated; the quality of content did not correlate with how easy it was to locate the site.[25] Price and Hersh have attempted to improve the results of consumer health queries with a prototype system in which web pages found by a search engine are ranked according to quality.[26]

Email messages to physicians

An October 2000 survey of 700 physicians showed a 200% growth in physicians' use of email with patients in less than one year. Ten per cent of the physicians communicated with their patients by email.[27] Yet nearly half of New Zealand GPs surveyed recently expressed concerns that the Internet could have unwelcome effects on the doctor–patient relationship.[28] Eysenbach and Diepgen have identified that patients with dermatological problems are increasingly seeking advice via email.[29] Eysenbach commented that it is unclear whether 'ask the doctor' forums and unsolicited email messages constitute medical practice and whether physicians have an ethical obligation to respond to unsolicited email messages sent by patients.[30]

Huntley has pointed out that it is relatively easy for patients to obtain the email address of physicians who appear to have some expertise.[31] The physician can attempt to answer the question, simply direct the patient to seek the care of a dermatologist using a standard reply or delete the message. Dispensing medical advice without performing a physical examination may lead to inappropriate diagnosis and treatment.

Ferguson has suggested that email should be seen as an opportunity to provide patients with the online information they want, delivered by the very people from whom they would most like to obtain it – their own physicians.[1] He has pointed out that most physicians are delighted to discover that email helps them save time (by avoiding telephone tag and interruptions), while being more accessible and supportive to their patients.[7] Some health insurers have agreed to pay physicians for email communications with some patients (an office.com report called 'You've Got Mail: Will Physicians Respond?' was published in November 2000, but is no longer online).

The American Medical Informatics Association has drawn up comprehensive guidelines regarding patient-provider email.[32] These do not address communication between providers and consumers in which no contractual relationship exists. The communication guidelines discuss patient privacy, what should be included in the text and what should be left out and the need to file the message in the patient's casenotes. Administrative guidelines suggest obtaining informed consent, giving the patient instructions about how and when to communicate, and also discuss security issues.

The New Zealand Medical Council has published guidelines for physicians offering telemedical consultations over the Internet.[33] The main concerns are medicolegal.

Although the medium has been thought inappropriate, inexpensive direct consultation services are inevitable. The Australasian consultation service DoctorGlobal (http://doctorglobal.com) receives about 5000 site visits each month (personal communication, October 2000). Popular topics include sexual health, mental health, pain management and asthma. DoctorGlobal is not yet offering dermatological consultations (June 2001).

Positive features of Internet information

There are many positive features of Internet information. These include:

▶ extensive and accurate information is available on a previously unimaginable scale;

▶ information can be found on rare as well as common conditions;

▶ current information includes new and unusual theories, conventional and alternative treatments;

▶ authors come from all parts of the industrialized and developing world;

▶ articles are frequently authoritative and written by worldwide experts;

▶ in such cases, there is often extensive biographical information about the author or consultant;

▶ the information is readily accessible.

Problems resulting from the Internet

Only a small proportion of the investment in healthcare information technology is focused on helping patients. The Internet is unregulated and unsupervised so that important information from trustworthy sources is transmitted side by side with unauthorized and unreliable information.[2] The patient may not know whether the medical expertise they are getting is reliable and from an appropriate and qualified source. Some patients may make decisions based on poor information.[34]

Other problems resulting from the Internet include:

▶ The patient depends on having the correct diagnosis to research a specific skin condition.

▶ It is difficult for an expert to determine the quality of the information – it is perhaps impossible for the average consumer.

▶ Much of the material is biased, non-evidence based, non-peer reviewed, anonymous and factually incorrect. This includes provocative, despicable, violent, criminal and pornographic material.[2]

▶ Poor site navigation and formatting may make information hard to find and its quality hard to assess.

▶ The material may be poorly written and is frequently unedited.

▶ Advice may be inappropriate, being geographically or culturally specific. This is a particular risk of interactive software tools that diagnose or manage disease.

▶ Recommended treatments may be fraudulent, unconventional, dangerous and unproven.[35]

> The question of claims upon negligence, privacy, confidentiality, copyright and intellectual property rights on the part of the provider and user are undefined and need further serious consideration. Who is liable if the patient self-manages illness on the basis of information found on the Internet?

We do not know what factors distinguish those people who use the Internet for health concerns from those who do not.[36]

Physicians sometimes feel threatened by the patient who presents with reams of material printed from the Internet. Perhaps they fear a loss of power or control – they are no longer the only source of diagnosis, management choices and information. Or they fear the patient ordering a 'cure' via the Internet is dissatisfied and distrustful.[37] However, such an interaction should be seen as an opportunity to improve the patient's self-respect by expanding the doctor's navigation skills. The patient's respect for the doctor will increase if he or she guides the patient towards authoritative information and appropriate online support groups.

The role of the physician is undergoing a subtle change, to a facilitator who can share decision making with his or her patient, guiding them through the quagmire of confusing information. The doctor should read the information carefully, as inaccurate or dangerous information puts the patient at risk. Good physicians should direct their own patients to high-quality health sites for their mutual benefit.

The informed patient should have a greater sense of autonomy regarding health choices. They no longer need to fear mysterious medical terms or hold suspicions about their healthcare provider's motives. The Internet should aid in compliance with treatment and strengthen the relationships between patient and health professional. This should reduce the desire to seek a second opinion or pursue unconventional routes.

A Dutch report of the possibilities and perils of the Internet in relation to health care was commissioned because of government concerns that prescription drugs could be procured from abroad on the Internet.[38] Some conclusions included:

> Not everyone has access to the Internet or knows how to use it (particularly the sick); investment in technology such as voice activation to help the illiterate, and public access should be a priority.

> Provision of health information remains patchy; the breadth and quality of content depend on the provider rather than the consumer. More information is needed on health, sickness and its treatment and healthcare facilities.

> Patients may be able to save money, obtain drugs otherwise unobtainable in their home country or one their doctor is unwilling to prescribe such as traditional remedies, 'miracle cures' of last resort or so-called lifestyle drugs (such as finasteride for hair loss). Not everyone can deal with products and services available on the Internet; the advent of e-commerce may result in sales of bogus medicines as well as inappropriate prescribing, dangerous drug interactions and toxicities. Diagnostic services provided offshore suffer from poor information gathering and lack of physical examination; counselling may be out of context and inappropriate culturally.

Not everyone can distinguish reliable from unreliable information. There is considerable incorrect, incomplete, out-of-date and misleading information including unsubstantiated claims of miracle cures. Patients need to be taught how to assess the reliability of information. Unbiased agencies should provide a health portal (such as the US Government HealthFinder.gov). Good sites could be certified (although information published on the Internet can easily be altered) or actively identified by government-sponsored banners or links. It is deemed too difficult to certify organizations.

Determining the quality of the health information on the Internet

An editorial in the *Journal of the American Medical Association* published in 1997 is subtitled *'Caveant Lector et Viewor – Let the Reader and Viewer Beware'*.[39] Silberg et al express concern that the Internet 'resembles a cocktail conversation' despite the core standards required to achieve these goals being 'not complicated' (authorship, attribution, disclosure and currency). The authors state that 'Internet sources of medical information that fail to meet at least these basic standards should be considered suspect'.

Wyatt referred to Silberg's criteria but also suggested that the reliability of a website depended on credibility and conflicts of interest; structure and content; functions; and impact. He suggested evaluating a site by first inspecting and comparing the information with current best evidence, and then performing laboratory tests with users to ensure that the content is easy to read. The web server statistics and results of online questionnaires should be examined to ensure that the site is easy to access. A field trial should be conducted to determine the effect on clinical practice and patient outcome.[40]

In 1998, Jadad identified 47 rating instruments for websites providing health information and concluded that it is unclear whether they should exist, whether they measure what they claim or whether they lead to more good than harm.[41] In 1999 Kim et al reviewed criteria for evaluating health-related websites. The most frequently cited criteria in 29 published rating tools were those dealing with content, design and aesthetics, disclosure of authors, sponsors or developers, currency of information, authority of source, ease of use, accessibility and availability.[42]

Eysenbach et al identified how patients may misinterpret even good information on the Internet because of 'context deficit' (e.g. not all treatment options listed), inappropriate context (e.g. designed for a health professional) or not viewing the cover page that includes disclaimers. They proposed 'automatic downstream filtering' where users and their software would rate the medical information.[43]

There are numerous websites that discuss how to evaluate other sites. Tillman compared the Internet with print publications. His generic criteria for evaluation were: stated criteria for inclusion of information, authority of author, comparability with related sources, stability of information, appropriateness of format and software/hardware/multimedia requirements. He discussed review tools such as the Lycos Top 5% and the Magellan Internet Guide. He advised those publishing via the Internet to consider the target audience – its access to the site, who they are and what they need.[44]

Kirk also offered practical steps in evaluating Internet resources, referring to authorship, publishing body, point of view or bias, referral to and/or knowledge of the literature, accuracy/verifiability of details and currency.[45] She referred to the Copyright website for explanations of fair use of copyrighted information.[46]

The Health on the Net Code of Conduct (HONcode) has eight principles or ethical guidelines which the HON Foundation (http://www.hon.ch/) consider indicate a high quality World Wide Web site containing medical and health information.[47] The HON receives a request from a site to be evaluated for HON certification and permission to display the HON seal. The check site tool helps assess a website's author credentials, date of last modification, confidentiality of data, source data reference and funding/advertising policy. It is quick to use and appears to be widely respected as authoritative but it does not evaluate the accuracy of the information presented.

The Health Information Technology Institute's Criteria for Assessing the Quality of Health Information on the Internet includes a more comprehensive and detailed instrument for assessing credibility, content, disclosure, links, design, interactivity and caveats.[48] I used this to review dermatology Internet sites with mixed results.[49]

The Internet Healthcare Coalition code of ethics regarding Internet-based health information is a framework upon which a health-related website should be constructed to ensure quality, safety and privacy or informed consent.[50] The intention is to self-police sites. The principles considered are:

- candour (full disclosure)
- honesty
- quality
- informed consent
- privacy
- professionalism
- accountability.

Emory University has created a WELLNESS instrument that health educators and clinicians can use to evaluate the appropriateness of websites for their clientele. It covers intended audience, objectives, content (information, purpose, bias, links) and accuracy (documentation of sources, subscribing to HONcode).[51] The University of California at San Francisco's Biosites guidelines cover scope, quality of content, functionality and ease of use, utility, stability and currency.[52] McGill University Health Library has selected good sites on the Internet using similar criteria.[53]

The American Medical Association has produced guidelines for its own Internet sites, which include the Medem.com health portal megasite.[54] The focus is the provision of authoritative content without conflict of interest and includes warnings to visitors that they are leaving the site, the kind of information that is gathered from them and why, and offers them chances to opt in or opt out of providing personal information.

Barrett's website Quackwatch.com identifies some characteristics of a website that indicate it is not a trustworthy information source. He includes sites marketing herbs, homoeopathic products, 'alternative' methods, and those promoting 'non-toxic', 'natural' and 'holistic' treatments; false statements about nutrition, 'alternative' methods and other issues such as fluoridation, immunizations and mercury-amalgam fillings.[55]

Implementing quality codes for medical sites on the Internet may be difficult, if not impossible. Conventional printed material may be of equally poor quality but the information is not required to comply with a specific standard. Organizations offering approval of websites could face legal challenges should they overvalue or undervalue certain sites.[16]

In 1998 the UK National Health Service Information for Health Strategy proposed a National electronic Library for Health to include Virtual Branch Libraries containing online knowledge about specific health-related topics. Well-defined appraisal criteria were found necessary when assessing the quality of a vast number of web resources, the best of which were to be included in the Dermatology Virtual Branch Library.[56]

Quality tools may also be applied to non-web-based consumer health information. The three principles of the UK Help for Health Trust's Centre for Health Information Quality are that good quality patient information is evidence based, clearly communicated and involves patients throughout production.[57] The Centre has devised a checklist (DISCERN) for patients, health providers and educators to appraise patient information about treatment choices.[58] It consists of 15 questions assessing the reliability of the publication and its specific information, and an overall quality rating.

There are few publications comparing web advice to published guidelines. Impicciatore et al compared the advice on 41 web pages on managing fever in children at home and found that only a few websites provided complete and accurate information.[59] Sandvik evaluated 17 websites with information about urinary incontinence and found most to be accurate and some to be excellent.[60] General quality criteria were partly based on those suggested by Silberg et al[39] and partly on the HONcode principles.[47]

Conclusion

Physicians should direct their patients to sources of good quality evidence-based consumer health information, and be prepared to write it themselves if it does not yet exist. However, this is a time-consuming process, following not only validated quality criteria but also involving patients in developing and testing materials.[61]

There is no doubt that information technology offers a huge font of knowledge for patients and will have far-reaching effects for those with skin diseases and their healthcare providers.

References

1 Ferguson T. Digital doctoring – opportunities and challenges in electronic patient–physician communication. *Journal of American Medical Association* 1998;**280:**1261–1262.

2 Wolf R, Ballan S. Virtual doctors – ready for launching. *International Journal of Dermatology* 2000;**39:**487–489.

3 About Us page of MedHelp. June 2001. (http://www.medhelp.org/AboutMedHelp/ABOUT_US_files/aboutus.html).

4 Med Help International: Where there's a Doctor on the Web. Electronic Journal of the US Department of State Office of International Information Programs, *Global Issues* 2000;**5:**(3). (http://usinfo.state.gov/journals/itgic/1100/ijge/gj05.htm).

5 US National Library of Medicine press release January 2001. (http://www.nlm.nih.gov/news/press_releases/medplus1.html).

6 Mastocytosis Society web site home page. June 2001. (http://mast.gil.com.au/).

7 Ferguson T. Online patient-helpers and physicians working together: a new partnership for high quality health care. *British Medical Journal* 2000;**321:**1129–1132.

8 Vandenberg T, Meads G, Engel J, et al. A randomized pilot study of the effect of computer-based information and support for women with newly diagnosed breast cancer [meeting abstract]. In: *Proceedings of the Annual Meeting of the American Society of Clinical Oncology; May 1997; Denver, Colorado.* Abstract 293. (http://asco.infostreet.com/prof/me/html/abstracts/asc/m_293.htm).

9 Jupiter Research page. (http://www.jup.com/) or (http://:www.jmm.com/xp/jmm/services/jup).

10 Onhealth/WebMD.com web site. October 2000. (http://onhealth.webmd.com/home/info/item,95217.asp).

11 Intelihealth's Press Room. March 2000. (http://www.intelihealth.com/IH/ihtIH/WSIHW000/24479/21204/236954.html?d=dmtContent).

12 DermNet NZ web page. About DermNet: sponsors. June 2001. (http://www.dermnet.org.nz/sponsors.html).

13 Allhealth.com web site, section 'Caring for your skin'. June 2001. (http://www.caringforyourskin.com/).

14 Jupiter Strategic Planning Services Market Module: Health Online landscape. MMH99-V2.September 1999.

15 Charatan F. DrKoop.com criticised for mixing information with advertising. *British Medical Journal* 1999;**319:**727.

16 Delamothe T. Quality of websites: kitemarking the west wind. *British Medical Journal* 2000;**321:**843–844.

17 Charatan F. Health websites in US propose new ethics code. *British Medical Journal* 2000;**320:**1359.

18 Healthcentral.com web site, Online press release. October 2000. (http://www.healthcentral.com/AboutUs/PressReleases/pr10242000_2.cfm).

19 Vitacost.com web site. June 2001. (http://www.vitacost.com/company/index.html).

20 Whois.net web site. June 2001. (http://www.whois.net).

21 BetterHealthUSA web site. June 2001. (http://www.urticaria-hives.net/; http://www.candida.net/; http://www.eczema-dermatitus.com/; http://www.skin-rashes.net/).

22 Lawrence S, Giles CL. Accessibility of information on the web. *Nature* 1999;**400:**107–109.

23 Larkin M. What's amiss with web search engines? *Lancet* 1999;**354**(9174):260.

24 Wu G, Li J. Comparing Web search engine performance in searching consumer health information: evaluation and recommendations. *Bulletin Medical Librarians Association* 1999;**87:**456–461.

25 Bykowski JL, Alora MB, Dover JS, Arndt KA. Accessibility and reliability of cutaneous laser surgery information on the World Wide Web. *Journal of the American Academy of Dermatology* 2000;**42**(5 Pt 1):784–786.

26 Price SL, Hersh WR. Filtering web pages for quality indicators: an empirical approach to finding high quality consumer health information on the World Wide Web. *Proceedings of the American Medical Informatics Association Symposium* 1999;911–915.

27 Medem Press Release. Medem.com. November 2000. (http://www.medem.com/corporate/press/corporate_medeminthenews_press023.cfm).

28 Eberhart-Phillips J, Hall K, Herbison GP, et al. Internet use amongst New Zealand general practitioners. *New Zealand Medical Journal* 2000;**113:**135–137.

29 Eysenbach G, Diepgen TL. Patients looking for information on the Internet and seeking teleadvice: motivation, expectations, and misconceptions as expressed in emails sent to physicians. *Archives of Dermatology* 1999;**135:**151–156.

30 Eysenbach G. Towards ethical guidelines for dealing with unsolicited patient emails and giving teleadvice in the absence of a pre-existing patient–physician relationship – systematic review and expert survey. *Journal of Medical Internet Research* 2000;2(1):e1. (http://www.jmir.org/2000/1/e1/).

31 Huntley A. The need to know. Patients, e-mail and the Internet. *Archives of Dermatology* 1999;**135:**198–199.

32 Kane B, Sands DZ. Guidelines for the clinical use of electronic mail with patients. *Journal of the American Medical Informatics Association* 1998;**5:**104–111.

33 Medical Council of New Zealand, Guidelines for Doctors Using the Internet. June 2000.

34 Gawande AA, Bates DW. The use of information technology in improving medical performance Part III Patient-support. Medscape General Medicine 2000; **22:**E12.

35 Gottlieb S. Health information on internet is often unreliable. *British Medical Journal* 2000;**321:**136.

36 Jadad AR. Promoting partnerships: challenges for the internet age. *British Medical Journal* 1999;**319:**761–764.

37 Curley KC. I'm not a doctor, but I play one on my website. *Cybermed Catalyst* 2000;(Summer). (http://www.amip.org/catalyst/webdoc_html).

38 Onno van Rijen. The patient and the Internet. *Cybermed Catalyst* 2000;(Summer). (http://www.amip.org/catalyst/vanrijen_html).

39 Silberg WM, Lundberg GD, Musacchio RA. Assessing, controlling, and assuring the quality of medical information on the Internet. *Journal of the American Medical Association* 1997;**277:**1244–1245.

40 Wyatt JC. Commentary: measuring quality and impact of the world wide web. *British Medical Journal* 1997;**314**(7098):1879–1881.

41 Jadad AR, Gagliardi A. Rating health information on the Internet: navigating to knowledge or Babel?. *Journal of the American Medical Association* 1998;**279:**611–614.

42 Kim P, Eng TR, Deering MJ, Maxfield A. Published criteria for evaluating health related web sites: review. *British Medical Journal* 1999;**318**(7184):647–649.

43 Eysenbach G, Diepgen TL. Towards quality management of medical information on the internet: evaluation, labelling, and filtering of information. *British Medical Journal* 1998;**317:**1496–1502.

44 Tillman HN. Evaluating quality on the Net. Babson College. 2000 (http://www.hopetillman.com/findqual.html).

45 Kirk EE. Evaluating information found on the Internet. Milton's Web. 1996. (http://milton.mse.jhu.edu:8001/research/education/net.html).

46 O'Mahoney B. The Copyright Website. 1995. (http://www.benedict.com/).

47 Health On the Net Code of Conduct. Version 1.6 April 1997. Health On the Net Foundation. (http://www.hon.ch/HONcode/Conduct.html).

48 Ambre J, Guard R, Perveiler FM, Renner J, Rippen H. Criteria for assessing the quality of health information on the Internet. Health Information Technology Institute. 1997. (http://hitiweb.mitretek.org/docs/criteria.html).

49 Oakley A. On-line patient information. 1999. (http://www.dermnet.org.nz/ptinfo.html).

50 Internet Health Coalition Code of Ethics. 2000. (http://www.ihealthcoalition.org/ethics/ehcode.html).

51 Teach L. Health-related web site evaluation form. Emory. 1998. (http://www.sph.emory.edu/WELLNESS/instrument.html).

52 Selection criteria for Internet resources. Regents of the University of California, San Francisco. 1996. (http://www.library.ucsf.edu/biosites/help/guidelines.html).

53 Lambrou A, Grant S. Internet resources selection criteria. McGill Health Library. June 2000. (http://www.health.library.mcgill.ca/resource/criteria.htm).

54 Guidelines for medical and health information sites on the Internet . May 2001. American Medical Association (http://www.ama-assn.org/ama/pub/category/1905.html).

55 Barrett S. How to spot a 'quacky' web site. June 2000. (http://www.quackwatch.com/01Quackery RelatedTopics/quackweb.html).

56 Kamel Boulos MN, Roudsari AV, Gordon C, Muir Gray JA. The use of quality benchmarking in assessing web resources for the Dermatology Virtual Branch Library of the National electronic Library for Health (NeLH). *Journal of Medical Research* 2001;**3**(1):e5. (http://www.jmir.org/2001/1/e5/).

57 Centre for Health Information Quality. (http://www.hfht.org/chiq/guidelines.htm).

58 Charnock D. DISCERN. Centre for Health Information Quality. 1998. (http://www.discern.org.uk/).

59 Impicciatore P, Pandolfini C, Casella N, Bonati M. Reliability of health information for the public on the World Wide Web: systematic survey of advice on managing fever in children at home. *British Medical Journal* 1997;**314**(7098):1875–1879.

60 Sandvik H. Health information and interaction on the internet: a survey of female urinary incontinence. *British Medical Journal* 1999;**319:**29–32.

61 Shepperd S, Charnock D, Gann B. Helping patients access high quality health information. *British Medical Journal* 1999;**319:**764–766.

14

An Online Dermatology Atlas

Carl R. Blesius, Uli Klein, Jörn Paessler, Gabriel Yihune and
Thomas Diepgen

Introduction

Dermatology is a visually oriented specialty. The majority of diagnoses in dermatology are made by optical inspection of skin lesions, appraisal of cutaneous biopsies, analysis of superficial ultrasound images and evaluation of skin tests. The visual component of dermatology makes the acquisition, storage and presentation of images crucial to practitioners and students at all levels. It also accentuates the importance of imaging technologies.

A dermatological atlas is an essential tool for the profession. In the years before photography, skin diseases were painstakingly recorded using the tools available at the time. The main tools were ink, paints, presses and paper. Other study aids were three-dimensional models moulded from plaster, wax or even papier-mâché. These specimens were originally created by artists, although subsequently wax casts started to appear. Although the casts helped speed up the production process they still required painting by hand. These three-dimensional aids came the closest to substituting for actual patients, but they were very expensive to produce.

In the second half of the nineteenth century Daguerre and others developed the process of photography. Dermatology atlases quickly became peppered with black and white photographic images. These images attained a realism rarely achieved by artistic means. Colour, which came later, remains one of the most important factors for a dermatological image. It is not surprising that many dermatologists of the past were artistically or graphically inclined.

The importance of colour and images in dermatology was obvious to Ferdinand Hebra, the physician who founded the New Vienna School of Dermatology (the basis of modern dermatology) around the same time that photography was slowly maturing. Hebra worked with two artistically talented physicians (Elfinger and Heitzmann) to put together one of the most beautiful dermatological publications ever created: the 'Atlas der Hautkrankheiten', first published in 1856 (Elfinger and Hebra). The Hebra Atlas is a work that reflects Hebra's understanding of the importance of the visual record in dermatology. In the preface and introduction he elucidated the motive of the atlas: 'The images should take the place of the patients and the text should take the place of the teacher'. Hebra wanted to make a large spectrum of skin diseases, which could only be found in a large dermatological clinic, accessible to a wider audience. The atlas was not bound in the way one would expect, but came in two parts: a collection of 59 × 45 cm prints on cardboard and a bound booklet with the descriptive text for each image. The prints showed each skin disease as a colour lithograph, printed using four plates, and a black and white lithograph (Fig. 14.1). The publisher of this unique piece of dermatological history was the Kaiserliche Akademie der Wissenschaften (Imperial Academy of Sciences) and it was printed in the K.K. Hof- und Staatsdruckerei zu Wien (Royal Imperial and National Printing Office of Vienna).

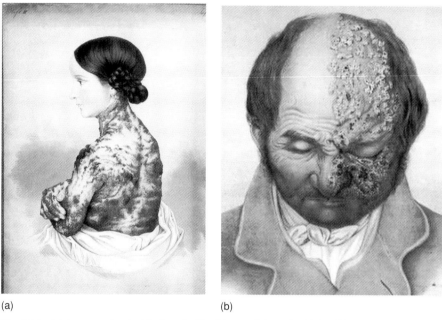

(a)
(b)

Fig. 14.1. (a) An example of a black and white lithograph from the Hebra Atlas. (b) An example of a colour lithograph from the Hebra Atlas (reproduced here in monochrome).

One of the main problems with dermatology atlases, today and in the past, has been the cost of printing coloured images. The publication of the highly detailed and colourful Hebra atlas, for example, was made possible through a substantial government grant. The costs involved in producing a modern colour atlas also impose constraints, usually limiting the number of diagnoses illustrated, the use of colour and the number of images per diagnosis. The variability in the individual manifestations of a single skin disease can be significant, which may necessitate a high number of images per diagnosis. Some factors that may cause variations in appearance are skin type, stage of disease and severity, as well as age, gender and location.

Just as the technologies progressed that made traditional photography an essential tool of dermatology, the digital revolution is changing the way that images of the skin and diseases of the skin are stored, retrieved and shared. Images taken with digital cameras are approaching the resolution that can be achieved with photographic film, high-speed Internet access is becoming common, and digital storage space has become cheap and plentiful. Dermatology is poised to profit more from these advances than from most other medical specialties. All of these factors are relevant to dermatology's potential for telemedical applications.

Our original goal in setting up a dermatological image atlas online was to facilitate access to a large number of images from a variety of sources, archive them in a logical manner and make them easily accessible through the Web. The atlas started as a collection of images and their hypertext descriptions but has grown into a resource for research, patient education and medical education.

Architecture of an online image database

The following features are important in an online image database:

▶ a library of digitized images

▶ corresponding descriptive text

▶ a system of integrating the information into a database

▶ a template-based interface for the input of images and their descriptions (for contributors) and to present images and descriptive text (to viewers).

The image library

Obviously any good atlas in dermatology depends on images of diseases of the skin, yet for traditional film and paper-based images, storage and presentation are usually restricting factors. As mentioned above traditional textbooks and atlases are limited in the number of images per diagnosis and the number of diagnoses overall due to the high cost of printing coloured images on paper. Printed materials also require a complex infrastructure for publication and distribution.

Digital images are ideal for dermatology as they eliminate many of the limitations of traditional photography. Digital images have the following advantages: they are inexpensive, easy to process, offer a safe form of storage, are of consistent quality, and allow quick search and retrieval, digital watermarking, easy duplication and distribution. In 1995 the quality of digital images had already been shown to be of similar clinical value to traditional photographs,[1] and the resolution of digital images has significantly increased since then. In studies evaluating the effectiveness of digital photography for dermatological diagnoses, there was over 80% agreement between diagnoses made in person and those made using digital photographs.[2] Some studies have shown that digital images can substitute for a dermatological examination in up to 83% of cases.[3]

Descriptive text

Although images may be the main component of an atlas, additional information about the dermatological disorders and patients being portrayed is required. It is important to collect as much information as possible when the image is captured and entered into the atlas framework. This facilitates future changes such as alternate forms of presentation or grouping of content. A wealth of meta-information makes images more valuable for manipulation and storage, and makes it possible to tailor the information for the user.

Database

The use of a database allows the atlas to be kept up to date and maintained easily. This is particularly important when dealing with a large dataset. These operations depend on careful database design and integration with existing information resources. Database entity-relationship model design should take place before the actual creation of tables or object-classes (an entity-relationship data model is a view of the real world as a set of basic objects or entities with basic relationships among themselves). The design is crucial to the consistency, integrity and accuracy of the information within the database. Well-thought-out database planning will result in improved efficiency in data storage and retrieval, accuracy of information and predictability. Poor database design quickly results in problems with maintenance and management. When creating the database one should always consider existing information resources and standards (e.g. the Unified Medical Language System).

In designing a database there are important steps that should be taken in order to complete the design process. The first step is to define the purpose of the database. In the process, one must consider the tasks that are to be performed by users. Second, one creates tables by determining the subjects and the data model used to store the information in the database (e.g. a relational or object-oriented scheme). The next step is to analyse and identify relationships that exist in the tables and connect them using links, primary keys and other keys, after which one sets the various characteristics for the relationships. One should also have a rough idea of the various ways that the users are going to be looking at, changing, inserting and deleting the information, and then create views for data input and output.

Time spent on database structural design is time well spent. It permits easy modification of the data, tables and fields within a database and it allows easy retrieval and input of information.

Input interface

An atlas requires high-quality images and information about the images, lesions and patients. The input interface is a very important factor in the success of an online atlas. The process of creating an atlas is not completed after taking some pictures, digitizing them and storing them on the file system; the images must be named, identified, classified and integrated into the database framework. The interface must be simple to use.

User interface

The ultimate goal of a dermatology atlas is to present the images and their information to the user, making the user interface even more important. The interface should help the user find the information that he or she is looking for. It should provide different ways to access the database and at the same time link existing information in logical and helpful ways. Each page should look similar. When all the pages of the atlas have similar navigational structure and organization, the user feels comfortable and confident in using it.

Dermis.net

A survey of online atlases on the Internet shows that there is a wide range of dermatological resources. At present almost all of these image collections are image and HTML files stored on web servers. There appear to be various approaches to the problem of storing and presenting the images. The dermis.net information service (http://www.dermis.net) is a practical example. Dermis.net is a comprehensive online dermatology information service for healthcare professionals and patients.

The dermis.net information service started as the Dermatology Online Image Atlas (DOIA), a collection of static HTML and images. DOIA has been online since 1994 and was originally funded by the DFG (German Research Foundation). The atlas began at the Department of Dermatology of the University of Erlangen-Nuremberg, Germany. It was originally published on the servers of the university computer centre. In 1997 the website was transferred to an independent server. As the atlas grew, other services started to appear, such as German language patient information for sufferers of atopic eczema. The store of images on the DOIA has grown by approximately 100 images per month.

The grant from the DFG ended in 1998, following which the coordination of the project moved to the University of Heidelberg's Institute of Clinical and Social Medicine (Professor Dr Diepgen). The cooperation with the University Dermatology Clinic in Erlangen (Professor Dr Schuler) persists and flourishes. Further collaborations have arisen (e.g. University of Nantes, France; Dermatology Clinic of Heidelberg, Germany) and the server hardware and software have been updated. The project is now financed by educational grants from industry.

In order to cope with the rapid growth and popularity of the atlas, server side technologies were introduced at the start of 1998. These allow a higher degree of actuality, interactivity, dynamic modularity and simplified maintenance. The dynamic nature of the new architecture made it possible to cater to different audiences using a shared database of images. The Pediatric Dermatology Online Atlas (PeDOIA) was established.

In the year 2000 the entire website was restructured and a large amount of new material was added. During this process, a site-wide navigational structure, global design and full text search were implemented. The redesign served to consolidate existing information and to provide visual unification. The large number of images on the site made performance on the server side important.

Server hardware and software

The present www.dermis.net web server is a double Pentium III-500 with 500 MBytes RAM and 17 GBytes of disk space. The server runs under Windows NT 4.0 with the

Internet Information Server 4.0. The generation of the HTML pages occurs dynamically using a combination of Active Server Pages (ASP), server side JavaScript and a relational database (Microsoft Access).

The image library

The DOIA image database contains approximately 5000 images linked to at least 650 different diagnoses. Most of the images originate from hospital slide archives, which have been digitized onto Kodak PhotoCDs and stored on a file system. Next to the original slides the CDs serve as an archive of high-quality images. The images are identified using a combination of CD number and image number (corresponding to the image numbers on the CDs themselves). These images are then reduced in size (to approximately 800×800 pixels) and compressed using the JPEG (Joint Photographic Expert Group) image compression algorithm at 30–40%, the average resulting image size being between 20 and 30 kBytes.

The majority of the DOIA images originate from the Department of Dermatology at the University of Erlangen, while many of the PeDOIA images originate from the University of Nantes in France. Some images are the result of other international contributions. Most of the images are clinical in nature, a few being histological. An increase in the number of histological images is planned.

Descriptive text

Descriptive text is entered into the image collection using the input interface and the descriptive fields in the database. Standardized information and image-specific information are recorded. This is discussed below in the description of the user input interface.

Database

Due to a lack of specific tools to describe dermatological images, a proprietary database was developed. The following fields are used:

- a diagnostic code based upon the 'Erlanger Diagnosis Code' (this was a 6-digit numerical code based upon ICD-9; subsequently these were mapped to the Unified Medical Language System – Concept Unique Identifiers[4,5])

- diagnosis (optional free text)

- disease location code, consisting of body part (e.g. arm, hand, finger, nail) and side (e.g. flexural side, palmar)

- patient skin type (e.g. black, Asian, white)

- patient age

- patient gender

- image technical quality (scale of 1 to 5; 1 being the best)

- image subject quality (scale of 1 to 5)

▶ image teaching quality (scale of 1 to 5)

▶ image specific information (height, width, size, photographer, creation date, creator)

▶ number of images per diagnosis (automatic)

▶ links specific to diagnosis.

Lesion description set:

▶ lesion type (e.g. nodule, plaque, ulcer)

▶ colour

▶ properties (e.g. verrucous)

▶ distribution (e.g. disseminated)

▶ demarcation (e.g. irregular, sharp)

▶ form (e.g. round, oval).

There are also tables to translate the user interface into multiple languages. All images are classified by a dermatologist in the final years of training and then reviewed by a senior dermatologist.

Integration with other information resources

In order to link our image database to other factual and bibliographic databases, we mapped the system to the CUI (unique concept identifiers) of the National Library of Medicine's Unified Medical Language System (UMLS) Metathesaurus. The UMLS Metathesaurus linked alternative names or similar concepts from different medical vocabularies to a unique concept identifier, and also provided the information regarding which term is to be used by which database for a given CUI. This mapping was accomplished by linking the Erlanger diagnosis code directly with the CUI numbers.

Thus, once we mapped our diagnoses to their CUIs we were able to use preferred terms automatically in order to look up the diagnoses in other databases. At present our database has been linked to three other databases:

▶ Medline (bibliographic database). With the implementation of a link to a publicly accessible version of Medline on the Internet at the US National Centre for Biotechnology Information, additional scientific information concerning a diagnosis can be searched. This happens automatically, due to the integration of the CUI in our database

▶ Physicians Data Query (PDQ). The dermatological diagnoses in the atlas are covered by PDQ, which is a factual/expert database from the US National Cancer Institute. Users of the atlas can query the PDQ Database by clicking on a hyperlink that contains the key used by PDQ for the given diagnosis

Online Mendelian Inheritance in Man (OMIM) is a factual/expert database about human and genetic disorders based upon the work of McKusick et al. Diagnoses with genetic associations hyperlink to the OMIM Database with an automatic search for the respective disease.

An additional advantage of linking to CUIs of UMLS is that the addition of other languages to the database is easier and more accurate.

Input interface

Image input into the system is achieved using a database interface that is independent of the web server itself. This is a very effective security measure, but it makes image input and database management difficult and unwieldy. Patient privacy is an important factor and certain information that is collected with the images should not be kept on a web server accessible to the public.

The interface is a program that runs under the Microsoft Windows operating system and was programmed using Delphi and Borland's Database Engine (BDE) as an Object-Oriented Database Connectivity (ODBC) front-end to a Microsoft Access database.

After the images have been digitized and saved, information about the images, the lesions and the patients is collected using this interface. In addition to the information that was listed in the previous section, there is a field in which descriptive text and information can be entered.

User interface

One can create a very nice atlas by fusing good content and good design to create a coherent sequential reference work. In a paper and printing world this would be the only goal, but the medium of the Web, which is permeating most areas of modern-day medicine, allows much more. Ideally content, presentation and logic should be separated, so that the user interface can be changed and expanded with little effort. There are various ways that a user can access the information that he or she is looking for.

The main menu of dermis.net (Fig. 14.2) links to the different areas of the site. The user is introduced to the navigational tools that are found throughout the site. The banner links to major sections and a trail of 'breadcrumbs'. These are links designating one's location on the website and the path taken to get there (the term comes from the Grimms' fairy tale in which a trail of breadcrumbs was left by Hansel and Gretel to find their way back home). From the main menu or the banner one can jump directly to the three different image resources on dermis.net: DOIA, PeDOIA and the Hebra Image collection.

The user interfaces of the DOIA and the PeDOIA are almost identical (Fig. 14.3). When entering the main pages there are different criteria with which to search the database.

One can browse the database by diagnoses alphabetically, by localization, by chapter in the PeDOIA and in a quiz mode. A full text search is also possible, with

Navigational Elements

Language

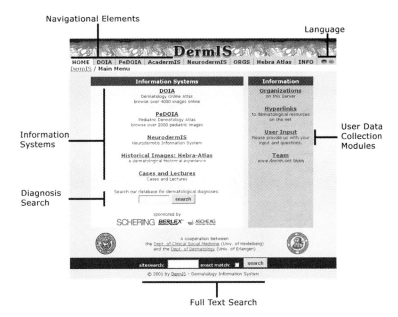

Information Systems

Diagnosis Search

User Data Collection Modules

Full Text Search

Fig. 14.2. The index page of http://dermis.net. The main elements of the site are accessible from this page.

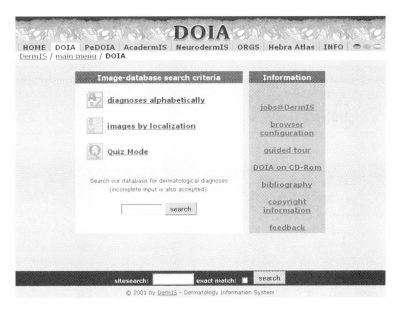

Fig. 14.3. The main menu of the DOIA (Dermatology Online Image Atlas) showing three modes of access: by diagnosis, by localization and by using the quiz mode (the paediatric version of the atlas has also been broken down into chapters).

which the user can search the atlases or the entire site for any phrase (incomplete input is also accepted).

When the alphabetical diagnosis search is chosen, an alphabetical listing of the diagnoses is requested using SQL (Structured Query Language) with limits according to what the user clicks.

The body browser tool allows a search by localization of the skin lesion (Fig. 14.4). This tool is an anterior and posterior representation of an adult male in the DOIA version and of an adolescent female in the PeDOIA version. Clicking on various parts of the diagram results in a menu specific to that area of the body, together with thumbnail images (miniature previews), e.g. all images relating to the legs. This option helps in differential diagnosis of lesions in a particular location.

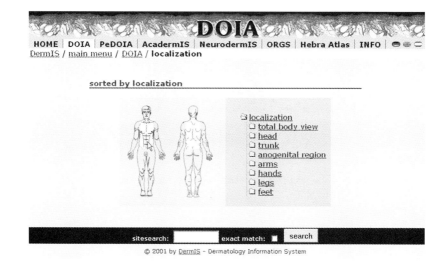

Fig. 14.4. A tool from the atlas that allows the user to search for images using the anatomical localization of the lesion.

In the PeDOIA, diagnoses have also been structured into 16 chapters with numerous subtopics.

All images can be viewed as thumbnails. These have reduced file size, and are very quickly loaded, which allows rapid preview of a group of pictures. After selecting a thumbnail, all image and diagnosis-related information is presented along with a large version of the image and thumbnails of other images with the same diagnosis (Fig. 14.5). The majority of images are specifically described and give the age of the patient, location and type of lesion as well as additional information. The images can be zoomed and also scrolled in the zoomed view. With this option special regions of interest can be viewed in detail.

It is possible to access related information using the tabs that appear between the breadcrumbs and image. In this area there are four tabs: 'info', differential diagnosis, images and hyperlinks. In the info tab page, synonyms for each diagnosis have been compiled and the majority of diagnoses include a definition. Furthermore UMLS terms in multiple languages have been included. The differential diagnosis page was implemented by grouping diagnoses according to morphology and querying the information to dynamically generate the pages. The image tab is the view shown in Figure 14.5. The hyperlinks page links to relevant external sites and to the databases described above.

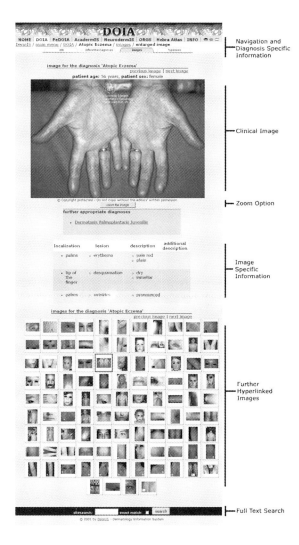

Fig. 14.5. An example of a page showing a single image and hyperlinked thumbnails of all images with the same diagnosis.

A quiz mode is available in both the DOIA and the PeDOIA to allow users to test and train their skills. The same basic techniques were used to create the quiz mode as were employed to present the images in the localization mode. Once the student has decided on a diagnosis the answer appears in a pop-up window along with the option of reading more about the diagnosis or continuing the quiz. The quiz feature is popular.

Patient survey

Due to its popularity and the fact that a large proportion of our visitors suffers from one of the diagnoses presented, the atlas has proved to be a valuable resource for research.

Since 1998 we have included an extensive questionnaire to measure quality of life for patients with various skin diseases. In the first 20 months of its existence it was completed by 9511 patients with dermatological diseases. Most questionnaires were filled out by patients between the ages of 18 and 55 years (63% female, 37% male). The patient population came from 112 different countries (58% USA, 16% Germany, 6.2% Canada, 4.1% UK, 2.5% Australia, 1.3% Netherlands, 1.1% Austria, 1% Switzerland). Skin diseases showing a very high adverse effect on quality of life included hidradenitis suppurativa, pruritic urticarial papules and plaques of pregnancy, scabies, acne vulgaris and atopic eczema.[6] We found the results of the Internet quality-of-life questionnaires were in general slightly better than those reported in the literature.

Conclusion

An online atlas with thousands of images of skin disorders that is free and readily accessible from anywhere in the world has wide-ranging educational and clinical implications. The medium itself is an exciting tool for health research and education. At present dermis.net receives 1.85 million page hits per month, and with the recently implemented Spanish version and the planned Portuguese version this number should rise considerably.

Originally a simple collection of images and descriptions, dermis.net has become an important web-based resource for healthcare professionals, students and patients. It not only serves as a tool for general practitioners and non-specialists, but also for specialists encountering patients with uncommon skin diseases. The potential for health education and the advantages of the separation of content, presentation and logic were not obvious when dermis.net was founded. Our future work aims to continue to separate these areas and expand the health education modules. At present we are developing a skin cancer information system. We will be able to collect and analyse data to evaluate the programme and measure outcomes. The Internet is proving to be a valuable and empowering information resource for patients, researchers, students and medical professionals alike.

References

1 Perednia DA, Gaines JA, Butruille TW. Comparison of the clinical informativeness of photographs and digital imaging media with multiple-choice receiver operating characteristic analysis. *Archives of Dermatology* 1995;**131**:292–297.

2 Kvedar JC, Edwards RA, Menn ER, et al. The substitution of digital images for dermatologic physical examination. *Archives of Dermatology* 1997;**133**:161–167.

3 Krupinski EA, LeSueur B, Ellsworth L, et al. Diagnostic accuracy and image quality using a digital camera for teledermatology. *Telemedicine Journal* 1999;**5**:257–263.

4 NLM. Unified Medical Language System. National Library of Medicine. 2001. (http://www.nlm.nih.gov/research/umls/).

5 Lindberg DA, Humphreys BL, McCray AT. The Unified Medical Language System. *Methods of Information in Medicine* 1993;**32**:281–291.

6 Eysenbach G, Paessler J, Diepgen T. Akquirierung von lebensqualitätsdaten dermatologischer patienten über das Internet. [The acquisition of quality of life data from dermatological patients over the Internet.] In: *Dermatology 2000 Symposium MEDICAL* (2 Freiburger Symposium 'Gesundheitsoekonomie in der Dermatologie', Freiburg im Breisgau, Germany 17–18 March 2000): 10–11.

15

Distance Teaching of Dermatohistology

Jörg Tittelbach, Andrea Bauer, Olaf Götz, Ruthild Linse and Peter Elsner

Introduction

Developments in information technology allow more rapid decision making, the accumulation of valuable information, and its evaluation and redistribution. The most common applications of the Internet are the World Wide Web and email. Internet-based technology is also used in internal company networks (called intranets), which allow the working process to be optimized on the basis of a closer interconnectivity and improved information sharing. In the medical field these new communication and interaction facilities have mainly been employed for information retrieval using the World Wide Web and for communication purposes using ordinary email.

In German primary healthcare facilities the equipment for these techniques already exists. Intelligent use of these tools will raise standards in health care and improve the teaching of students and medical staff. However, many patients and physicians do not understand the possible applications of modern information technology (IT) to medical practice. There is a wide range of IT that can be used in telemedicine. A new way of interacting and a new quality of medical service brought to the patient by the exchange of the patient's medical data between different healthcare providers are two of the most obvious advantages. The opportunity of 'second opinion consulting' offers an improved service and better standards for the patient. In addition, telemedicine can be used for the education of both the patient and the doctor. In this way the medical information on the World Wide Web creates a group of patients with a high degree of medical knowledge, which is sometimes even more profound on a specific topic than the doctor's expertise. Therefore it becomes more and more important that the doctors are trained to use this source of knowledge as well.

We are conducting a teledermatology project that is focused on the education of students and doctors in training. The project involves the exchange of histological data in expert conferences to discuss common and rare diagnoses. The focus on dermatohistology resulted from the following circumstances. Until now the bandwidth of Internet connections has been limited. However, the exchange of images can easily be carried out at high quality and with acceptable speed using modern compression algorithms. Therefore, histological diagnoses that are based on the evaluation of visual information are possible using the Internet.

The cooperation described in this chapter is based on historical developments in Thuringia, which is located in the centre of Germany covering an area of 16 170 km with about 2 500 000 inhabitants. There has been longstanding teaching cooperation between the Departments of Dermatology and Allergology of the Friedrich-Schiller University in Jena and the Department of Dermatology at the Erfurt Hospital, which has specific expertise in dermatohistology.

Jena (100 000 inhabitants) is located in the East of Thuringia and has been a university town since 1558. The Medical Faculty of the Friedrich-Schiller University of Jena is the only one in Thuringia. Erfurt (500 000 inhabitants), the capital of Thuringia, does not have a medical faculty but has a teaching hospital of the Friedrich-Schiller University of Jena involved in training students and doctors.

Distance teaching is an excellent tool. To use the clinical and dermatohistological cases of both clinics for teaching purposes provides the best possible education for medical students and doctors in training. The exchange of histological images can be carried out using a simple (and slow) modem or ISDN Internet connection – transmitting images as an email attachment. In order to provide the best possible learning environment we decided to use an interactive exchange of histological pictures as well, enabling students to interact with the speaker during the lecture. Therefore we added a whiteboard function to imitate the normal lecture environment. Moreover, patients benefit from this cooperation by getting immediate expert knowledge from both clinics. The aim of the project was to optimize the technology for the exchange of dermatohistological data. The effect of the project on teaching quality was evaluated in an open controlled trial.

Methods

Technology

The following equipment was used (Fig. 15.1):

- codec – used for receiving and for transmitting video pictures
- Pentium III 600 MHz 128 MByte RAM, MPEG-2 encoder/decoder card, 10/100 Mbit/s network card, Windows NT
- Graphics PC – used for presentation/application-sharing/ whiteboard functionality
- Pentium III 500 MHz, 128 MByte RAM, Windows NT, 10/100 Mbit/s network card, presentation software, e.g. 'MS PowerPoint', whiteboard software.

Video pictures were compressed using MPEG-2 compression.[1] This allowed the real-time exchange of histological images, video pictures of the lecturer, whiteboard content and voice. The high-speed Internet connection used the B-WIN network.[2] This is a fast (155 Mbit/s) backbone connecting universities and other educational institutions in Thuringia and Germany (Fig. 15.2).

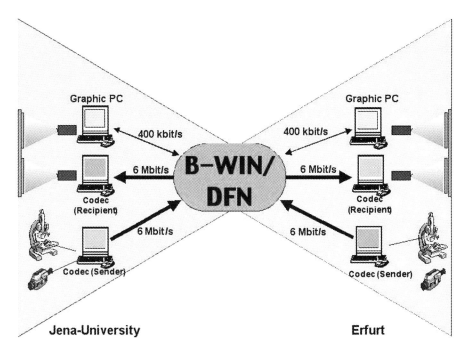

Fig. 15.1 Technical architecture for the teledermatohistological cooperation between Jena and Erfurt.

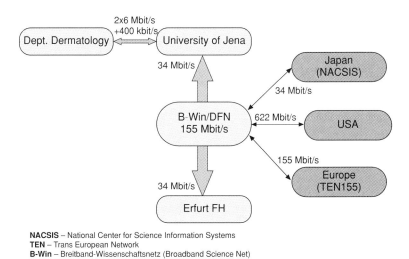

NACSIS – National Center for Science Information Systems
TEN – Trans European Network
B-Win – Breitband-Wissenschaftsnetz (Broadband Science Net)
DFN – Deutsches Forschungsnetz (German Research Net)

Fig. 15.2 Connections between Jena and Erfurt and with other international networks.

Student lectures

In the dermatological education of medical students the explanation of the histological background of the different dermatological diseases is difficult in a clinical setting. We decided to implement extra lessons focusing on dermatohistology. The lecturer presents the history of two or three different dermatological cases (Fig. 15.3). First, clinical findings and the results of technical investigations, blood samples and swabs are discussed. Second, dermatohistological findings are presented and discussed in detail. During these interactive lectures the lecturer communicates using a radiomicrophone and the whiteboard for a bidirectional exchange of written or drawn information. We plan to conduct five teledermatohistological lessons each term (they have not yet begun).

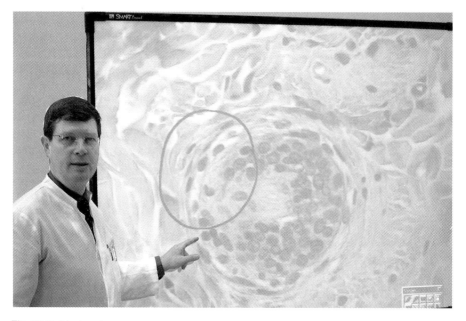

Fig. 15.3 A lecture in progress.

Medical specialist education

During these lessons the same technology is used. Rare cases are presented to the remote partners as well as to the local colleagues. A discussion about the cases follows, a standardized diagnostic procedure is worked out and plans for treatment are outlined. Visiting experts temporarily staying in Jena or Erfurt explain and discuss interesting cases.

Evaluation strategy

To evaluate our teleteaching project we plan to determine the opinion of students and lecturers. We will assess the following items:

Students:

- quality of transmitted histological images

- quality of transmitted video/audio of the lecturer

- quality of the lesson (presentation, quality of slides and figures, content of the lesson)

- opinion about interaction between students and lecturer, or between students in different lecture halls

- preference for traditional or new teaching models.

Lecturer:

- effort required to prepare a lesson (e.g. to create PowerPoint slides or to scan macroscopic photographic slides)

- effort to establish the connection and the degree of technical assistance needed

- distracting effect of the technology

- interaction between the lecturer and the local and remote students

- usability of the whiteboard.

Results

The aim of the present study was to evaluate the technical requirements for data transmission. We found the following to be necessary. For adequate video quality 25 frames per second using the CIF (Common Intermediate Format) picture format (352 × 288 pixels) or the 4CIF format (704 × 480 pixels) are desirable. For synchronous transmission of voice and video data the MPEG-2 standard has to be used. This standard uses a 24-bit colour depth (16 million colours). This resolution and colour depth guarantees an appropriate image quality. Using IP videoconferencing (H.263 standard[3]), audio and video data are transmitted in different data packets resulting in a desynchronization of spoken content and transmitted video pictures. For our purposes we found the optimum data-rate to be 6 Mbit/s and the minimum data rate to be 3 Mbit/s. The B-WIN backbone does not guarantee quality of service so that the actual data-rate achieved depends on the other activities in progress on the network. If the bandwidth needs to be shared with too many other participants the usable data-rate falls below 3 Mbit/s leading to pixel-artefacts or the total breakdown (and re-establishment after a few seconds) of the connection.

For the application sharing and whiteboard functions a connection using the T.120 conferencing standard[4] with a data-rate of 400 kbit/s was found to meet our needs. Using this as the graphics channel it is possible to transmit prepared slides or to draw on the whiteboard with sufficient quality. The two-way projection of video-images and graphics channel information allows a high level of interactivity.

During the installation of the necessary infrastructure problems arose in setting up a high-speed link to the B-WIN network. Most difficulties were caused by the configuration of the local computer network. To maintain adequate transmission quality a minimum network speed of 2×6 Mbit/s + 400 kbit/s was required, as described above. Major parts of the local network infrastructure are still based on the 10 Mbit/s standard so that the required speed could not be achieved. Another problem is the use of firewalls which control all outgoing data traffic.[5,6] For security reasons a computer scans each Internet-protocol (IP) packet for sender, recipient and content. If the outgoing traffic is low and the firewall is fast enough no harm is done to the connection. However in times of heavy traffic all outgoing packets get placed on a stack (buffered) and are processed in order of arrival. This can lead to a delay in the delivery of the packets for a teleteaching lesson. Depending on the delay the results are pixel artefacts or a (temporary) breakdown of the connection.

The acoustics of the lecture hall can be another problem. In halls with bad acoustic design the noise of the speakers is reflected and again recorded. With a delay of 500 ms, echos occur which make it difficult to follow the lecturer's talk. We also integrated all the control devices for the audiovisual equipment (video, audio, presentation, room-lights and window blinds) into the speaker's desk. For lecturers not familiar with the equipment the management of all these devices turned out to be very difficult.

Until now the evaluation of our project has focused on the technical issues described above. In the future we will concentrate on evaluating the quality of the lessons.

Despite the unavoidable problems in planning and carrying out teledermatology lessons there have been several positive outcomes. The telemedical cooperation offers the chance of providing high-quality medical education to students and residents. Beside this, students and medical staff get trained to work with the new technologies that are necessary to obtain suitable skills and knowledge for telepractice.[7,8] The telemedical infrastructure provides an easier and quicker way of sharing valuable medical expertise.[9,10]

Even the patient can benefit: first, a better educated medical staff will provide a more reliable medical service; second, difficult dermatological cases can be discussed between doctors who are specialists in the respective field.

Conclusion

Although the influence of the Internet is growing in all parts of daily life, the effect on medical practice is still small. Many physicians are not yet aware of the opportunities provided by new technology. In visual specialties such as radiology and dermatology the application of technology provides a greatly improved medical service. On the one hand, the interaction with the patient can be intensified. On the other hand, implementation of Internet technologies can take medical education a great step forward.

Our cooperation focuses on the dermatohistopathological education of our students and staff. Therefore we have established a conferencing system together with the

Department of Dermatology of Erfurt which has a high level of expertise in this field. This system uses a high-speed network connecting universities and other educational institutions, which permits the sharing of histological image information, voice and video pictures of the lecturer, as well as whiteboard functions.

We have defined the technical requirements for establishing a conference at an acceptable quality. We believe that these new ways of educating our students represent a better way of teaching. We hope to fill them with enthusiasm and for this reason increase their dermatological knowledge. This may also be seen as a good way to make our university more attractive to students and to assistant physicians. Further investigations will show to what extent these hopes are realized.

References

1   International Organisation for Standardisation. *ISO 13818-1: Coding of Moving Pictures and Audio.* 1995. (http://www.cselt.it/mpeg/ [last checked 29 July 2001]).
2   DFN Geschäftsstelle Berlin. (http://www.dfn.de/win [last checked 29 July 2001]).
3   International Telecommunication Union. *ITU-T Rec. H.263 Video coding for Low Bitrate Communication.* 1995.
4   International Telecommunication Union. *ITU-T Rec. T.120 Data Protocols for Multimedia Conferencing.* Geneva: International Telecommunication Union, 1996.
5   Cheswick WR, Bellovin SM. *Firewalls and Internet Security: Repelling the Wily Hacker.* Reading, MA: Addison Wesley, 1994.
6   Chapman DB, Zwicky ED. *Building Internet Firewalls.* Sebastapol, CA: O'Reilly and Associates, 1995.
7   Picot J. Meeting the need for educational standards in the practice of telemedicine and telehealth. *Journal of Telemedicine and Telecare* 2000;**6**(suppl 2):59–62.
8   Blignault I, Kennedy C. Training for telemedicine. *Journal of Telemedicine and Telecare* 1999;**5**(suppl 1):112–114.
9   Filler TJ, Jerosch J, Peuker ET. Live interdisciplinary teaching via the internet. *Computer Methods and Programs in Biomedicine* 2000;**61**:157–162.
10   Demartines N, Mutter D, Vix M. Assessment of telemedicine in surgical education and patient care. *Annals of Surgery* 2000;**231**:282–291.

Section 4: The Future

16

The Development of Standards in Teledermatology

Marta J. Petersen and Margretta A. O'Reilly

Introduction

The need for standards as they relate to exchange of information in health care is well recognized. According to a recently published report[1] by the National Committee on Vital and Health Statistics, 'the greatest impediment to the adoption of information technology is the lack of complete and comprehensive standards for patient medical record information'. The report defined standards as a prescribed set of rules or conditions related to systems that: classify components; specify materials, performance or service; or delineate procedures. As telemedicine services become further integrated into the delivery of health care, the development of standards for each element of the encounter are important in order to facilitate the exchange of information and seamless integration between systems. Standards can be applied to each component of a teledermatology consultation, ranging from the technical (image capture, videoconferencing protocols, transmission speed for real-time consultations) to patient data including content (such as images, identifiers or clinically relevant text) and the lexicon employed to convey this information.

This chapter discusses hardware standards and issues related to standards as they apply to patient medical record information. Standards pertaining to image acquisition are discussed elsewhere in this book. Very few specific standards have been developed for teledermatology, in contrast to radiology where the DICOM (Digital Imaging and Communication) Standards Committee has been in existence for almost 20 years. It should also be noted that technical standards in telemedicine, telecommunications and electronic data interchange are rapidly evolving.

Network and hardware standards

'Interoperability' and 'open architecture systems' are terms used to describe the design of telemedicine networks. Interoperability is defined as 'the condition achieved among communications-electronics systems when information or services can be exchanged directly and satisfactorily between them and/or their users'.[2] An open architecture system is one that complies with and uses readily available standards in order to promote interoperability within and between networks. So-called 'proprietary' systems use algorithms developed by a specific manufacturer that might work properly only when interfaced with equipment from the same company. However, the use of standards-based hardware does not guarantee interoperability between systems in all cases, i.e. conformance to standards is a necessary, but not sufficient, condition for interoperability.

In the USA, both state and federal governments have begun to mandate 'open systems' when taxpayers' money is used to fund network development.[3] Interoperability and compatibility are stressed in a set of guidelines developed by the Office for the Advancement of Telehealth (OAT).[4] In its 1999 Final Report, the Alaska Telehealth Advisory Commission established four guiding principles for the development of telehealth technologies, the second of which states 'All entities participating in telehealth must assure that their systems meet interconnectivity and interoperability standards'.[5]

Videoconferencing is an area where there has been significant progress in the development and adoption of industry-wide standards. Until the mid-1990s, proprietary compression algorithms hindered interoperability between videoconferencing units from different manufacturers. Today, standards set by the International Telecommunication Union[6] have been adopted almost worldwide. The main standards that apply to videoconferencing are: H.320 for circuit-switched transmission (e.g. ISDN lines); H.323 for packet-switched transmission (e.g. Internet Protocol (IP) video on local area and wide area network lines); and H.324 for transmission over ordinary telephone lines.

Teleradiology is an area of telemedicine in which standards have been developed and widely adopted by industry. The so-called DICOM standard was developed jointly by the American College of Radiology (ACR) and the National Electrical Manufacturers Association (NEMA). The aim was to provide 'an interface between imaging equipment and whatever the user wanted to connect'. When initially developed, the DICOM standard included specifications for hardware connections, plus a dictionary of 'data elements needed for proper display and interpretation'.[7] Newer versions of the standard include specifications for radiology, ultrasound and visible light images. The current version, DICOM 3.0, is an object-oriented model using SNOMED (Systematized Nomenclature of Human and Veterinary Medicine) International as the vocabulary for coded data.

With regard to teledermatology, organizations such as the American Telemedicine Association, the American Academy of Dermatology and the OAT have formed committees, task forces or special interest groups focusing on telemedicine and telehealth issues. These committees have issued sets of recommendations or guidelines regarding hardware, transmission modalities and room setup as it relates to telemedicine[4,8] and teledermatology[9,10] (see Appendix 16.1). However, these are only recommendations. Since they were not developed in collaboration with manufacturers or standards organizations (e.g. the American National Standards Institutes, ANSI), they are not in a position to be uniformly adopted, either by the users or the manufacturers.

Patient medical record information standards

Electronic exchange of patient information, while more easily grasped on an intuitive level than hardware standards, is a very complicated process. The National Committee on Vital and Health Statistics (NCVHS) is a statutory public advisory committee to the Secretary of Health and Human Services. The NCVHS issued the 'Report on Uniform Data Standards for Patient Medical Record Information'[1] in July 2000. The report emphasized that privacy, confidentiality and security were integral to the development of standards for electronic exchange of medical records. The report also emphasized the need for a broader health information infrastructure in order to move forward with electronic data exchange. Information infrastructure refers to the laws, regulations, standards, business practices and technologies required in order to share patient data in a secure manner. Information infrastructures have been widely developed and implemented in other industries such as banking. The report acknowledged that the healthcare industry has lagged behind in developing an industry-wide information infrastructure. In response to the problem, the NCVHS began to develop a separate set of recommendations about a national information infrastructure.

The NCVHS report recognized three levels of interoperability relating to the exchange of patient data: basic, functional and semantic. Basic interoperability allows the message (patient data) to be exchanged between computers but does not require the receiving computer to be able to interpret the data. Functional interoperability defines the structure, or format, of messages. By defining the syntax of the message, functional interoperability ensures that messages between computers can be interpreted at the level of data fields, but does not ensure that the meaning of the data fields is understood. Semantic interoperability provides common interpretability of data contained within the specific message fields. Semantic interoperability necessitates the use of standard message formats in conjunction with a standard vocabulary, such as SNOMED.

Message development organizations were formed in the early and mid 1980s to define standards for the electronic exchange of clinical data, in order to reduce the cost of interfacing different systems. At present, more than 80% of medical interfaces adhere to one of the most common message standards.[11] DICOM and HL7 (Health Level 7) are examples of two widely adopted message standards used in telehealth applications. HL7, an ANSI-accredited standard, standardizes how messages are defined in regard to healthcare services, including: patient administration (admit, discharge, transfer, demographics); orders for clinical observation, pharmacy, diet and supplies; accounting and charges; appointment scheduling and referrals.[12] It is the most commonly used standard for numerical, textual and coded clinical data in the USA and has a number of international affiliates in Australia, New Zealand, Canada, England, Germany and the Netherlands. Extensible Markup Language, XML, is a computer markup language for documents containing structured information. It is an organizing program that both formats information and allows processing and transmission of data. It was developed in order that richly structured documents could be used over the Internet. XML is expected to be incorporated into the new HL7 v. 3.0 specification.

Teledermatology case presentation standard

Clinicians practising teledermatology have recognized the need for practice standards for all aspects of a teledermatology consultation, from image acquisition and resolution to historical data supplied to the consultant from the referring practitioner.[13,14] Examination of the literature and telemedicine websites reveals that many teledermatology programmes have developed their own teledermatology consultation forms for their own use.[15] However, the lack of a standard format for consultations has compromised analysis of the efficacy and usefulness of teledermatology in general.

The need for a general or standard case presentation format for teledermatology was discussed in May 2000 at a meeting of the Teledermatology Special Interest Group of the American Telemedicine Association. The group decided to survey existing forms in use by teledermatology providers and create a standard case presentation format. Protocols from seven teledermatology programmes (San Francisco, Travis Air Force Base, Uniformed Services University of the Health Sciences, University of Arizona, University of Miami, University of Utah and the Walter Reed Medical Center) were reviewed. The core components, present in all protocols, were identified (Box 16.1).

The case presentation format was created from these core components. Both a Short Form for routine cases and a Long Form for more complex cases were developed. A simple form for use in busy primary care settings (Short Form) was considered

---

Box 16.1. Core components of case presentation

Consultation information
Date of consultation request
Name of referring provider
Address of referring provider
Contact information for referring provider (e.g. phone and fax, email address)

Patient information
Patient name
Date of birth/age
Unique patient identifier (e.g. social security number, medical record number)
Sex
Ethnicity

Problem information
Reason for consultation: chief complaint
Location of skin lesions/rash
Onset and duration of problem
Precipitating, exacerbating and palliative factors
Associated signs, symptoms – character, severity
Prior diagnostic/therapeutic measures, outcomes
Number of images sent (store-and-forward consultations)

Box 16.2.   Case presentation – short form

Patient identifiers {space for imprint}	**Entry field**
Date	yyyy/mm/dd
Patient name	[text box]
Date of birth:age	yyyy/mm/dd:age
MRN/SSN/identifier	[text box]
Sex	M/F
Ethnicity	{census pick list}
Referring physician/provider	[text box]
Location	[text box]
Contact phone/email	[text box]
Chief complaint/reason for consultation	[text box]
History	
History of present illness (HPI):	[text box] or { disease-specific HPI pick list}
Past dermatology/medical/surgical/ family/social history/review of symptoms (ROS):	Select non-contributory/relevant If relevant, enter data in [text box]
Medications (topical/systemic)	[text box] or attach list
Allergies	[text box] or attach list
Physical examination	
Physical examination	[text box], attach diagrams if pertinent
Clinical images	Enter number of images, other pertinent information [text box]
Other data	
Biopsies	Yes/no [text box – date, results] or attach document(s)
Pertinent laboratory data	Yes/no [text box – date, results] or attach document(s)
Provisional diagnosis:	[text box]

important, and was limited to one page in order to facilitate its use (Box 16.2). For more complex cases, and those with significant teaching value, the more detailed Long Form was developed (Box 16.3). Patient identifiers, demographic information and the presenting problem are common to both Short and Long Forms. The History of Presenting Illness (HPI) may be entered in an open text box, or entered by selecting from a list for disease-specific dermatological HPI. Past history is collapsed in the Short Form and may be omitted if not relevant. By contrast, each section of the past history can be answered individually, when relevant, in the Long Form. Ideally, information already available electronically (e.g. medication lists, allergies, problem lists/history, laboratory data, pathology and radiology results) will be attached to the document to avoid re-entering data. Since digital images will constitute the major part of the physical examination data, the number of images is a required field. The Case Presentation Forms have yet to be tested in clinical teledermatology settings.

Box 16.3. Case presentation – long form

Patient identifiers {space for imprint}	**Entry field**
Date	yyyy/mm/dd
Patient name	[text box]
Date of birth:age	yyyy/mm/dd:age
MRN/SSN/identifier	[text box]
Sex	M/F
Ethnicity	{census pick list}
Referring physician/provider	[text box]
Location	[text box]
Contact phone/email	[text box]
Chief complaint/reason for consultation	[text box]
History	
History of present illness (HPI)	[text box] or {pick list of disease-specific HPI, e.g. acne HPI, pigmented lesions HPI, alopecia HPI, urticaria HPI, rash HPI}
Past dermatology history:	[text box], or select from atopic history (asthma, allergies, eczema, hayfever, family history), none, unknown
Past medical history – systemic illness/hospitalizations immunocompromise	[text box] or attach list
Past surgical history:	[text box] or attach list
Family history:	Select non-contributory or [text box]
Social history/employment/activities	[text box]; {S, M, D, W}; tobacco, alcohol; [text box]
Review of symptoms (ROS):	Select non-contributory/relevant; if relevant, {pick list of organ systems}, [text box]
Medications (topical/systemic)	[text box] or attach list
Allergies	[text box] or attach list
Physical examination	
Physical examination:	
general patient description	{well-developed white male (WDWM),
vital signs	acutely ill, chronically ill}
description	[text box]
	[text box], attach diagrams if pertinent
Clinical images	Enter number of images, other pertinent information [text box]
Other data	
Biopsies	Yes/no [text box – date, results] or attach document(s)
Pertinent laboratory data	Yes/no [text box – date, results] or attach document(s)
Provisional diagnosis:	[text box]

Conclusions

Development and implementation of standards in teledermatology and telemedicine in general have lagged behind both the technology and the delivery of healthcare services. Various organizations (including the American Telemedicine Association and the American Academy of Dermatology) and government agencies (such as the Office for the Advancement of Telehealth) have formulated guidelines and recommendations for teledermatology. However, unlike the situation in radiology, working groups consisting of clinicians, medical informaticists and industry representatives have not established an ANSI-accredited Standard Development Organization such as DICOM.

In the USA, implementation of the Health Insurance Portability and Accountability Act (HIPAA) within the next two years has and will continue to push the development of standards and requirements for electronic transmission of health information. The National Committee on Vital and Health Statistics is currently developing recommendations for patient medical record information standards and has previously recommended funding to accelerate the development and adoption of such standards.[1] Adoption of patient medical record information standards will greatly facilitate the development and adoption of more case presentation standards in teledermatology, and telemedicine in general.

References

1   *Report on Uniform Data Standards for Patient Medical Record Information.* National Committee on Vital and Health Statistics. 6 July 2000. (http://www.cpri-host.org/events/meetings/2000annual/ppt/blair-cohn/ [last checked 29 July 2001]).
2   Federal Standard 1037C. *Telecommunications: Glossary of Telecommunications Terms.* (http://www.its.bldrdoc.gov/fs-1037/ [last checked 29 July 2001]).
3   H.B. 72, Utah Telehealth Commission, 2000 General Session, State of Utah. (http://www.le.state.ut.us/~2000/bills/hbillenr/HB0072.htm).
4   Office for the Advancement of Telehealth. Telehealth Technology Guidelines, 1999. (http://telehealth.hrsa.gov/pubs/tech/techhome.htm [last checked 29 July 2001]).
5   State of Alaska, Department of Health and Social Services. Alaska Telehealth Advisory Commission: Final Report, June 1999. (http://www.hss.state.ak.us/atac/ [last checked 29 July 2001]).
6   International Telecommunication Union. (http://www.itu.int/ITU-T/index.html [last checked 29 July 2001]).
7   http://medical.nema.org/dicom.html [last checked 29 July 2001].
8   Simmons SC, Craft R, Balch D, Bath PE. American Telemedicine Association, Special Interest Group White Paper. (http://www.atmeda.org/icot/technologysigrec.htm [last checked 29 July 2001]).
9   Tracy J, Sprang R, Burgiss S. Office for the Advancement of Telehealth. Telehealth Technology Guidelines: Dermatology. (http://telehealth.hrsa.gov/pubs/tech/derm.htm [last checked 29 July 2001]).
10 Telemedicine Task Force, American Academy of Dermatology, Position Statement on Telemedicine. 2000. (http://www.aad.org/Members/telemedicine.html) [available only to members of the American Academy of Dermatology]).
11 Huff SM. Clinical data exchange standards and vocabularies for messages. In: *American Medical Informatics Association Symposium, 1998.* (http://www.amia.org/pubs/symposia/D005239.PDF [last checked 29 July 2001]).
12 Health Level 7. (http://www.hl7.org/ [last checked 29 July 2001]).
13 Zelickson BD, Homan L. Teledermatology in the nursing home. *Archives of Dermatology* 1997;**133**:171–174.
14 Vidmar DA. Plea for standardization in teledermatology: a worm's eye view. *Telemedicine Journal* 1997;**3**:173–178.
15 Norton SA, Burdick AE, Phillips CM, Berman B. Teledermatology and underserved populations. *Archives of Dermatology* 1997;**133**:197–200.

Appendix 16.1 American Academy of Dermatology Position Statement on Telemedicine: 2001

The Task Force on Telemedicine and its consultants have put considerable effort into determining what telemedicine issues affect dermatologists and recommending courses of action for those issues. They are as follows:

I. Qualifications, credentialing and privileging

Recommendation: Because of the emphasis on clinical slide conferences in dermatology residency training programs, dermatologists are eminently qualified to render diagnoses from images. For this reason, dermatologists who perform telemedicine consultations should have completed an ACGME-accredited dermatology residency program or the international equivalent for dermatologists outside of the United States. Dermatologists should adhere to credentialing and privileging requirements of institutions for whom they perform telemedicine consultations.

II. Ancillary telemedicine personnel

Recommendation: Ancillary telemedicine personnel should have an appropriate medical background so that they understand the need for privacy and confidentiality and have a knowledgeable and professional manner with telemedicine encounters. Such personnel must be trained to operate telemedicine equipment and perform user level maintenance.

III. Medical records

Recommendation: Appropriate medical records should be available to the consulting dermatologist prior to or at the time of the telemedicine encounter. This information should include specific questions that the referring physician wishes answered. A copy of the record generated by the telemedicine consultation should be subsequently available at both the consultant and referral sites. These records should be maintained according to regulations at each site.

IV. Privacy and confidentiality

Recommendation: Privacy and confidentiality must be maintained at a level comparable to face to face physician/patient encounters. The patient's dignity must be protected throughout the consultation. Informed consent should be obtained prior to all telemedicine encounters.

V. Patient safety

Recommendation: All telemedicine equipment coming in physical contact with the patient during a telemedicine examination should be Underwriter Laboratory (UL) approved (or the international equivalent). Specific safety protocols for telemedicine equipment should be developed for telemedicine examination rooms by institutions serving as referral sites for telemedicine consultations.

VI. System capabilities

Recommendation: Imaging and communications hardware used for telemedicine consultations should possess at least the following minimal capabilities. The color rendered by the monitor and camera should represent true colors. To ensure this, equipment should be calibrated for color correction according to their specifications, including such techniques as a 'color wheel' if appropriate.

Analog color display:

▶ 450 TV lines of resolution.

Analog color camera output:

▶ 450 TV lines of resolution.

Digital display:

▶ .28 dot pitch

▶ 640 × 480 pixel spatial resolution

▶ 24 bit color depth.

Digital color output:

▶ Single chip camera

▶ 1 K × 1 K spatial resolution

▶ 24 bit color depth.

Three chip camera:

▶ output equivalent to spatial resolution of a 1 K × 1 K single chip camera

▶ 24 bit color depth.

Video conferencing systems:

▶ adhere to standards developed by the International Telecommunications Union (ITU)

▶ capable of providing a resolution of 14 line pairs per mm resolution documented by use of a high contrast test object such as a 1951 United States Air Force test pattern (this should be obtainable without requiring the use of a contact microscope peripheral device)

▶ capable of accurately producing a full range of human skin tones.

Adoption of standards for compression are difficult at this time because research in their use for dermatology is limited. Standards for creation and transmission of clinical information are also in a state of flux. No national or international policy has evolved as it relates to transmission of medical information over telecommunication networks, particularly the Internet. For the present it is recommended that at least two layers of security be implemented (including passwording and encryption) for non-dedicated lines. Access to dedicated lines through multi-point control units and other switching devices should also be appropriately protected. The Board of Directors of the American Medical Informatics Association have developed explicit guidelines for the clinical use of E-mail (appendix A). Adherence to these guidelines is recommended.

VII. Clinical examination environment

Recommendation: Qualities of the telemedicine examination area directly impact the effectiveness of telemedicine consultations. For interactive full-motion consultations, ambient light of uniform color temperature throughout the room is important. For all types of telemedicine consultations, light should be of appropriate intensity to provide the greatest possible depth of field for imaging devices. Directional lighting should be available in order to provide a sense of dimensionality to skin lesions.

VIII. Licensing

Recommendation: Laws vary from state to state, and the AAD advises all dermatologists to be in compliance with all regulatory directives. However, telemedicine at this time is an inherent consultative activity. The situation is analogous to a patient being sent to another physician's office for consultation, as the patient's image is being sent. In the classic model where the patient travels, this may or may not be within the boundaries of a particular state. The consulting is done in the consultant's office, and therefore the physicians state licensure is accepted at the site where the consultant is rendering their opinion. The AAD supports the position that during a telemedicine consultation, the physician is rendering his/her opinion from his/her place of practice and therefore the consultant should be licensed in the state where she/he is rendering her/his opinion and NOT in the state where the patient is located.

IX. Reimbursement

Recommendation: In the interest of making dermatologic expertise available to all patients, reimbursement for telemedicine consultations by public (Medicare and Medicaid) and private third party payors is supported at least at the same level as an office consultation. Although this is recognized to be predominantly an American problem, it may have international dimensions. Each healthcare funding system will need to resolve reimbursement issues locally.

X. Becoming involved in telemedicine

Recommendation: Many telemedicine programs are intra-state serving natural geographic referral areas. It is recommended that dermatologists living in these areas investigate the possibility of participating in one of these programs in an effort to assist patients with limited access to specialist care. Limited access may be due to geographic reasons, physical infirmity, transportation difficulties, incarceration or occupational factors.

XI. Telemedicine research

Recommendation: The Telemedicine Task Force recommends that the American Academy of Dermatology take a lead role in encouraging studies that document the effectiveness of the teledermatology encounters as compared to the effectiveness of face to face patient encounter. The focus for these studies should include patient outcomes.

The Task Force also supports the position that the American Academy of Dermatology keep open communication channels and develop interactions with other specialties and appropriate organizations such as the American Telemedicine Association and the Association of Telemedicine Service Providers. These interactions should greatly assist the Academy with its responsibility to keep the membership informed of pertinent changes or evolving issues in telemedicine.

Acknowledgment

The Regulations Sub-Committee wishes to thank Phyllis F. Granade of Kilpatrick

Stockton LLP, Atlanta, GA, for her assistance in the preparation of this material. Ms. Granade serves as legal consultant to the Task Force. In addition, the task force members have been listed for their contributions.

1998–1999 Telemedicine Task Force Members:

Robert Schosser, MD 1998 Chair

Anne Burdick, MD

Rachel Clarke, MD

Scott Dinehart, MD

Rhett Drugge, MD

Clark Julius, MD

Charles Phillips, MD

Gary Rogers, MD

P. Robert Rigney, MD

Jack Lesher, Jr., MD

Mark Lowitt, MD

Kenneth Neldner, MD

Scott Norton, MD

Nolan Parsons, Jr., MD

Marie L Johnson, MD

Joseph Kvedar, MD

William Stoecker, MD

1999–2000 Telemedicine Task Force Members:

Anne Burdick, MD Current Chair

Rhett Drugge, MD

Jack Lesher, MD

Scott Norton, MD

Charles Phillips, MD

M. Joyce Rico, MD

Robert Weiss, MD

Armand Cognetta, MD

Joseph Kvedar, MD

Mark Lowitt, MD

Douglas Perednia, MD

Harold Rabinovitz, MD

Gary Rogers, MD

James Grichnik, MD

17

DICOM (Digital Imaging and Communications in Medicine) in Dermatology

Timothy K. Chartier

Introduction

There has been an upsurge in interest in telemedicine over the past decade. In 1998, it was estimated that there were over 130 active telemedicine programmes in the USA performing nearly 58 000 teleconsultations.[1] Important and often underappreciated foundations to this activity are the underlying protocols and standards. Communications standards are those standards that address the exchange of information by specifying, among other things, the form and flow of the exchanged data.

Telecommunications in medicine has been no exception to the fundamental issue of communications standards, and there is little doubt that they will play an increasingly important role in the success of telemedicine. This was evident during the development of digital imaging and radiology information systems (RIS). During these years the American College of Radiology together with the National Electrical Manufacturers created what has become the de facto international standard for the transfer of radiology digital images between image acquisition devices, display workstations, picture archiving and communications systems (PACS), printers and radiology information systems (RIS). This is the DICOM standard (Digital Imaging and Communications in Medicine). Until the DICOM standard had been agreed, each manufacturer and institution had independently developed proprietary systems for transferring digital imaging information between devices. As upgrades, new technology and new manufacturers were introduced the components did not interface properly thereby creating a chaotic environment. DICOM imposed order on this situation by creating a communications protocol that ensured interoperability of DICOM-compliant equipment.

Nowadays every major manufacturer of radiology imaging equipment and software incorporates the DICOM standard into their design, allowing easier integration of old and new equipment. It is expected that telemedicine systems will also need to develop their own set of standards to ensure their success as well. Several medical societies and telemedicine special interest groups are beginning to explore the issue of telemedicine standards. It is almost certain that in future telemedicine systems will require a set of standards by which they operate, and will also have to interface with other hospital information systems (HIS) including radiology information systems, picture-archiving computer systems, image information systems, as well as electronic patient medical record systems to ensure the exchange of necessary information. As telemedicine will undoubtedly include the acquisition and transmission of digital images, such systems will need to interface with existing DICOM-based image information systems.

DICOM overview

History of DICOM

With rapid advances in digital medical imaging acquisition, display, archiving and radiology information systems over the past three decades, it became clear by the early 1980s that a standard was necessary to ensure interoperability. In 1983, the American College of Radiology (ACR) joined forces with the National Electrical Manufacturers Association (NEMA) to create a standard protocol for transferring medical images and related data between medical devices regardless of the device manufacturer. Their goals were to promote the electronic communication of medically related digital imaging information (irrespective of manufacturer), to facilitate the development and expansion of image archiving computer systems and their interface with other hospital information systems, and to allow the creation of diagnostic information databases that could be interrogated by a wide variety of medical information systems regardless of location.[2]

The original ACR–NEMA Standards Publication was published in 1985 as version 1.0. Subsequent revisions over a 3-year period led to the publication of ACR–NEMA Standards Publication No. 300-1988, known as version 2.0, in 1988. At this point the standard, designed for radiology systems, specified a hardware interface using point-to-point interconnection, a minimum set of software commands, and a consistent set of data formats to which radiology-based imaging systems would adhere to ensure interoperability. Major revisions were made over the next few years, which led to version 3.0 in the early 1990s. Perhaps the most significant change related to networked environments based on the ISO (International Organization for Standardization) OSI (Open Systems Interconnection) Network Reference Model and TCP/IP (Transmission Control Protocol/Internet Protocol). It previously only supported point-to-point connections. Other important changes included restructuring the DICOM Standard into a multipart document thereby facilitating its future extension, the introduction of DICOM conformance standards, and the creation of new data structures to represent studies, series, reports, patients and the like as part of the DICOM Information Model.

The standard had clearly become more robust. However, as a standard developed for the field of radiology, it was largely only applicable to radiology. In 1993, the American National Standards Institute (ANSI) organized the Endoscopic Image Exchange Ad Hoc Committee with the aim of extending the DICOM Version 3.0 standard to include support for (colour) visible light imaging modalities such as endoscopy, microscopy and photography. In addition, a flurry of industry and medical specialty interest in the standard occurred between 1993 and 1998 (Box 17.1), which culminated in the development of Supplement 15 ('Visible Light Image for Endoscopy, Microscopy and Photography').[3] This supplement incorporated changes that affected every specialty involved in medical imaging. In addition, it provided a platform for the creation of telemedicine systems that involved networks, telecommunications, medical imaging and patient-related data.

Box 17.1. Medical society contributors to the development of the DICOM standard (partial listing)

American College of Radiology
American Society for Gastrointestinal Endoscopy
College of American Pathologists
American Dental Association
European Society for Gastrointestinal Endoscopy
Organisation Mondiale d'Endoscopie Digestive
American Academy of Ophthalmology
American Academy of Dermatology
American Association of Oral and Maxillofacial Radiologists
American College of Surgeons
International Association of Dentomaxillofacial Radiology
Society of American Gastrointestinal Endoscopic Surgeons
American Gastroenterological Association
American College of Chest Physicians
American Urological Association

In addition, Supplement 23 ('Structured Reporting'), introduced in 1997 by the DICOM Working Group 8 (see below for a discussion on DICOM Working Groups), further extended the DICOM Standard to support semantically rich interpretative reports.[4] Such reports can include text, codes, numerical measurements and waveforms, and allow a dermatologist or dermatopathologist, for instance, to convey a report of clinical or histological findings, including annotations and labels, measurements and text descriptions of significant findings. Furthermore, these findings can be linked to DICOM-image or waveform coordinates. To extend its support for standardized terminology, Supplement 23 introduced significant changes to the area of structured terminology using coded terminology mapping such as the SNOMED (Systematized Nomenclature of Medicine) DICOM Microglossary (SDM), the Health Level 7 (HL7) Vocabulary, and the Terminology Resource for Message Standards (TeRMS). These changes further enhanced the applicability and flexibility of the DICOM standard.

At present there are over 20 Supplements (and many more proposed changes) to the DICOM Base Standard (Box 17.2). These changes address various issues and their effect on medical imaging and information systems such as multimedia storage devices, the Internet, the World Wide Web, data compression, security and interfacing with other national and international standards relating to telecommunications and health information systems. In addition, the DICOM Committee (Working Group 20), together with HL7, the Radiological Society of North America (RSNA), and the

---

Box 17.2. DICOM Standard Supplements (partial listing)

Supplement 9: Multibyte Character Sets
Supplement 10: Worklist Management
Supplement 11: Radiotherapy

Supplement 15: Visible Light
Supplement 23: Structured Reporting
Supplement 29: Radiotherapy Treatment
Supplement 30: Waveform Interchange

Supplement 31: Security Enhancements One
Supplement 33: Grayscale Soft Copy
Presentation State Storage
Supplement 36: Codes and Controlled
Terminology
Supplement 40: DVD using UDF Media

Supplement 41: Security Enhancements Two
Supplement 45: Ultrasound Protocol Support
Supplement 48: Intravascular Ultrasound
IOD and Application Profile
Supplement 50: Mammography CAD
Supplement 51: Media Security
Supplement 52: Interpretation Worklist
Supplement 53: DICOM Content Mapping
Resource
Supplement 54: DICOM MIME Type
Supplement 55: Doppler Audio

Supplement 58: Hanging Protocols

Healthcare Information Management Systems Society (HIMSS), is actively involved in trying to integrate various medical information systems (RIS, HIS, image acquisition devices, network workstations and image archiving systems).

DICOM organizational overview

The DICOM Standards Committee is administered by the NEMA Diagnostic Imaging and Therapy Systems Division. As a standards development organization, it is devoted to creating and maintaining standards for the communication of biomedical images and associated information. It does this in conjunction with national and international members from a variety of standards organizations, professional organizations, manufacturing companies, trade associations and government agencies. The standard is developed in conjunction with other standards organizations including the American National Standards Institutes–Healthcare Informatics Standards Board (ANSI–HISB), the International Organization for Standardization (ISO), the Japan Industries Association of Radiological Systems (JIRA), the European Committee for Standardization (CEN), the Health Level 7 (HL7), the Systematized Nomenclature of Medicine (SNOMED), the JAMI (Japan Association of Medical Informatics) and more recently the Internet Engineering Task Force (IETF). It is composed of 21 working groups (Box 17.3). The Committee and its working groups meet several times each year. As new issues are identified, the working groups petition the Committee for work items. These work items take the form of either supplements or change proposals, and as they are completed they are sent to the Base Standards Working Group (WG6) for review, then to all interested parties for public comment, and from there to letter ballot once approved by the DICOM Committee. Once in letter ballot, DICOM members vote to approve the change, and if successful, the change becomes a part of the official DICOM Standard.

Box 17.3. DICOM Committee Working Groups

WG 1: Cardiac and Vascular Information	WG 12: Ultrasound
WG 2: Digital X-ray	WG 13: Visible Light
WG 3: Nuclear Medicine	WG 14: Security
WG 4: Compression	WG 15: Digital Mammography
WG 5: Exchange Media	WG 16: Magnetic Resonance
WG 6: Base Standard	WG 17: 3D
WG 7: Radiotherapy	WG 18: Clinical Trials and Education
WG 8: Structured Reporting	WG 19: Dermatologic Standards
WG 9: Ophthalmology	WG 20: Integration of Imaging and Information
WG 10: Strategic Advisory	Systems
WG 11: Display Function Standard	WG 21: Computed Tomography

DICOM technical overview

DICOM is a non-proprietary communications protocol that specifies how imaging devices transmit digital images and information related to these images. It defines the form and flow of these interactions by specifying: (i) the information content, including both its structure and encoding; (ii) a set of DICOM services for managing the information; and (iii) a messaging protocol. Applications written to the DICOM Standard (DICOM applications) will be able to establish a communications session and exchange information reliably regardless of the source of hardware or software.

DICOM information model

The DICOM information model is a model of real-world entities (e.g. patients, images, visits and reports) and their relationship. The information model represents the important entities and relationships in medical imaging, not insurance billing, patient medical records or other medical information domains, although there is a certain degree of overlap. The entity-relationship diagram provides the foundation on which the DICOM standard is built, and lays the framework for DICOM data structures and their relationships.

Using this model and an object-oriented design approach, DICOM builds a series of data structures (called information object definitions, or IODs) to represent real-world entities such as a CT scan or a photographic image, and allows applications conforming to the DICOM standard to exchange, and to manage, these IODs using a set of defined DICOM services, called DIMSE services. Both IODs and DICOM services are discussed in more detail below. At this point it is important only to understand this division of information from services, and their relationship. Furthermore, DIMSE services can be grouped together as service groups and combined with IODs to build a set of service object pair (SOP) classes useful to accomplish a given task, such as image management or printing. For instance, an IOD representing a 'CT scan' might be combined with the DICOM service 'STORE' for storing a CT scan on a networked storage device such as a network hard drive or a PACS system.

DICOM information object definitions

Information object definitions (IODs) represent the data (information) component of DICOM. They are templates of 'attributes' that represent real-world entities (such as a digital CT scan or a photographic picture), or a related group of information (such as patient name, patient ID or data describing under what conditions an image was collected). To make the design more logical and modular (for reuse and extensibility purposes), collections of related attributes are combined into 'modules', and IODs are, in turn, built from these. An IOD is, therefore, a collection of related attributes (similar to 'structures' in computer programming). An example of the visible light supplement (VL) photographic image IOD is shown in Figure 17.1. Also shown is an expansion of the 'general image module' to illustrate both the attributes of the module and the object-oriented design of the IODs. DICOM defines numerous generic modules and

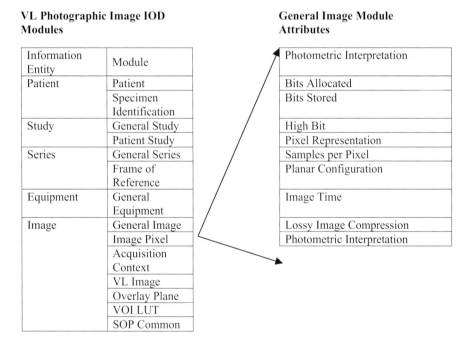

VL Photographic Image IOD Modules

Information Entity	Module
Patient	Patient
	Specimen Identification
Study	General Study
	Patient Study
Series	General Series
	Frame of Reference
Equipment	General Equipment
Image	General Image
	Image Pixel
	Acquisition Context
	VL Image
	Overlay Plane
	VOI LUT
	SOP Common

General Image Module Attributes

Attribute
Photometric Interpretation
Bits Allocated
Bits Stored
High Bit
Pixel Representation
Samples per Pixel
Planar Configuration
Image Time
Lossy Image Compression
Photometric Interpretation

Fig. 17.1. The visible light photographic image information object definition with expansion of the general image module to illustrate both the module's attributes as well as the modular nature of IODs.

IODs for a variety of radiological images (e.g. CT scan, MRI, nuclear medicine and ultrasound) and visible light images (e.g. endoscopy, photography and microscopy) as well as for patient, visit, study, results, interpretation and printer information management.

DICOM IODs are classified as either 'normalized' or 'composite'. (The term normalized here bears no relationship to its use in databases.) Normalized IODs are used to denote IODs that contain attributes describing a single real-world entity in the DICOM information model such as patient information, visit information and study information. A composite IOD, on the other hand, is an IOD that contains attributes describing information about related real-world entities that is not inherent in the real world entity itself. Examples of composite IODs include the CT IOD, MRI IOD, ultrasound IOD, and VL photographic image IOD. These IODs contain not only the image information, but also important information related to, but not inherent in, the image. Composite IODs are the ones most often employed for image management applications.

It is important to realize that the image data (the actual, or raw, image) are merely a component of the (photographic) image IOD and are represented by the 'pixel data' attribute of the 'image pixel' module (not shown). Therefore, when two DICOM applications exchange an image, they actually exchange an IOD. This IOD contains, in addition to the actual raw image data, other image-related information. This additional information is sometimes called 'meta-data' and is one of the important differences between a mature communications protocol such as DICOM and other more rudimentary communications protocols such as the file transport protocol (FTP), email or hypertext transport protocol (HTTP) that can be used to exchange medical images in simple telemedicine systems. Although one could easily use any of these protocols to transfer an image, none of them require, or provide, a standardized and consistent method of including image-related 'meta-data'. As such, systems built on these protocols need to have custom-built interfaces for incorporating these data, and are fraught with potential data integrity and interface problems. Furthermore, without consistent representation of the image and its meta-data, it is difficult to build robust information systems that allow sophisticated queries and data retrieval. In addition, without incorporating appropriate measures aimed at protecting the integrity and quality of the data, such systems create the potential for violating patient confidentiality (as patient X's image inadvertently becomes associated with patient Y).

Therefore, DICOM image IODs contain not only the image data, but also important information about the image. For instance, the example composite image IOD contains information about the patient (the subject of the image) represented by the 'patient information entity' (patient IE), the study ('study IE'), the series of images collected ('series IE'), and the equipment ('equipment IE') used to generate the image(s). In addition, important information about the physical image itself is also incorporated into the IOD including the acquisition context ('acquisition context' module), number of bits allocated per pixel ('bits allocated' attribute), number of samples per pixel ('sample per pixel' attribute), and whether or not a lossy compression algorithm has been employed ('lossy image compression' attribute), as well as others. In this way, the DICOM standard promotes data quality and integrity by ensuring that important structured information about the image is coupled with the image, and that the image and its 'meta-data' travel together.

Another important point about the DICOM standard is that it does not impose restrictions about the resolution or colour depth of the image. Instead, it leaves these details to those who implement the applications. Therefore, if in dermatology it is necessary for diagnostic accuracy that an image must be acquired at a minimum resolution of 800×600 pixels, for example, then the DICOM standard does not restrict this. It does, however, require that the DICOM applications communicate this resolution information ('meta-data') as part of the image data (IOD) so that the applications and users are aware of this important piece of information.

Attributes contain the values used to describe an entity. For instance, in a transaction between two DICOM-compliant applications, the 'bits allocated' attribute of an exchanged VL photographic image IOD may contain the value 8. The value contained by an attribute can be a major source of incompatibility between disparate computer systems. To avoid such incompatibility issues, the DICOM committee, with the help of the ANSI, IEEE (Institute of Electrical and Electronic Engineers) and ISO organizations, has specifically addressed this by specifying: (i) what type of data (data type) the attribute is (e.g. character string, date, name, unsigned integer, double precision floating point); (ii) the encoding of each data type (i.e. how many bytes long the data type must be and how the bytes are ordered); and (iii) how the attributes (the form) are transmitted. Therefore, a great deal of technical detail is included at every level to ensure reliable communications between computer systems.

DICOM services

DICOM services play an important role in the DICOM information model. Also called DICOM message service elements (DIMSE), these services operate on (perform functions on) DICOM IODs. They are used to perform a variety of data management functions, such as transferring and storing images (in the form of IODs) from an image-acquisition device to an image-archiving system. In the DICOM model, services are grouped together with an IOD to form a service object pair (SOP) class. SOP classes are created to accomplish a specific purpose (such as image retrieval and management) and are specified within service classes according to their purpose. In addition, similar to IODs, SOP classes are broken down into composite and normalized types depending upon whether they are composed of composite or normalized IODs, respectively. Examples of both normalized and composite DICOM services are shown in Box 17.4.

Before requesting any DIMSE services, DICOM-compliant applications must first establish a connection, or association. This is done using the association management services, A-ASSOCIATE and A-RELEASE. During association establishment information is exchanged between DICOM-compliant applications that allows the DICOM applications to arrive at an understanding on what information will be exchanged, the structure and encoding of that information, and the services requested and offered. Association management is handled by an upper layer protocol (called the

Box 17.4. DIMSE services

Normalized:	Composite:
N-ACTION	C-ECHO
N-CREATE	C-FIND
N-DELETE	C-GET
N-EVENT-REPORT	C-MOVE
N-GET	C-STORE
N-SET	

association control service element) that fits logically between the DICOM application and the TCP/IP stack, or lower level OSI layers.

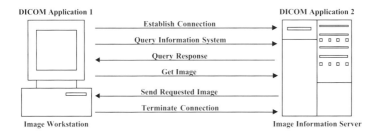

Fig. 17.2. Example of the interaction between two DICOM applications, applications 1 and 2. The diagram depicts an image display workstation retrieving an image from an image information system and the general sequence of events involved in such a transaction.

To illustrate how this works, Figure 17.2 shows the general sequence of events that occurs as application 1 queries and retrieves an image from application 2, the image archiving system. Before any image-related information can be exchanged, the two applications must first establish an association (A-ASSOCIATE). Once an association is established, application 1 queries application 2 (C-FIND) for image X on patient Y. Application 2 returns a response to application 1 indicating the success of the search request. Assuming a successful match was found, application 1 then sends another request to application 2 requesting retrieval (C-GET) of the image record from the repository. Application 2 sends the image to application 1 (C-STORE), and the association is terminated (A-RELEASE) in the final step.

Throughout the communications process, requests and responses are exchanged using a well-defined DICOM messaging protocol that is composed of service commands (such as C-STORE or C-GET) together with DICOM data structures (IODs). For instance, in the final C-STORE command sent from application 2 to application 1, the command was sent together with an IOD that contained, among other things, the image requested. Furthermore, to ensure reliable communications the syntax and structure of the exchanged message is precisely defined. By combining IODs and DIMSE services in this way, DICOM provides a series of SOP classes that support a broad range of image management functions including network image management, network image interpretation management, network printer management, imaging procedure management and off-line storage media management.

In addition, an important aspect of DICOM is that it operates independently of the underlying network – providing that the network conforms to existing TCP/IP or OSI network standards. Therefore, DICOM applications can communicate using a wide range of network types.

DICOM and dermatology

With the creation of the 'Visible Light Supplement' to DICOM (Supplement 15) for photographic and microscopic digital images, the DICOM standard became relevant to other specialties, including dermatology. Until this time dermatology had no real need for an electronic image communications protocol. For this reason the dermatology community was not involved in the early work of DICOM. Even the creation of the 'Visible Light Supplement' was done with very little input from the dermatology community.

Dermatology's lack of need for a digital imaging communications protocol stems from the fact that dermatologists did not take clinical pictures using digital cameras until recently. Furthermore, they have not traditionally needed to send digital images between providers or other parties, and have not needed to manage the resulting repositories of digital images. Even within the area of teledermatology, where digital imaging and digital communications are more common, most systems have been based on proprietary non-digital technology employing a combination of live videoconferencing systems or printed photographs (e.g. Polaroid) together with some other information exchange mechanism such as fax, telephone or ordinary mail.

Recently, however, there has been a change in the technology used to take clinical photographs and to implement teledermatology. Digital cameras and imaging are becoming more common, and piecemeal telemedicine systems are beginning to give way to more reliable, more cost-efficient, and more easily managed digital systems. All this information is transmitted over widely accessible electronic telecommunication networks such as the Internet.

Because of these changes, the American Academy of Dermatology (AAD) commissioned the Task Force on Telemedicine in 1998 to evaluate telemedicine issues as they relate to dermatology. In addition to addressing important telemedicine issues such as physician qualifications, credentialling and licensing, patient privacy and confidentiality, reimbursement, and telemedicine research, an analysis of telemedicine system capabilities was undertaken including electronic transmission protocols such as DICOM. As a result of this review and the likely future effect of the DICOM standard on telemedicine, the AAD joined the DICOM Committee as Working Group 19 in late 1998 and an official Telemedicine Position Paper was released in late 1999.[5]

For reasons relating to both the number of medically related electronic communication protocols and the state of flux of many of these standards, an official statement regarding such standards was withheld from the Position Paper. It can be expected that some official AAD guidance will be provided in future.

DICOM, telemedicine and information systems

The DICOM standard was originally developed for radiology. What relationship, if any, does DICOM have to telemedicine and teledermatology? The answer to this question requires first examining how telemedicine is developing and how it will fit into hospital and national healthcare information system infrastructures.

As mentioned previously, traditional telemedicine systems have largely depended upon the acquisition of data in a variety of different forms including paper documents, printed photographs and digital media. Furthermore, reports sent back to the referring physician have been largely generated in paper form, and management of this information has been done through the creation of a paper-based medical record, perhaps with small components (such as the images and/or live interactive video clips) stored in digital format.

The availability of digital technology and more efficient information management systems is changing this. As telemedicine systems become popular and begin to take advantage of digital technology, telemedicine information systems (TIS) will be created to manage this information. These information systems will need to fit within the framework of hospital and national healthcare information infrastructures (HII). Such infrastructures incorporate all aspects of information technology that pertain to the management of electronic patient information including patient demographics and insurance information, medical history (e.g. problem lists, medical reports, diagnostic tests and laboratory studies), drug/pharmacy information, patient admissions and discharge information, patient scheduling and billing. Successfully integrating with such a large and complex HII will require that telemedicine information systems communicate via data-exchange protocols such as DICOM, as well as others (Fig. 17.3). Communication with radiology information systems and picture archiving and communications systems (PACS) will require the use of the DICOM standard. Box 17.5 lists the main medical exchange standards development organizations that develop relevant communication protocols.

Another role for DICOM in telemedicine involves its potential use as a telemedicine information exchange protocol (TIEP). Currently telemedicine does not have such an exchange protocol. DICOM could serve this role in one of two ways; either as a method of managing, and providing an interface into, the image components of a broader telemedicine information system, or as a larger exchange protocol for managing the entirety of the telemedicine encounter information. In the former role, telemedicine systems would simply employ DICOM as the communications protocol for managing the image component of the telemedicine information system. This could include managing reporting features offered through the 'Structured Reporting Supplement' (Supplement 23). Retrieving, moving, storing and manipulating images and their related

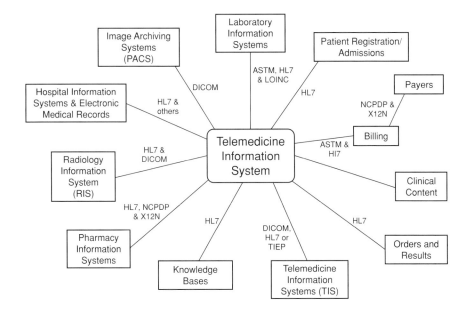

Fig. 17.3. Healthcare electronic information exchange standards and their relationship to future telemedicine information systems. ASTM, American Society for Testing and Materials; X12N, Accredited Standards Committee X12; DICOM, Digital Imaging and Communications in Medicine; HL7, Health Level Seven; LOINC, Logical Observation Identifier Names and Codes; NCPDP, National Council for Prescription Drug Programs; TIEP, (hypothetical) Telemedicine Information Exchange Protocol. (Modified from Murphy GF, Hanken MA, Waters KA, eds. *Electronic Health Records: Changing the Vision*. Philadelphia: W.B. Saunders Company, 1999.)

data within the TIS would, therefore, be done using DICOM. In addition, the TIS would provide a DICOM interface allowing other healthcare information systems, as well as other remote telemedicine systems, access (presumably in a secure manner) to the image components of the larger TIS. The DICOM standard appears to be important, given the image-centric nature of much of telemedicine.

In the latter scenario DICOM would be used, probably with some modifications, to meet the larger data communications and management needs of telemedicine systems. These arise from the larger dataset that telemedicine information systems will need to manage. This includes not only images and the related data, but also patient demographic information, insurance/payor information, provider information and structured components of a larger patient electronic medical record (EMR) such as problem lists, medication histories, adverse drug and allergy information, discharge summaries, progress notes and others. These needs mirror those of information systems concerned with managing the complete patient EMR. DICOM provides few direct ways of managing this type of information, without perhaps using elaborate structured reporting methods. Other exchange protocols are better designed to handle this type of information.

Box 17.5. Summary of major healthcare information exchange standards

Accredited Standards Committee (ASC) X12N (Insurance Subcommittee) – an ANSI-chartered committee that is concerned with developing electronic data interchange (EDI) standards for transactions between health insurance providers (payors) and healthcare providers

American College of Radiology–National Electrical Manufacturers Association (ACR-NEMA) – an ANSI-accredited organization that has developed the national and international standard Digital Imaging and Communications in Medicine. The DICOM standard permits the transfer of digital biomedical and medical images as well as associated information between computer systems

American Society for Testing and Materials (ASTM) Committee E31 – an ANSI-accredited organization, the various ASTM E31 subcommittees have developed several standards addressing the transfer of data from laboratory and other clinical instruments to computer systems and the exchange of digital neurophysiological data between computer systems. In addition, they have produced several standards addressing electronic health records

Health Level Seven (HL7) – an ANSI-accredited and US Department of Health and Human Services (DHHS) designated standards maintenance organization, HL7 is a standards development organization that has developed the national and international de facto standard for the electronic exchange of clinical, administrative and financial data between computer systems

Institute of Electrical and Electronic Engineers (IEEE) – an international society that has developed a set of standards for communicating between bedside medical devices and computer systems

National Council for Prescription Drug Programs (NCPDP) – a standards development organization that creates data exchange standards for pharmacy transactions

---

Such a complete TIEP may be better served by another protocol altogether such as HL7, or a hybrid protocol that incorporates aspects of several communication protocols. Alternatively, future telemedicine information systems may need to utilize one of several different communications protocols depending upon the data transfer needs of the particular situation. This may ultimately be what occurs. The answer will only be known when the requirements of telemedicine can be compared with the capabilities of DICOM and other communication protocols.

There are two closely related efforts that have emerged recently in healthcare informatics that are likely to have a major effect on future telemedicine information systems and TIEPs. The first of these efforts addresses exchange protocols, and is represented by the growing national and international interest in integrating and harmonizing the various domain-specific healthcare-related exchange protocols. Groups leading these efforts include various government agencies, several standards development organizations such as the joint DICOM-HL7 Image Management Special Interest Group, and industry and medical society groups such as the joint Radiologic Society of North America–Healthcare Information and Management Systems Society (RSNA–HIMSS) sponsored Integrating the Healthcare Enterprise

(IHE) Project, as well as efforts between HL7 and the National Council for Prescription Drug Programs (NCPDP) and Accredited Standards Committee Insurance Subcommittee (ASCX12). The goals of these efforts are to support the seamless, consistent and accurate exchange of medical information in a manner that also safeguards data integrity and confidentiality. The resulting protocols may be able to serve as a comprehensive TIEP.

A second closely related effort addresses medical information representation, encoding and structure. Although individual protocols provide detailed specifications for the data structures pertinent to their own application, there is growing interest in developing a uniform set of standards for representing all patient healthcare-related information and electronic medical records. Within the USA, several government agencies are championing this effort. In response to the HIPAA (Health Insurance Portability and Accountability Act, 1996) mandate, the National Committee on Vital and Health Statistics (NCVHS) recently reported the need for uniform standards for patient-related medical information as a way of improving healthcare quality and productivity, managing healthcare costs and safeguarding data.[6] Fundamental to this effort is the creation of an electronic medical record (EMR) that incorporates all components of the patient healthcare record. Other groups involved in this and similar efforts include the American Medical Informatics Association (AMIA), the International Medical Informatics Associations (IMIA), the ANSI Health Informatics Standards Board (ANSI-HISB), the ASTM Committee E31, the National Library of Medicine, the Computer-based Patient Record Institute, the Medical Record Institute, ISO Technical Committee (TC) 215, the CEN TC 251, the JAMI, the Internet Engineering Task Force (IETF) and the American Telemedicine Association (ATA) among others. The ATA has acknowledged that a 'critical aspect of the ideal telemedicine system will be the seamless integration with the EMR'.[7] Therefore, as these standards are developed, telemedicine systems will need to incorporate them into their design.

Conclusion

DICOM is the non-proprietary de facto standard for the exchange of digital medical images. The DICOM standard is constructed around an image-based information model, and uses highly organized and precisely defined data structures to represent various image types and related information. It combines these with DICOM services to provide a mechanism of managing images across a network, point-to-point connections, or offline storage devices to ensure interoperability and consistent data representation. Although originally developed for radiology images, the DICOM standard has recently been extended to other medical specialties, including dermatology, through the incorporation of the 'Visible Light Supplement 15'. In addition, robust reporting features have been added through the 'Structured Reporting Supplement 23'.

As telemedicine moves to become a standard healthcare practice, there will emerge a need to manage and exchange telemedicine information between healthcare providers. In addition, telemedicine information systems will need to fit seamlessly into the hospital, national and possibly international healthcare information infrastructure. This will require that telemedicine systems incorporate data format and exchange standards, including DICOM as well as others, into their design.

References

1   Grigsby B, Brown NA. *1999 Report on U.S. Telemedicine Activity.* Portland, OR: Association of Telemedicine Service Providers, 2000.
2   *Digital Imaging and Communications in Medicine (DICOM).* NEMA Publications PS 3.1–PS 3.14. Rosslyn, VA: National Electrical Manufacturers Association, 1998
3   *Digital Imaging and Communications in Medicine (DICOM).* NEMA Publications PS 3, supplement 15: *Visible Light Image for Endoscopy, Microscopy, and Photography.* Frozen Draft, Version 1.11. Rosslyn, VA: National Electrical Manufacturers Association, 1997.
4   *Digital Imaging and Communications in Medicine (DICOM).* NEMA Publications PS 3, supplement 23: *Structured Reporting Storage SOP Classes.* Rosslyn, VA: National Electrical Manufacturers Association, 2000.
5   American Academy of Dermatology Task Force on Telemedicine. *Position Statement on Telemedicine.* Schaumberg, IL: American Academy of Dermatology, 1999.
6   National Committee on Vital and Health Statistics. *Report to the Secretary of the US Department of Health and Human Services on Uniform Data Standards for Patient Medical Record Information,* 6 July, 2000. (http://ncvhs.hhs.gov/hipaa000706.pdf).
7   *Technology Special Interest Group White Paper.* Washington, DC: American Telemedicine Association, 1998. (http://www.atmeda.org/ICOT/TechnologySIGRec.htm [last checked 27 July 2001]).

18

Teledermoscopy – Experience from Switzerland

Ralph Peter Braun and Jean-Hilaire Saurat

Introduction

In the last two decades the incidence of malignant melanoma has been rising.[1–8] Due to a lack of adequate therapies for advanced metastatic melanoma, the best treatment is still early diagnosis and surgical excision. Dermoscopy (also known as epiluminescence microscopy or ELM, auflichtmikroskopie, dermatoscopy, dermatoskopie or amplified surface microscopy), is a simple, easy to use *in vivo* method that has been reported to be useful for the early recognition of malignant melanoma. The performance of dermoscopy has been investigated by many authors. Its use increases diagnostic accuracy by 5–30% over clinical visual inspection, depending on the type of skin lesions and the experience of the physician.[9–30]

Dermoscopy uses an immersion technique to render the skin surface translucent and has been shown to increase diagnostic accuracy for pigmented skin lesions, especially for malignant melanoma.[12,27,31–34] The technique allows structures to be visualized, so-called ELM criteria which are not visible by clinical examination alone, and which facilitate the diagnosis of pigmented skin lesions.[35,36]

Digital dermoscopy uses two-dimensional pictures of pigmented skin lesions which can also be dealt with by telemedicine. Most of the commercially available devices for digital dermoscopy offer the possibility for live examination, storage and retrieval of images as well as patient data. Telemedine allows medical consultations at a distance. This can be real-time consultation with live examination of the patient, or a simple email-based store-and-forward consultation. Since telemedicine is progressing and since devices for digital dermoscopy (DD) have become affordable, a critical evaluation of this method under routine conditions is required. Most studies which have been published so far have been based on selected pictures that have been exchanged via new electronic media (mainly email) between groups of experts. Our aim was to evaluate the feasibility and the benefit of a telemedicine approach in the setting of private practice.

Methods

All participating dermatologists in private practice used the same equipment for macro pictures. They all used a commercially available DD system (in Germany: Foto Finder Derma, Teachscreen AG, Bad Birnbach; in Switzerland: Dermanet System, Arpage AG, Zürich).

Hardware

The system is based on a commercially available PC, which was equipped with a standard PCI graphic card (4 MByte RAM, 24-bit colour depth at 600×800 resolution), and a 43-cm Sony screen. As a frame grabber the Fast Screen Machine II was used (physical resolution 768×586 pixels and an apparent resolution of 1024×768 pixels after interpolation). A Mitsubishi CCD camera which was adapted for dermatological purposes and which is commercially available (MediCam, Teachscreen AG, Bad Birnbach, Germany) was added to the system. This camera has a resolution of 768×567 pixels and allows macro pictures as well as DD examination. For the DD pictures an additional ELM lens was added. This lens includes the incident light source (4 × LED cold light source). The camera has a built-in zoom function so that the view can be easily adapted to the size of the lesion. The ELM lens has a built-in scale (see Figs 18.1–18.5). The distance between two lines of the scale is 1 mm.

Software

The Foto Finder System as well as its Swiss version (Dermanet System) is a software package that has been developed by a group of experienced dermatologists for both private practice and university hospitals. It is a patient-oriented database which allows the management of the patient's data and easy storage and retrieval of digital images. The digital images can be acquired directly with a camera or be imported from other sources such as scanners or files. In addition, it offers several possibilities for communication and information exchange such as a videoconferencing module and integrated email software. Pictures can be exchanged via a secure national network for dermatologists which is called dermanet. The Foto Finder System uses a simple drag and drop technique and was therefore judged as very user friendly by the participants.

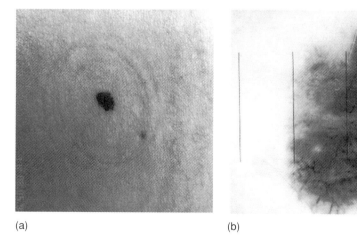

(a) (b)

Fig. 18.1. Case S.G., 35 years old, acquired lesion, right hip, histopathology: dysplastic naevus. (a) Clinical picture. (b) Dermoscopy.

Fig. 18.2. Case D.S., 32 years old, histopathology: SSM in situ. (a) Clinical picture. (b) Dermoscopy without oil. (c) Dermoscopy with oil. SSM = superficial spreading melanoma.

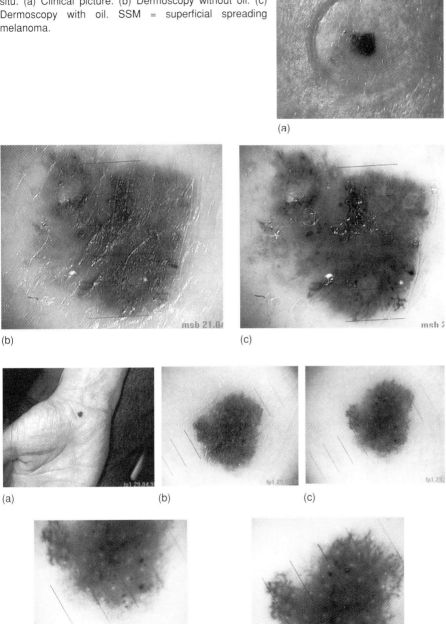

(a)

(b)

(c)

(a)

(b)

(c)

(d)

(e)

Fig. 18.3. Case V.G., 48 years old, acquired lesion, histopathology: ALM, Clark II, Breslow 0.47 mm. (a) Clinical picture. (b) Dermoscopy without oil. (c–e) Dermoscopy with oil; ALM = acrolentiginous melanoma.

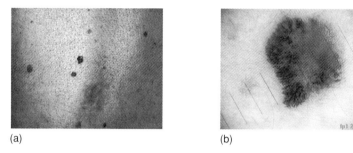

(a)   (b)

Fig. 18.4. Case D.G., 35 years old, acquired lesion, histopathology: inflamed junctional naevus. (a) Clinical picture. (b) Dermoscopy.

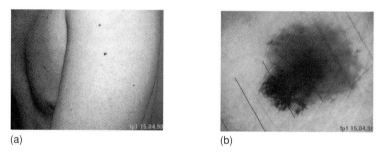

(a)   (b)

Fig. 18.5. Case A.S., 19 years old, acquired lesion, histopathology: junctional naevus. (a) Clinical picture. (b) Dermoscopy.

Study design

The system was used by eight dermatologists in private practice under routine conditions, i.e. they experienced the time pressure of their normal consultation schedule. All participants were familiar with dermoscopy but had different levels of experience. However, none of them had used a system for digital dermoscopy before. To become familiar with the camera and especially the features concerning the use of the new electronic media (email and videoconferencing), all participants met for a 1-day training session in Basel.

The lesions were stored in a JPEG graphic format with 40% compression ratio. At the beginning of the study we asked the participants to add clinical data such as age, sex, localization, Fitzpatrick's phototype, history of melanoma, history of atypical naevi, other risk factors for melanoma, acquired lesion, congenital lesion and recent changes of the lesion.

Over a period of 10 months, the participants used the system for the examination of pigmented skin lesions, for patients who had already been scheduled for routine excision due to suspicion of malignancy or on patients who requested the procedure. For complete documentation a macroscopic as well as a digital dermoscopy picture with and without immersion oil were taken from every lesion. The patients were informed about the experimental nature of the study and gave oral consent to participate. Based on the consultation, including past medical history, physical and DD examination of the patient, the dermatologists in private practice established a diagnosis which was called *diag1*.

The pictures were sent as attached documents to email messages to the Pigmented Skin Lesion Unit of the University Hospital, Geneva. After they arrived, they were evaluated by a physician with experience in dermoscopy. A diagnosis based on the digital pictures was made and transmitted to the participant. This diagnosis was called *diag2*. In a second step the quality of the pictures was evaluated by two independent physicians. Because the quality of a digital image is subjective and depends on the application, it was evaluated on a four-point scale (+++, ++, +, -). After the lesions were removed, histopathology was performed by the participant's local dermatopathologist, and a copy of the histological report was sent to a third physician who only collected the data (*diag1*) and who was otherwise not involved in the study. The physician involved in teledermoscopic diagnosis (*diag2*) did not have access to these data until the end of the study.

After 6 months, the two different approaches were compared, using the histopathology diagnosis as the 'gold standard'. In case of doubt the original histopathology slides were reviewed.

Results

After the initial training all participants were able to take pictures of good quality, to store and retrieve the images, to send them as attached documents to email messages and to perform videoconferences. Based on the feedback from the participants, the system was well accepted and integrated into their daily routine.

Picture quality was evaluated as good (+) or very good (++) in 92% of the DD pictures and in 95% of the macroscopic pictures (Table 18.1). During the 10-month study period, a total of 87 lesions were collected. Four lesions had to be excluded from the study because they had not been removed or because the histopathology report was not accessible. The analysis was therefore based on 87 lesions on 76 patients (Table 18.2). The number of cases submitted was 4–16 per month. Most of the cases were sent during the second and third month of the study. Clinical data were only available in approximately 15% of all cases, so that the diagnosis was based on the images in the majority of the cases.

Table 18.1. Evaluation of picture quality

Quality	Macro		Dermoscopy	
	N	%	N	%
–	7	8	4	5
+	23	26	17	20
++	54	62	61	70
+++	3	3	5	6
Total	**87**	**100**	**87**	**100**

The lesions were divided into two different groups, according to the algorithm of Stolz et al: melanocytic lesions ($n = 64$) and non-melanocytic lesions ($n = 23$).[13] According to the ABCD rule of dermoscopy the melanocytic lesions were divided into benign ($n = 34$), suspect ($n = 14$) and malignant melanocytic skin lesions ($n = 16$). The diagnostic accuracy of teledermoscopy was superior to the conventional diagnosis for benign melanocytic lesions (71% compared to 56%). For the malignant melanocytic lesions it was even better, 94% compared to 75% for the conventional approach (Table 18.2). The diagnostic accuracy for suspect melanocytic skin lesions was 86% compared to 64%. For the non-melanocytic skin lesions the diagnostic accuracy of teledermoscopy was similar to the traditional approach, with the exception of Kaposi's sarcoma (Table 18.2). In these cases, the diagnosis was made in 100% with the conventional approach but none of the cases was diagnosed with teledermoscopy.

To measure the agreement between the observers, Cohen's kappa statistics was calculated using SPSS statistical software (SPSS for Windows v. C9.0, SPSS Inc.). Cohen's kappa measures the agreement between two evaluations: a value of 1 indicates perfect agreement, while a value of 0 indicates that agreement is no better than chance. For the agreement of the clinical diagnosis (*diag1*), we obtained a kappa value of 0.57 compared to 0.74 for the remote diagnosis (*diag2*).

Table 18.2. Diagnostic accuracy of dermoscopy (*diag1*) and teledermoscopy (*diag2*)

	Diagnosis 1	%	Diagnosis 2	%	Histological diagnosis
Melanocytic lesions					
Benign					
Lentigo	1	33	3	100	3
Junctional naevus	5	56	6	67	9
Compound naevus	11	55	13	65	20
Congenital naevus	2	100	2	100	2
Benign (total):	**19**	**56**	**24**	**71**	**34**
Suspect:					
Atypical naevus (dysplastic)	9	64	12	86	14
Suspect (total)	**9**	**64**	**12**	**86**	**14**
Malignant					
SSM	9	75	11	91	12
ALM	1	100	1	100	1
NLM	3	100	3	100	3
Malignant (total)	**12**	**75**	**15**	**94**	**16**
Non-melanocytic skin lesions					
Basal cell carcinoma	5	71	6	86	7
Seborrheic keratosis	11	100	10	91	11
Kaposi's sarcoma	2	100	0	0	2
Angioma	3	100	3	100	3
Non-melanocytic skin lesions (total)	**21**	**91**	**19**	**83**	**23**
Total	**61**	**70**	**70**	**78**	**87**

Discussion

All participants were dermatologists in private practice and performed the documentation under routine conditions in between their consultations. Even though most of the participants were not familiar with computers and had never used a system for digital dermoscopy before, they were able to integrate a system for digital imaging and DD into their daily routine. After an initial short training period, they were able to take pictures of good quality, to store and retrieve them easily and to send them as attached documents to email messages.

The participants collected 87 lesions over a period of 10 months. At the very beginning of the study we received only a few lesions. This was probably because the participants had to become familiar with the system and were still in a 'learning phase'. After this phase, which took approximately four weeks, most of the participants entered a 'curiosity phase' where they sent every lesion scheduled for routine excision. The duration of this phase depended on the participant. In some cases it persisted until the end of the study. Towards the end of the study fewer and fewer lesions were sent. After the 'curiosity phase' we had the impression that the participants sent selected cases instead.

The principle of telemedicine in general is that a consultant at a distance is involved in the diagnostic process. This consultant only has access to images and the data provided by the consulting physician. In an interactive teleconferencing system the consultant has the possibility of interacting with the consulting physician and will be able to obtain additional information and documents. Such a system needs coordination because consultant and consulting physician have to communicate and to interact at a precise moment at the same time. In academic settings this might be possible but in private practice this is not feasible. In a store-and-forward system the consultant depends completely on the material provided by the consulting physician. Direct interaction is not possible, but the consultation is independent from any time schedules. A hybrid development such as an 'e-room' (Instinctive Technology Inc.) may be useful. An e-room provides password-protected access to a number of virtual rooms. The participant can place any kind of information in a virtual room (e.g. still images, sound recordings, video clips). The e-room provides a text chat function so that the contents of the room can be discussed between two or more participants. It also contains a pager function to invite all potential participants to join online at a particular moment.

Dermoscopy is a non-invasive method for the differential diagnosis of pigmented skin lesions and the early diagnosis of malignant melanoma. The method itself is based on a two-dimensional picture and therefore ideal for telemedicine purposes. Physicians using this method are used to two-dimensional pictures. This is not the case in clinical examination in dermatology where the appreciation of the three-dimensional aspect of the lesions has an important effect on the diagnostic process.

The evaluation of a pigmented skin lesion by dermoscopy and DD mainly depends on the experience of the physician and has been shown to be increased by formal training.[32] As this is a relatively new method not all dermatologists will have developed this experience yet and therefore a consultation by teledermoscopy might be beneficial. The diagnostic accuracy of the teledermoscopy approach was always superior to the DD approach of the consulting physician. Ninety-four per cent of all malignant melanocytic skin lesions were identified with the teledermoscopic approach while four were not diagnosed as such in the conventional approach (75%). This could have had an effect on the therapy modalities such as the surgical margins.

Because clinical information such as age, sex, risk factors for melanoma and phototype was only available in 15% of cases, we are unable to comment on the effect of this on our study. However, the diagnostic accuracy of teledermoscopy suggests that experience in the field of ELM seems to have more effect on the diagnosis than clinical information, particularly for non-pigmented lesions. If clinical data had been available to the consultant in all cases, it would probably have had an influence on the diagnostic accuracy. However, typing text files such as clinical data on a keyboard of a computer is a time-consuming procedure in private practice settings and turned out to be difficult in our study. The possibility of attaching voice-recorded text to email messages instead of typing might be helpful.

We have confirmed the feasibility of consultations by teledermoscopy but consider our study to be exploratory, since it lacks the appropriate controls necessary to make general conclusions. Further large-scale controlled studies are therefore required.

References

1   MacKie RM. Strategies to reduce mortality from cutaneous malignant melanoma. *Archives of Dermatological Research* 1994;**287**:13–15.
2   Schneider JS, Moore DH, Sagebiel RW. Risk factors for melanoma incidence in prospective follow-up. *Archives of Dermatology* 1994;**130**:1002–1007.
3   Brozena SJ, Fenske NA, Perez IR. Epidemiology of malignant melanoma, worldwide incidence and etiologic factors. *Seminars in Surgical Oncology* 1993;**9**:165–167.
4   Kelly JW, Yeatman JM, Regalia C, et al. A high incidence of melanoma found in patients with multiple dysplastic naevi by photographic surveillance. *Medical Journal of Australia* 1997;**167**:191–194.
5   Elwood JM, Koh HK. Etiology, epidemiology, risk factors, and public health issues of melanoma. *Current Opinion in Oncology* 1994;**6**:179–187.
6   Kopf AW, Salopek TG, Slade J, et al. Techniques of cutaneous examination for the detection of skin cancer. *Cancer* 1995;**75**(2 suppl.):684–690.
7   Elder D. Human melanocytic neoplasms and their etiologic relationship with sunlight. *Journal of Investigative Dermatology* 1989;**92**:297s–303s.
8   Elwood JM. Recent developments in melanoma epidemiology. *Melanoma Research* 1993;**3**:149–156.
9   Kelly JW, Crutcher WA, Sagebiel RW. Clinical diagnosis of dysplastic melanocytic nevi. *Journal of the American Academy of Dermatology* 1986;**14**:1044–1052.
10   Wolf IH, Smolle J, Soyer HP, Kerl H. Sensitivity in the clinical diagnosis of malignant melanoma. *Melanoma Research* 1998;**8**:425–429.
11   Argenziano G, Fabbrocini G, Carli P, et al. Epiluminescence microscopy for the diagnosis of doubtful melanocytic skin lesions. Comparison of the ABCD rule of dermatoscopy and a new 7-point checklist based on pattern analysis. *Archives of Dermatology* 1998;**134**:1563–1570.
12   Kreusch J, Rassner G. *Auflichtmikroskopie pigmentierter Hauttumoren.* [Dermoscopy of Pigmented Skin Lesions.] Stuttgart: Thieme, 1991.
13   Stolz W, Braun-Falco O, Bilek P, Landthaler M. *Farbatlas der Dermatoskopie* [Colour Atlas of Dermoscopy], 1st edn. Berlin: Blackwell Wissenschaft, 1993.
14   Lorentzen H, Weismann K, Secher L, et al. The dermatoscopic ABCD rule does not improve diagnostic accuracy of malignant melanoma. *Acta dermato-venereologica* 1999;**79**:469–472.

15 Hartge P, Holly EA, Halpern A, et al. Recognition and classification of clinically dysplastic nevi from photographs: a study of interobserver variation. *Cancer Epidemiology, Biomarkers and Prevention* 1995;**4**:37–40.

16 Cascinelli N, Ferrario M, Tonelli T, Leo E. A possible new tool for clinical diagnosis of melanoma: the computer. *Journal of the American Academy of Dermatology* 1987;**16**:361–367.

17 Morton CA, MacKie RM. Clinical accuracy of the diagnosis of cutaneous malignant melanoma. *British Journal of Dermatology* 1998;**138**:283–287.

18 Grin CM, Kopf AW, Welkovich BA, et al. Accuracy in the clinical diagnosis of malignant melanoma. *Archives of Dermatology* 1990;**126**:763–766.

19 Kang S, Barnhill RL, Mihm MC, et al. Melanoma risk in individuals with clinically atypical nevi. *Archives of Dermatology* 1994;**130**:999–1001.

20 Stanganelli I, Bucchi L. Epiluminescence microscopy versus clinical evaluation of pigmented skin lesions: effects of operator's training on reproducibility and accuracy. Dermatology and Venereology Society of the Canton of Ticino. *Dermatology* 1998;**196**:199–203.

21 Kerl H, Wolf IH, Sterry W, Soyer HP. [Dermatoscopy. A new method for the clinical diagnosis of malignant melanoma.] *Deutsche medizinische Wochenschrift* 1995;**120**:801–805.

22 Lorentzen H, Weismann K, Petersen CS, et al. Clinical and dermatoscopic diagnosis of malignant melanoma. Assessed by expert and non-expert groups. *Acta dermato-venereologica* 1999;**79**:301–304.

23 Argenziano G, Fabbrocini G, Carli P, et al. Epiluminescence microscopy: criteria of cutaneous melanoma progression. *Journal of the American Academy of Dermatology* 1997;**37**:68–74.

24 Benelli C, Roscetti E, Pozzo VD, et al. The dermoscopic versus the clinical diagnosis of melanoma. *European Journal of Dermatology* 1999;**9**:470–476.

25 Pehamberger H, Binder M, Steiner A, Wolff K. *In vivo* epiluminescence microscopy: improvement of early diagnosis of melanoma. *Journal of Investigative Dermatology* 1993;**100**:356S–362S.

26 Stanganelli I, Seidenari S, Serafini M, et al. Diagnosis of pigmented skin lesions by epiluminescence microscopy: determinants of accuracy improvement in a nationwide training programme for practical dermatologists. *Public Health* 1999;**113**:237–242.

27 Steiner A, Pehamberger H, Wolff K. Improvement of the diagnostic accuracy in pigmented skin lesions by epiluminescent light microscopy. *Anticancer Research* 1987;**7**(3 Pt B):433–434.

28 Schulz H. Auflichtmikroskopische differenzierung maligner melanome. [Diagnosis of malignant melanoma using dermoscopy.] *Aktuelle Dermatologie* 1991;**17**:134–136.

29 Schulz H. Maligne melanome in der auflichtmikroskopie. [Malignant melanoma as seen by dermoscopy.] *Der Hautarzt; Zeitschrift fur Dermatologie, Venerologie, und verwandte Gebiete* 1994;**45**:15–19.

30 Schulz H. Epiluminescence microscopic characteristics of small malignant melanoma. [Epiluminescence microscopic characteristics of small malignant melanoma.] *Der Hautarzt; Zeitschrift fur Dermatologie, Venerologie, und verwandte Gebiete* 1997;**48**:904–909.

31 Ascierto PA, Satriano RA, Palmieri G, et al. Epiluminescence microscopy as a useful approach in the early diagnosis of cutaneous malignant melanoma. *Melanoma Research* 1998;**8**:529–537.

32 Binder M, Schwarz M, Winkler A, et al. Epiluminescence microscopy. A useful tool for the diagnosis of pigmented skin lesions for formally trained dermatologists. *Archives of Dermatology* 1995;**131**:286–291.

33 Menzies SW, Crotty KA, Ingvar C, McCarthy WH. *An Atlas of Surface Microscopy of Pigmented Skin Lesions.* Sydney: McGraw Hill, 1996.

34 Puppin D, Salomon D, Saurat JH. Amplified surface microscopy. Preliminary evaluation of a 400-fold magnification in the surface microscopy of cutaneous melanocytic lesions *Journal of the American Academy of Dermatology* 1998;**28**:923–927.

35 Bahmer FA, Fritsch P, Kreusch J, et al. Diagnostische kriterien in der auflichtsmikroskopie. [Diagnostic criteria in dermoscopy.] Konsensus-Treffen der Arbeitsgruppe Analytische Morphologie der Arbeitsgemeinschaft Dermatologische Forschung, 17 November 1989 in Hamburg. *Der Hautarzt; Zeitschrift fur Dermatologie, Venerologie, und verwandte Gebiete* 1990;**41**:513–514.

36 Fritsch P, Pechlaner R. Differentiation of benign from malignant melanocytic lesions using incident light microscopy. In: Ackerman AB (ed) *Masson's Monograph in Dermatopathology.* New York: Masson, 1998: 301–311.

19

Where the Basics are Lacking – Teledermatology in Developing Countries

Peter Schmid-Grendelmeier, Prosper Doe, Lorenz Kuehnis, Laura Milesi and Günter Burg

Introduction

Telemedicine in developing countries is very different from telemedicine in the industrialized world. While practitioners in the northern hemisphere talk about communication rates of Megabits per second, most developing countries do not have ISDN lines. In Africa, basic needs such as a reliable power supply or telephone access cannot be taken for granted. Therefore telemedicine of a sophisticated kind, for example requiring videoconferencing, is something that developing countries can ill afford – at least at the moment.

The probability of a child dying before age 5 years is ten times greater in developing countries than in industrialized countries. Some developing countries have less than US$40 to spend on health care per person per year. Does telemedicine make sense for developing countries under such conditions? And if so, how should it be delivered? These are not easy questions to answer.[1] And what about teledermatology in these areas, where skin diseases are common but are almost neglected by many public health services?

The question of teledermatology in developing countries is worth discussing. Our contribution is based on our experience with a teledermatology link between Tanzania and Switzerland. We have learnt that there is a need for improved communication between healthcare professionals who care for skin diseases in rural areas. The simplest telecommunication link can significantly improve medical education of isolated nurses or doctors, facilitate the exchange of vital information about epidemics, provide useful material about prevention, and promote cooperation between remote health centres and urban hospitals. Many people have the impression that telemedicine involves the use of sophisticated, expensive and complicated equipment, but some applications require no more than an ordinary telephone and a computer. With recent advances in communications and information technology, the cost of telemedicine equipment and services has been falling rapidly, which means that its potential can be extended to many more people.

Telemedicine in developing countries

While there are still very few reports about teledermatology in developing countries, there have been reports about other telemedical activities. There are excellent reviews summarizing these, written mostly by Wright.[2-4] They contain a survey of telemedicine in 60 countries, half of which are from the so-called third world. These papers highlight telemedicine activities in and for developing countries and are strongly recommended to the interested reader. A Study Group of the International Telecommunication Union (ITU) made recommendations for telemedicine in developing countries in the form of a report.[4] The report also examined types of telemedicine services, the technologies for diffusion of telemedicine, the costs and benefits of different solutions and the prospects for global standards.

Two organizations are worthy of note: Inmarsat and the Midjan group. Inmarsat was a partner in the production of the ITU Report and was also a participant in the European Telemedicine Corporation Group. Inmarsat provides satellite telephone systems which can be used almost anywhere on earth (see http://217.204.152.210/index.cfm [last checked 29 July 2001]). The latest Inmarsat satellite phone is the size of a laptop computer and can be purchased for less than US$3000. This is less than one-tenth of the cost of the terminals used a decade ago. The cost of operation has also dropped, with rates for some voice and data services of under US$3 a minute. One early telemedicine case in 1984 involved a young Swazi boy who was examined remotely by physicians in London's Great Ormond Street Hospital. The boy was diagnosed as having Crouzon's disease. Inmarsat invited journalists to witness the use of its satellite system and the resulting press coverage led to the boy being brought to London for treatment.

The Midjan group was formed as a result of an initiative of the French Ministère des Affaires Sociales, the Telecommunication Development Bureau (BDT) of the International Telecommunication Union (ITU) and Inmarsat. The Midjan Group took their name from telemedicine demonstrations which its members gave at two major development conferences in the **Mid**rand, South Africa, and Abid**jan**, Côte d'Ivoire in 1996. Using an Inmarsat-B mobile earth station, doctors in Abidjan and Midrand were able to exchange views and discuss cases with their counterparts at the European Institute of Telemedicine in Toulouse (France) and the Politecnico di Milano (Italy).

The Midjan Group organized a number of conferences about telemedicine in developing countries. The last meeting was the Second World Telemedicine Symposium for Developing Countries, which took place in Buenos Aires, Argentina in June 1999. Over 190 delegates from North and South America, Africa, Asia and the Pacific, Arab countries, Western and Eastern European countries took part. Representatives of the World Health Organization, the ITU and the Midjan group were present at this meeting.

At the meeting there were reports from the following countries about various experiences with telemedicine: Argentina, Australia, Canada, Colombia, Congo, England, France, Japan, Jordan, Kenya, Korea, Mali, Mauritius, Nepal, Peru, Senegal, Spain, Ukraine, USA and Uruguay.

The main conclusions from the conference were:

▷ Telecommunications is a dynamic sector, which has proved to be important to development as well as to building wealth.

▷ The major application areas of telematics are in sectors such as health, education and agriculture.

▷ The significant progress made in telehealth and telemedicine is reflected in the differences between the first and second world symposia.

▷ Telemedicine and related activities in care and education should be defined in order to respond to the needs of health professionals.

The final conclusion outlined strategies for introducing telemedicine in developing countries, and for finding appropriate technology and international partners (such as the World Health Organization). These meetings and guidelines reflected the upsurge in telemedicine activity that has occurred in the last few years.

The situation is rather different for teledermatology, as discussed below.

Teledermatology in developing countries

Dermatology is not a focus of governmental or non-governmental health policies in most developing countries. Except for some infectious diseases affecting the skin such as leprosy and onchocerciasis, very little priority is given to dermatological problems in these regions. The overwhelming health problems caused by the major killing diseases such as malaria, tuberculosis and the HIV/AIDS epidemic leave few resources for skin conditions.

The International League of Dermatological Societies (ILDS), amongst others, has recognized this lack of skin care. The ILDS developed a project to focus on providing health care to developing nations (see http://www.who.int/ina-ngo/ngo/ngo090.htm [last checked 29 July 2001]).[5,6] Through the International Foundation for Dermatology (see http://www.ifd.org [last checked 29 July 2001]), it operates two Regional Dermatology Training Centres, serving rural community nurses in Tanzania and Guatemala. A third Regional Dermatology Training Centre is under development. The ILDS provides liaison and communication services linking dermatological societies throughout the world and assists in the organization of the 5-yearly World Congress of Dermatology.

As dermatology is not a primary focus of health care in developing countries, there is little emphasis given to teledermatology in these areas. But teledermatology has been shown to be a useful tool for providing skin care to underserved populations such as in Canada or the Hawaiian islands,[7] the Azores[8] or Taiwan.[9] It offers great potential in a region like sub-Saharan Africa, which suffers a scarcity of dermatologists as well as limited communications and transportation. Although the potential use and projects are discussed,[10] reports about established teledermatology connections in this area are still rare.

We have had experience with teledermatology at the Regional Dermatology Training Centre (RDTC) in Moshi, Northern Tanzania, which aims to promote knowledge for allied health professionals in dermatology, leprosy and sexually transmitted diseases[11] (Fig. 19.1).

Using the experience of the Swiss Dermatologists' Telenetwork (see http://www.dermanet.ch/ [last checked 29 July 2001]), a complete computer package was installed at the RDTC (desktop PC Pentium 133 MHz, still digital camera, 28.8 kbit/s modem) (Fig. 19.2). A telephone line had to be established for the purpose, since there are few telephone lines in Tanzania. It was not possible to use cellular or satellite phones at that time in Tanzania, as the costs would have been much higher than a conventional fixed telephone line. Because of voltage instability and repeated power cuts, an uninterruptible power supply had to be installed to prevent damage to the equipment. A mobile computing system based on a laptop would have been preferable to the desktop PC, but the camera we used required a desktop PC. Although it was only protected by dust covers, the system proved to be astonishingly resistant to heat and humidity. Repeated attacks by termites feeding on telephone and power wires were an unexpected problem. There was also a high risk of theft, which had to be reduced by multi-lockable doors and iron-protected windows.

In a first attempt to obtain safe, guaranteed access we tried to get connected directly to our Internet service provider in Switzerland. However, connection between the modems in Tanzania and Switzerland was not possible because of poor line quality. Eventually we were able to establish access using an Internet service provider in Tanzania.

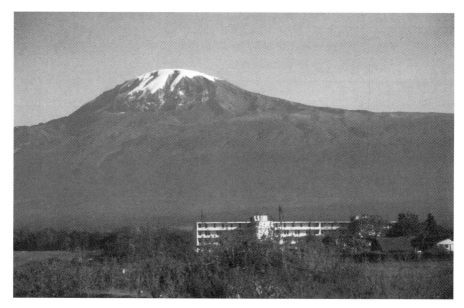

Fig. 19.1. The Regional Dermatology Training Centre at the slopes of Mt. Kilimanjaro in Moshi, Tanzania.

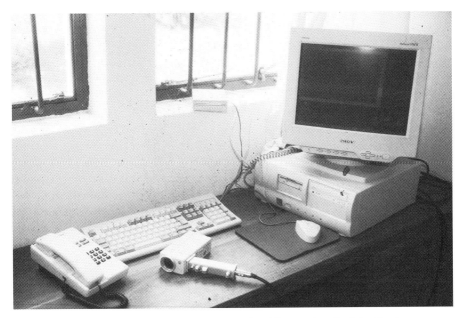

Fig. 19.2. PC and video equipment used at the Regional Dermatology Training Centre.

Taking video pictures of patients required relatively extensive counselling beforehand, because most patients were not used to being photographed or seeing themselves on a computer screen. Light conditions (sunlight or fluorescent ceiling lights) caused strong reflections from coloured skin and this had to be managed before pictures of sufficient quality could be obtained. Thus patients had to stand at an appropriate distance from the window to avoid too strong or too weak sunshine falling on their skin. Finally, clinical images and digitized histopathology slides of skin conditions were discussed by videoconferencing, which allowed interactive discussion with colleagues from Switzerland and other countries.

Expertise was also received by sending digital pictures to colleagues as email attachments. The speed of transmission was limited to a maximum of 19 kbit/s, but this was sufficient to transmit a compressed image in 1–2 minutes. The software (Dermanet Communication Suite) allowed safe, password-protected connections with colleagues all over the world who had the necessary hardware and Internet access.

Image transfer was done after normal clinic hours. This was due to the fact that all the patients had to register before 09:00 to be seen the same day (a rule of the hospital authorities). Often 100–150 patients were waiting outside the outpatient clinic to be seen for skin problems – and sometimes there were only one or two dermatologists available to attend to them. Therefore there was little time left to take digital pictures of interesting cases. Also, pictures could not be taken in the examination room. As the camera was linked by cable to the PC, the patients had to be sent to the room with the PC and video equipment. Hence documenting the patients with digital images was rather time consuming – in periods of sudden power-cuts sometimes even a matter of luck.

In the first year clinical or histopathology images of 30 patients were taken and then saved, on a PC hard disk or on a ZIP drive. Eighteen cases were discussed during a total of four videoconferences; other images were exchanged via email. Due to the fact that there was only a 1-hour time difference between Zürich and Moshi, a convenient time for videoconferencing was at about 13:00. This time also allowed reasonably fast data transfer via the Internet, although in the evening, when the Web was more heavily used by people from Europe and North America, the exchange speed rapidly declined in Moshi. The exchange of images had always to be agreed to first, because any Swiss picture sent during the transfer of a picture from Tanzania interrupted the transfer of the latter probably due to the much slower telephone lines.

Skin diseases sent from Moshi mostly involved four types of diagnosis:

> Typical tropical skin diseases, such as chromoblastoma, lepromatous and tuberculoid leprosy, onchocerciasis and tungiasis.

> Very extensive or advanced skin diseases seen also in Europe, such as impetiginized eczema or psoriasis, huge keloids or late-stage syphilis (Fig. 19.3).

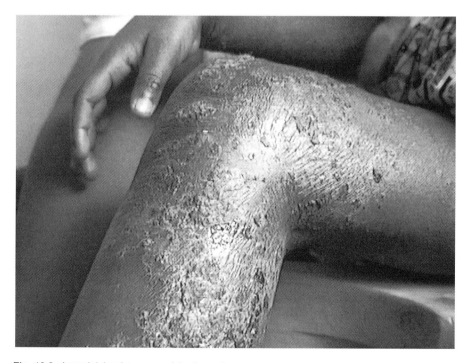

Fig. 19.3. Impetiginized eczema of the lower leg.

▶ Diagnostically challenging cases (clinically or histologically), such as unidentifiable infectious or blistering disorders or, due to the expertise at our clinic in Zürich, of cutaneous lymphomas.

▶ Images of patients who required sophisticated treatment unavailable in Tanzania.

We were able to obtain retinoids to treat two patients with extensive disorders of keratinization. Pictures of a 17-year-old patient suffering from a very severe congenital ichthyosiform non-bullous erythroderma were transferred. The unpleasant smell of the massive layer of scales isolated the patient completely in the social context of his tribe. A very generous donation of acitretin resulted in massive improvement in the patient's skin condition. For the first time for years he could participate in the social life of his village – a miracle for him and his family (Fig. 19.4). We also managed to obtain chemotherapy drugs for patients with lymphoma.

Colleagues from Europe started to ask the RDTC for expert opinions about patients with coloured skin or possible tropical skin diseases. We sent images of travellers returning from beach holidays in East or West Africa who had presented with ulcerating lesions on the feet or neck. Thanks to the expertise of the local African

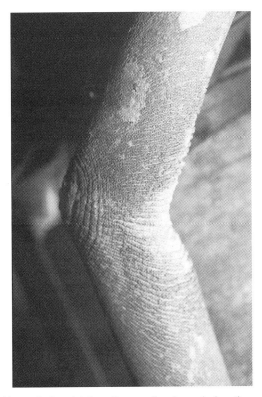

Fig. 19.4. Patient with non-bullous ichthyosiform erythroderma before therapy with acitretin.

health workers these lesions were identified as due to tunga penetrans in the toe webs, and beetle dermatitis due to contact with the paederus fly. Nodular lesions on the abdomen of a Swiss patient returning from the Kenyan coast were recognized by the RDTC students as furuncoloid myiasis caused by the 'tumbu fly', *Cordylobia anthropophoga*.

So a mutual exchange of knowledge was started, which continues three years later, although to a very limited extent with the exchange of digital images once every one or two months. The software normally needs to be updated once a year. The equipment is still working after three years, although it has suffered several severe crashes during massive power fluctuations and an impressive termite invasion. Communication has been very dependent on certain individuals at the RDTC. Some members in Tanzania still doubt if there is a need for teledermatology equipment costing several thousand dollars while it remains difficult to buy effective drugs urgently needed for the treatment of skin diseases as common as scabies or superficial fungal infections. In telemedicine links of this sort, the industrialized partner needs an advanced knowledge of tropical skin diseases and a basic idea of the limited possibilities in a developing country. Communication between various centres in developing countries with similar conditions would allow teledermatology to realize more of its potential. 'Horizontal exchange' might be more beneficial than 'vertical' exchange. However, vertical teledermatology can be beneficial to both partners if they can see the potential for learning and widening their understanding of each other.

Technical needs

Due to the fact that skin conditions can usually be discussed with still images, real-time videoconferencing does not seem to be essential in teledermatology of the sort under discussion. To develop reliable teledermatology, some basic requirements are essential. These include:

- a computer, including the necessary software
- a source of digital images (digital camera, video camera, flatbed or slide scanner)
- an uninterruptible power supply
- access to the telephone network
- access to an Internet service provider.

Computer

Obviously a computer is essential to exchange digital information. Although becoming more common, computers are still not used daily in many developing countries. Access to a computer is very limited and is a great privilege in many places. Computer knowledge is accordingly still very limited. The price of computers makes them mostly unaffordable for an individual, who may have a monthly income as low as US$40–80 per month. Most computers are found in the offices of government or other authorities. Using second-hand computers imported tax free from Western nations might help to alleviate this problem.

In general mobile computers (notebooks or laptops) are more useful than desktop computers, since they allow at least a few hours of autonomy from power supply interruptions. For a desktop computer, an uninterruptible power supply is essential. While the speed of the processor is less important, there should be enough hard disk space to store images, otherwise additional storage devices have to be added.

Digital image source

Sources of digital images include digital video and still image cameras. Standard resolution (e.g. 1600×1200 pixels) is usually enough to meet most of a dermatologist's needs. It has been shown that a 720×500 pixel image can be considered equivalent to a 1490×1000 pixel image for most store-and-forward teledermatology consultations.[12] Compressed images of this size can also be transmitted reasonably quickly, even with low data transfer rates.

Portable cameras are easier to use than desktop systems. A close-up function should be available. Devices to store images should be replaceable. Cameras linked to the computer are still advantageous for high-quality dermoscopy – a feature rarely needed in tropical areas.

Software

Software should be easy to use and stable. Whenever possible it should be available in the mother tongue of the users. It should not need too much hard disk space or processing capacity, since computers in developing countries are rarely the newest models. Software updating should be possible via the Internet or CD-ROM and should not need computer professionals, as these may be many hundreds or even thousands of kilometres away.

The system we used for the Tanzania–Switzerland connection was created primarily for Swiss dermatologists, who are well equipped and familiar with modern computers. It was certainly not designed to serve as a teledermatology tool in developing countries. However, the system proved to be functional, efficient and enriching for both parties. If communication was simpler (such as the exchange of digital images via email) and mobile computer and telephone equipment were integrated, the potential of teledermatology would remain, while the restrictions and costs would be reduced. Such systems are already available and in use (e.g. for the military), although rarely used for teledermatology.

In developing countries, as elsewhere, computers, especially those with Internet access, are vulnerable to viruses. Up-to-date antivirus software is therefore crucial. Data should always be backed up, even in developing countries.

Electrical power

Electricity cannot be taken for granted in developing countries. In rural and remote areas there is sometimes no power supply at all and a petrol-driven generator may offer the only power source.

In semi-rural or urban areas there is usually some power available, albeit of rather dubious stability. Power cuts due to natural, technical and man-made problems can be frequent. In addition the voltage often fluctuates. Power surges and failures can be harmful to computers, monitors and digital cameras. Uninterruptible power supplies are absolutely crucial.

Access to the telephone network and an Internet provider

A few years ago, lack of access to the telephone network and to an Internet service provider limited the exchange of digital information in developing countries. Recently there has been a significant change. Not only have public telephone lines become easier to obtain and more reliable, even in rural areas, but mobile phones are rapidly spreading in urban areas of developing countries and offer a much more reliable connection. For example, in Tanzania public telephone calls are increasingly using the more reliable mobile phone network. In addition there is the possibility of direct access to a satellite telephone network such as Inmarsat. This medium offers access to the telephone network and the Internet even from the remotest part of the world, albeit at relatively high cost.

Despite these new possibilities it must be remembered that a very limited section of the population in developing countries has access to such facilities. The costs of telephone rental or even an Internet provider are simply out of reach. If a person earns about US$50–100 per month, a monthly rate of around US$20–30 (the average for Internet access in east Africa) is simply unaffordable. An alternative is free access to the Internet during a limited time each day, which is offered by the United Nations and the World Health Organization. These systems are mainly used by international organizations, government authorities and military groups.

Sustainability

Sustainability is one of the principal requirements for all assistance given to developing nations. In most countries health care is considered a public service. The provision of teledermatology or telemedicine services in general meets an important social need to extend health care to remote and rural areas in developing countries.

While there are potential advantages and benefits from telemedicine, evidence for cost-effectiveness and sustainability has been limited until recently. Even in industrialized nations these aspects of telemedicine are controversial.[13–15] Teledermatology undoubtedly yields cost savings in certain circumstances, but few providing this service have found a way to recover their costs (and make a profit) from those to whom they offer their service. This is even true for industrialized countries, but weighs more heavily in developing countries, where the resources of healthcare providers are much more restricted. With low expenditure per person, developing countries face huge challenges in making public health services sustainable. Pilot projects like our Tanzania–Switzerland connection may be a first step in demonstrating the benefits and cost-effectiveness of telemedicine, but such projects should also be sustainable. Sponsors of such pilot projects must have a clear plan from the start about how the project can continue after the sponsorship comes to an end.[16,17] Some financial participation from the recipients should be included from the beginning, according to their ability to pay. Otherwise such a project risks becoming just a nice toy, for which no one feels responsibility. The sponsor must care about sustainability, which not only includes the generous donation of the equipment in the beginning, but also continuous support for hardware and software, technical assistance and training in the long term.

Education of local staff can be very difficult, as even basic knowledge about computers is often almost completely lacking. This is now changing. Continued support remains difficult, due to long distances and limited transportation facilities. The chance of obtaining technical help within hours or even days – something taken for granted in industrialized nations – is very small or non-existent in many areas of developing countries. Technical assistance via the Internet or telephone line can help resolve a considerable number of problems, but not all of them.

Ethical and educational aspects

The same ethical considerations for teledermatology exist in developing countries as in industrialized nations – possibly in an even more profound sense. Patients in these areas are rarely well informed about their rights. In areas where a classical photograph is rare and an encounter with a computer may be the first in a patient's lifetime, a digital image is sometimes beyond the patient's understanding. How can this patient, who has to travel perhaps several hours to the next large village, understand that his image can reach another expert somewhere far away within seconds? Also religious beliefs have to be considered among those who may not be allowed to be photographed. Therefore the patient needs correct information and an explanation so that he or she can really agree to this method of communication. Everyone transferring digital pictures from such patients must be careful that no information is misused. It should be absolutely obvious that the same rules of keeping the patient's identity anonymous should be applied as in industrialized nations.

There are two ways to conduct teledermatology in the so-called third world: consultations between developing and industrialized regions, and consultations among different centres within the developing nation. Both offer great potential for education.

Information exchange between developing and industrialized nations can be highly beneficial for both partners. Dermatologists in Europe and the USA are often unfamiliar with tropical skin diseases, although these are increasingly being seen in their home countries because of tourism and global migration. Here the expertise of colleagues living in the tropics can be most useful.

Colleagues in developing countries may benefit from their partners in more privileged areas by the additional use of technical, laboratory or pharmaceutical resources. The African saying 'many Western doctors are interested in tropical diseases, but few are interested in the patients with tropical diseases' should be contradicted by the use of teledermatology. The opposite should become true: by the exchange of digital information, Western dermatologists should become sensitized to the problems of their colleagues and their patients in underprivileged areas. We found this aspect of teledermatology between Tanzania and Switzerland particularly rewarding.

In developing countries the main focus is public health. Infectious diseases such as tinea capitis, scabies, impetigo and HIV-related skin problems dominate by far.[18] But the general knowledge of those responsible for primary health care is often very poor. So these simple conditions are often misdiagnosed, and the limited drug supply is wasted. A consultation with a person with expertise in skin diseases using selected digital images can be cost saving.

Teledermatology and the Internet are useful for teaching. Scientific journals are not readily available in many countries with limited resources, due to cost and restricted delivery. Symposiums and meetings are hard to attend because of long distances. Dermatology is a visually orientated discipline and is particularly suitable for online teaching.

Yellowlees formulated seven general principles for the successful development of telemedicine.[19] Adapted to teledermatology these principles are:

1. Teledermatology applications and sites should be selected pragmatically, rather than philosophically.

2. Clinicians and teledermatology users must own the system (or have at least permanent access).

3. Teledermatology management and support should originate from the bottom up (such as the community health worker) rather than from the top down. It should meet a need felt in the community and by the patient.

4. The technology should be as user friendly as possible.

5. Teledermatology users must be well trained and supported, technically and professionally.

6. Teledermatology applications should be evaluated in a clinically appropriate and user-friendly manner.

7. Information about the development of teledermatology must be shared.

These principles are also valid in developing nations and might be even more important.

Conclusion

In our experience, teledermatology is a highly beneficial and efficient tool in the diagnosis and management of challenging dermatology patients – at a consultant hospital level – in a country with limited resources such as Tanzania. Sustainability and basic requirements should be checked very carefully before investing in such facilities. At the RDTC it was necessary to upgrade the software and hardware once a year, which was made possible by repeated visits of Swiss colleagues to Tanzania. Locally enthusiastic, technically knowledgeable and reliable colleagues are essential and extensive training of local staff to enable self-reliance is crucial. Also back-up by a company or an organization able to cover the costs for new hardware and software is necessary but creates another form of dependence.

There is a tremendous lack of care and knowledge for patients with skin diseases in these areas. However modern communication has the potential to improve things.

If the technology is simple, easy to use and not too expensive, we are convinced that the advantages of teledermatology in developing countries outweigh the possible risks and possibly exaggerated expectations. The more a basic dermatology service and knowledge is lacking, the more a health system can benefit from consultation with experts located elsewhere. Teledermatology in developing countries makes absolute sense. The larger the distance to overcome to consult a person experienced in the care of patients with skin diseases, the more teledermatology can be justified. Simple, efficient solutions are mandatory – but they are increasingly available and have been shown to be useful in underserved areas.[11] Growing access to a high-quality mobile phone network in developing countries and progress in digital image capture are rapidly enabling teledermatology to be used more widely in these countries.

Teledermatology will certainly not solve all the health problems in countries with limited resources. But it can be an additional factor in assisting with these problems, especially in the care of skin diseases. Despite all the difficulties encountered, teledermatology in the third world is probably much less of a 'toy' than its use in industrialized nations. Teledermatology does imply fun and professional enrichment – but it is also a necessity for people working in remote or rural areas.

We would like to find ways to provide appropriate teledermatology services in these areas. Communication between colleagues caring for patients with skin diseases can be improved by teledermatology. Our final aim is to use teledermatology to improve the still very restricted care for patients suffering from skin diseases in many parts of the world.

Acknowledgements

We thank Luzi Gilli, Swiss dermatologist volunteering at the RDTC, now in private practice in Reinach, Basle, Switzerland and Andreas Haeffner, consultant dermatologist and computer expert at the Department of Dermatology in Zürich, who both contributed to the success of the Tanzania–Switzerland teledermatology link. We are also indebted to Henning Grossmann, Principal of the RDTC in Moshi, for providing the facilities to use the system, including a safe room and separate telephone line. The computer equipment used in Tanzania was provided by Roche Pharmaceuticals, Switzerland and free software support was given by Arpage Systems AG, Switzerland. The whole project was supported by the Department of Dermatology of the University of Zürich.

References

1 Wootton R. The possible use of telemedicine in developing countries. *Journal of Telemedicine and Telecare* 1997;**3**:23–26.

2 Wright D. Telemedicine delivery to developing countries. *Journal of Telemedicine and Telecare* 1997;**3**(suppl 1):76–78.

3 Wright D. The International Telecommunication Union's report on Telemedicine and Developing Countries. *Journal of Telemedicine and Telecare* 1998;**4**(suppl 1):75–79.

4 Wright D. Telemedicine and developing countries. A report of study group 2 of the ITU Development Sector. *Journal of Telemedicine and Telecare* 1998;**4**(suppl 2):1–85.

5 Kopf AW. International Foundation for Dermatology. A challenge to meet the dermatologic needs of developing countries. *Dermatologic Clinics* 1993;**11**:311–314.

6 Donofrio LM, Millikan LE. Dermatologic diseases of eastern Africa. *Dermatologic Clinics* 1994;**12:**621–628.

7 Norton SA, Burdick AE, Phillips CM, Berman B. Teledermatology and underserved populations. *Archives of Dermatology* 1997;**133:**197–200.

8 Goncalves L, Cunha C. Telemedicine project in the Azores Islands. *Archives d'Anatomie et de Cytologie Pathologiques* 1995;**43:**285–287.

9 Wu YH, Su HY, Hsieh YJ. Survey of infectious skin diseases and skin infestations among primary school students of Taitung County, eastern Taiwan. *Journal of the Formosan Medical Association* 2000;**99:**128–134.

10 Wright D, Androuchko L. Telemedicine and developing countries. *Journal of Telemedicine and Telecare* 1996;**2:**63–70.

11 Schmid-Grendelmeier P, Masenga EJ, Haeffner A, Burg G. Teledermatology as a new tool in sub-saharan Africa: an experience from Tanzania. *Journal of the American Academy of Dermatology* 2000;**42:**833–835.

12 Vidmar DA, Cruess D, Hsieh P, et al. The effect of decreasing digital image resolution on teledermatology diagnosis. *Telemedicine Journal* 1999;**5:**375–383.

13 Wootton R, Bloomer SE, Corbett R, et al. Multicentre randomised control trial comparing real time teledermatology with conventional outpatient dermatological care: societal cost–benefit analysis. *British Medical Journal* 2000;**320:**1252–1256.

14 Oakley AM, Kerr P, Duffill M, et al. Patient cost–benefits of realtime teledermatology – a comparison of data from Northern Ireland and New Zealand. *Journal of Telemedicine and Telecare* 2000;**6:**97–101.

15 High WA, Houston MS, Calobrisi SD, Drage LA, McEvoy MT. Assessment of the accuracy of low-cost store-and-forward teledermatology consultation. *Journal of the American Academy of Dermatology* 2000;**42:**776–783.

16 Taylor P. An assessment of the potential effect of a teledermatology system. *Journal of Telemedicine and Telecare* 2000;**6**(suppl 1):74–76.

17 Wright D. The sustainability of telemedicine projects. *Journal of Telemedicine and Telecare* 1999;**5**(suppl 1):107–111.

18 Schmid-Grendelmeier P, Mahé A, Poennighaus J, Welsh O, Stingl P, Leppard B. Periodical synopsis: tropical dermatology. Part I. *Journal of the American Academy of Dermatology* 2001(in press).

19 Yellowlees P. Successful development of telemedicine systems – seven core principles. *Journal of Telemedicine and Telecare* 1997;**3**:215–222.

20

Online Teledermatology Consultations from Private Doctors

Christopher Clay

Introduction

Much, if not most, of the teledermatology carried out so far concerns patients in the public sector. I have set up an Internet-based teledermatology system in Western Australia for private work. My conviction is that at least for the foreseeable future, only distance between the patient and specialist can justify office teledermatology in the private setting.

Particular features of private office practice include limited ability to bear the cost of the required infrastructure,[1,2] and the need to make a profit. The economics of telemedicine should be considered by publicly funded institutions as well, but are particularly important in the small business setting.

Geography

Western Australia constitutes one-third of the landmass of Australia. A large proportion of the outback is desert and distances are enormous. Once every 2 months, I do an outreach clinic in Kalgoorlie. This has a population of 30 000 in the town and about the same number in the far-flung surrounding districts. The town is just over 500 km from Perth (the state capital of Western Australia) and the trip takes an hour by jet (Fig. 20.1). The Australian Federal Seat of Kalgoorlie (a voting district of the Australian House of Representatives) is the largest voting district in the world and is mostly desert.

Population and distribution

The population of Western Australia is 1.8 million, and the people live mainly in the metropolitan area of Perth. The majority of the remainder live in small communities near the coast, except for those in the wheat belt in the southern and western part of the state and those in mining communities. Although this low population density represents an extreme, even in Australia, similar problems exist in much of the continent.

Disease patterns

Work in the country areas revolves around primary industries, mainly mining, agricultural and associated industries. There is a high incidence of industrial skin

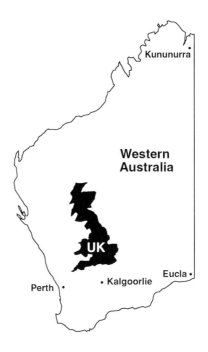

Fig. 20.1. Map of Western Australia showing the size relative to the UK.

problems particularly in the mining sector. The older generation of outdoor workers, who are mainly fair skinned and work in areas of high sun exposure, have an extremely high incidence of skin neoplasia.

The indigenous population have dermatological disease patterns resembling those in developing countries, with infections predominating. There can be some difficulties in diagnosing dermatological problems in patients with heavily pigmented skin.

The medical culture

Australia has a two-tier healthcare system with general practitioners (GPs or primary care physicians) and specialists. Most dermatology is practised as an office specialty in the private sector. There is a reasonably efficient and very popular compulsory, comprehensive, monopsonistic government health insurance system called Medicare (the Australian version). It is illegal even to offer 'top up' insurance for office-based treatment. This has kept fee increases well below the general rate of inflation over the past two decades. Patients cannot receive the full rebate allowable for a specialist unless referred by a GP, the gatekeeper into the healthcare system. This combination of circumstances ensures that except for non-subsidized treatment such as cosmetic work, specialists see the overwhelming majority of patients only by referral. There are implications for private teledermatology practice since consultations are held between GP and specialist. Because the patient does not approach a dermatologist directly, store-and-forward teledermatology can be characterized as a management support system, which reduces the apparent medicolegal risk. There is always a medical practitioner at the distant end (the GP) who implements and monitors any management proposals made by the specialist. The disadvantage is the absence of a direct relationship between the specialist and the patient which can render obtaining payment from the patient more difficult. Failure to convince the relevant authority to reimburse any teledermatology service makes fee-for-service private practice teledermatology unattractive.

Rural general practitioners

At least in Australia, rural GPs are vigorously individualistic and independent. They do not like having to hand over patients to others for management. However, it has been shown that dermatologists perform significantly better than GPs at diagnosing skin disease.[3–5] The rugged self-reliance so essential in a remote practitioner can be disadvantageous to the patient. Store-and-forward teledermatology may provide a satisfactory support for the GP without having to 'relinquish' the patient.[6]

A problem looking for a solution

Government imperatives and popular expectations

Political movements have greatly increased the importance of the rural vote to both major parties in Australia. As a consequence, politicians are laying increasing stress on the provision of health care to rural populations. The expectations of the rural community have risen partly for this reason and partly because of a general increase in the level of education and the ease of communication compared with the past. Simultaneously, rural populations have diminished because of automation in primary industries making the provision of services (including specialist dermatological services) even less economical. These factors have led to increased reliance on electronic communication. Most communities of any size have access to the Internet for the cost of a local telephone call. This has increased the expectation that medical services will be delivered electronically as well. It seems likely that similar considerations are driving the adoption of these techniques in other parts of the world.

Current specialist coverage

At present, specialist dermatologists visit some of the larger country centres in the state periodically, attending from once a week to once every 6 months. The localities with less frequent visits are usually too sparsely populated to warrant more personal attention. Teledermatology is the ideal method for the specialist to give advice or interim treatment for urgent cases which can be seen face-to-face on the next visit.

Once a specialist service has been supplied to an area, there is a natural expectation that it will be continued. Teledermatology can satisfy that expectation[7] to some degree, particularly if the discontinuance of service is only to be temporary.

Other options for rural patients

Apart from teledermatology, there are three options for rural patients:

1. Financial travel assistance. In some states, partial travel assistance is provided for patients referred to metropolitan specialists provided the journey is deemed necessary. The subsidy does not compensate for lost income or family dislocation. Teledermatology may offer considerable savings to the patient and the state.[8]

2. Telephone consultations. These have been the mainstay of assistance to country practitioners in the past but have drawbacks. Apart from being unable to see the skin lesion, the calls are usually ad hoc and can disrupt a busy session of consulting or operating.

3. The Royal Flying Doctor Service (RFDS). On a few occasions, patients with severe acute skin problems such as toxic epidermal necrolysis and cerebral melanoma metastases have needed evacuation to a major hospital in Perth.

Two solutions

In planning a teledermatology service in Western Australia, the main initial decision was whether to use real-time telemedicine or store-and-forward. As bandwidth on the Internet increases, it is becoming easier to combine modalities where necessary.

Real-time

Videoconferencing was the modality of much of the early teledermatology work. It has the advantage that the dermatologist can communicate directly with the patient for history-taking and management. The latter in particular can contribute positively both psychologically and by allowing detailed instructions regarding the use of medications and general treatment.

The American Academy of Dermatology has published a Position Statement on Telemedicine outlining the basic requirements.[9] See Chapter 16 for further details.

Store-and-forward

In a sparsely populated region, there will be large numbers of small centres making occasional requests for consultation. These are difficult to schedule efficiently in private office consulting. For our needs, in line with the concept of management support, a store-and-forward approach appeared adequate for initial contact. Videoconferencing or ordinary telephone contact could be used if necessary to discuss details of management with the referring doctor or the patient. Country patients are adept at transacting business of all types by telephone; presumably, this skill will transfer to the Internet with time.

Store-and-forward teledermatology also allows the dermatologist to consult online support such as Medline and CD-ROM publications. This is obviously possible following a videoconferencing consultation but store-and-forward operation facilitates reference to Internet resources. There have been suggestions that failure to consult such resources may be considered a breach of the standard of care in the future.

Some workers have suggested better concordance between videoconferencing teledermatology and face-to-face consultation when compared with store-and-forward.[10] The methods used for the store-and-forward teledermatology have been less sophisticated than for the videoconferencing, but the store-and-forward was found to be cheaper.[11]

Golden rules

Experience suggests some simple rules to ensure satisfactory teledermatology.

Keep it simple

Particularly in the area of private practice, but also as a general rule, it is best to achieve any end by the cheapest, simplest and least dangerous means. This may be self-evident but doctors seem to be easily seduced by bells, whistles and blinking lights. Of any technologies that can achieve a desired result, the one with the lowest infrastructure costs, the gentlest learning curve, and the least requirement for technical support is to be preferred. Another consideration is the use of an open architecture, meaning that the software will run on equipment from different manufacturers. Practitioners should look for the most cost-effective equipment, upgrade individual items as necessary and use equipment already available in the practice.[12]

Face to face is the gold standard

Face-to-face consulting represents the 'gold standard' against which any form of teledermatology should be judged. This is self-evident and it is difficult to envisage this changing.

Teledermatology needs a justification

This rule is a corollary of the previous one. The only obvious justification seems to be distance. There are some situations such as medical problems at the Australian Antarctic Base during winter when there is no alternative to telemedicine. Within Australia, the availability of the RFDS and other forms of transport means that any case can be brought to a metropolitan centre. However, this is so inconvenient and expensive in most circumstances that other forms of consultation should be considered. The precise distance required to justify teledermatology to the courts in the event of a lawsuit is unknown!

Communicate with the centre of first referral

Ideally, teledermatology cases should be directed to a dermatologist who can see the patient face to face should this become necessary. It might be a dermatologist who attends the country centre or a metropolitan specialist who could see the patient for follow-up.

One possible difficulty is the temptation to acquire several opinions for every case. An appropriate fee scale should discourage multiple 'simultaneous' consultations by telemedicine, just as it does in current practice. In the Australian context, Medicare maintains a watch on overservicing.

The initial attempt

The initial configuration for our system was a PC-based graphical user interface (GUI) program, using Visual Basic.[13] The program needed installation from disks sent by post. It was difficult to offer support and maintenance of the program for a large number of users, since this would have been expensive and time consuming. There would have had to be a charge for the program or the not inconsiderable costs would have needed to be recovered in the fees charged, making teledermatology less competitive.

The original configuration also resulted in problems relating to the transfer of data to the dermatologists. They would have to leave a computer running and attached to a telephone line or the sending doctor would have to ring and ask for a computer to be made available. The system was used on one occasion with a GP who was able to set up communications between two personal computers over the telephone network using proprietary software. It was clear that the majority of practitioners would not be able to manage this system.

Technological advances outpace development

Spread of the Internet

The rapid advance of technology seems to be the major problem in making predictions about the future of teledermatology. Whilst trying to organize the initial system described above, Internet availability spread throughout Western Australia and it immediately became the preferred option for telecommunication. The initial attempt at a website used the original program translated into a Java Applet. As Applets cannot access files on the client disk without special authorization, this system was also considered too complex for most doctors.

Digital photography

Digital photography has also progressed considerably over the last few years. It is difficult to recommend a specific camera, as new and greatly improved models appear on the market so quickly. At the time of writing, the most suitable models in our experience include the Nikon Coolpix 990 and the Olympus 2500. There are others of similar quality but a particular requirement is excellent close-up capabilities. More expensive professional cameras provide even better quality. As the referring doctors each need a camera, cost is important. One of the great advantages of digital photography is immediate access to the final result – it is even quicker than instant (Polaroid) photography.

The quality of images that a reasonable amateur photographer can obtain using cameras such as those mentioned makes the operator the limiting factor in obtaining adequate picture quality for practical purposes.[14–17] Conversely, it is possible to obtain a very unsatisfactory image with a very sophisticated camera. The best principle is the 'eyeball' test. The referring doctor should ask the question, 'Is the image I have produced a satisfactory representation of what I can see with the naked eye?' There is little point in having advanced colour indicators but substandard images as a result of poor technique. The variation in picture quality between doctors using the same model of camera is a striking feature of our experience to date.

The same remarks apply to lighting. Operators can adjust the ambient light until a satisfactory image is obtained using cameras with a digital viewfinder. In office practice, this process complies with the 'keep-it-simple' principle. It is preferable to have the operator concentrate on obtaining the optimum image than rely on standard conditions. The conditions are likely to vary with the background, skin type and the lesions in question (see Chapter 4).

The current configuration

Internet based

The Internet provides the most convenient communications medium for store-and-forward teledermatology at present and it is hard to see this changing. Internet-based videoconferencing may become common in due course, with increasing bandwidth. The Internet has the advantage of worldwide reach, constant availability, ease of use, familiarity, and reasonable acceptance by doctors and the general public. Internet technology is progressing at an enormous pace. This is mainly advantageous but does leave the private practitioner with the task of keeping up. Because the Internet is widely used by the general public, most of the facilities are readily understood and relatively easily mastered by non-technical operators, especially teenagers.

The homepage for our teledermatology system is located at http://www.theteledermatologist.com (Fig. 20.2). Rural practitioners access the site to send cases to dermatologists in their home state and currently, replies are returned by email.

Internet problems include inadequate bandwidth and security. The modem connection speed at our centre is 56 kbit/s, which is adequate for current operations. Bandwidth will improve as the public network is modernized. ISDN was considered to be too expensive for the likely advantage in speed. In fact, ordinary telephone lines have proved quite adequate, as the system is not used in real time. We have approached

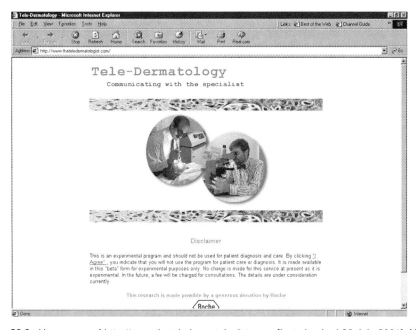

Fig. 20.2. Homepage of http://www.theteledermatologist.com. [last checked 26 July 2001]. Note the disclaimer.

the security issue by transmitting anonymized cases only but this will need to change if fees are to be charged, as is intended. (The service has been free of charge to date as it is still experimental.) The Australian Government is introducing a Public Key Infrastructure for all health-related electronic communications.

Graphical user interface

A graphical user interface is the preferred method of interacting with computers. It has the advantage of uniformity. No matter what the application, the method of achieving 'house-keeping' activities (such as opening and closing programs) is the same. This uniformity of access and the aesthetic appearance of the interface are sometimes described as its 'look and feel'. Most doctors are not rapid typists and even if they were, it is uneconomical to have doctors performing clerical tasks in private practice – they are a very expensive resource. Effective voice-input software may be available in the future but current systems do not appear to satisfy most medical users.

The website uses a form to obtain history from referring doctors (Fig. 20.3) and this is sent as an HTML document together with the digital photographs as a compressed email attachment to the dermatologist nominated by the referring doctor. The dermatologist considers the history displayed by browser software, and having formed an opinion, replies by email to the referring doctor.

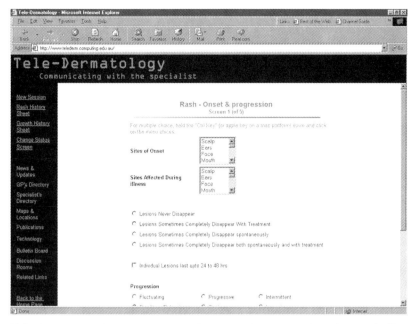

Fig. 20.3. An example of the forms used to obtain an orderly history. The aim is to facilitate use by non-typists.

Organization

In office practice, referral patterns are important. Telemedicine is more likely to be successful if it fits into existing patterns. In our situation, referring doctors select a specific dermatologist willing to take cases from a list on the website. Otherwise practitioners unfamiliar with computing are faced with the added problem of trying to find a specialist capable of responding to a request for a teledermatology consultation.

The need to make a profit will shape the way that private store-and-forward teledermatology is practised. This is discussed more fully in the section on 'Remuneration' below.

Experience to date

The response has been slower than expected. We receive an average of two requests for consultations per week, which is considerably less than would be expected for the size of population if teledermatology were a well-established method of accessing dermatological expertise. Most of the cases are inflammatory conditions. Anecdotally, the service has been helpful – but the early adopters are likely to be enthusiasts, and may therefore be unrepresentative of doctors as a whole.

The slow uptake is related to a number of factors. There is already an established pattern of referral and a number of country areas are visited by dermatologists. Use of a store-and-forward teledermatology site involves some effort and there is a learning curve. Until there is a definite incentive, learning to use digital cameras and the website may continue to be postponed by busy rural practitioners. It is easier to use current referral channels even though they may not be as convenient for the patient.

A potential incentive may be pressure from patients following advertisements that the service is available. We are about to commence a trial in the form of a quality assurance exercise. These are carried out by groups of GPs as part of their continuing professional development (which determines levels of government remuneration). We are hoping that this will introduce the concept to practitioners and particularly to patients in the rural area chosen.

Problems

A number of problems are always raised when telemedicine is mentioned. The following discussion refers largely to store-and-forward teledermatology via the Internet in private practice.

Lack of computer expertise

For teledermatology to become a mainstream medical activity, rural doctors need to be comfortable with day-to-day computer operations. The Internet has made this easier.

Time requirement

Time and effort are needed to prepare a store-and-forward referral. One solution is to have parts of the forms completed by a nurse or assistant. The referring doctor should still check the final result on the web page.

Medicolegal problems

Potential medicolegal issues are often a concern in telemedicine generally.[18] A recent report by Robert Milstein[19] commissioned for the Victorian Government sets out some medicolegal problems. A particular difficulty is Common Law jurisdictions where it is not really possible to know how courts will react ahead of time. There have been few precedents in telemedicine. It may be helpful to look at other areas such as banking.

An interesting point made by Milstein is that new technology may raise the expectations of the public and encourage litigation if these are not met. Teledermatology practitioners have a responsibility to avoid excessive claims for telemedicine. He also makes some other points:

> Liability often turns on the facts. The capacity to ascertain "who said what to whom and when" is often the critical issue. Communication – or its absence – is often at the heart of medical liability claims. The availability of contemporaneous documentation of a relevant encounter – or its absence – is often critical to the determination of liability and the resolution of factual disputes.

This raises three points in relation to store-and-forward teledermatology:

1. standard of care
2. attitude of medical defence organizations
3. registration.

Standard of care

Would a standard less than that of face-to-face dermatology be acceptable? The specialist does not have full access to the patient and is relying on the referring practitioner to ensure an adequate and representative view of the problem. Milstein makes this point about the standard of care:

> Reasonable care and skill in the provision of medical treatment and advice is the standard of care imposed by law. The doctor owes a single, comprehensive duty covering all aspects of practice, including diagnosis, the taking of a proper case history; listening to and, when appropriate, responding to patient complaints; treatment, whether medical or surgical; postoperative care; and the provision of information and advice. Although the duty is often divided for convenience into different areas such as diagnosis, treatment and advice, it is in fact the same duty to which the same principles apply.

Essentially, the standard of care is the same although influenced by certain factors:

> Location does not qualify the level of skill, although there may be features peculiar to the locality which ought to be taken into account in the overall assessment of the appropriate level of skill.

and:

> The ability of the courts to formulate a reasonable standard of telepractice will be impaired by the relative novelty of telemedicine and the absence of formal guidelines and input from peak bodies. It is likely that this situation will change over time.

It is incumbent upon us as teledermatologists to ensure that we set good, but reasonable, standards. The comment that the situation will change over time is ominous in a Common Law jurisdiction as one suspects that some of us may be involved with the evolution of the precedents.

However, it may be that teledermatology will be included as standard care and in remote areas under the appropriate circumstances, failure to obtain a teleconsultation will constitute negligence.

Private practitioners should be cautious. The advice is to avoid being dogmatic, always give a differential diagnosis, and err on the side of over-investigation particularly in relation to biopsy.

The absence of direct contact may increase the risk of litigation although this may be balanced by access to otherwise unavailable expertise in rural areas.

I use the following disclaimer. I am not sure of its legal status but I feel that it expresses my intentions:

> NOTE This advice is proffered on the basis of the information provided electronically by the referring doctor. As the teledermatologist is not physically

present, the advice must be interpreted by the referring doctor in the light of standard history-taking and examination by the attending doctor. This advice can only assist in managing the patient and should not override clinical judgement by the doctor "on the spot".

Attitude of medical defence organizations

The prudent private practitioner will approach the relevant indemnity carrier for a ruling on what is acceptable.

Registration

Is the doctor registered where he is practising? Milstein summarizes the problem:

> ...the question is whether the doctor is effectively being transported to the patient (in which case he is practising medicine in the patient's State) or whether the patient is being electronically transported to the doctor's State (in which case the doctor is simply practising medicine in the one and only jurisdiction in which he is registered).

Some US jurisdictions have addressed these problems explicitly. Perhaps as in all matters relating to private practice and in any jurisdiction, caution is the best policy as suggested by Milstein for the Australian situation:

> While the jurisdictional issue is yet to be resolved in Australia, it is submitted that medical practitioners would be taking a significant risk if they assumed that cross-border telemedicine did not require them to obtain multi-State registration via the mutual recognition procedures.

Our web site lists the states in which each dermatologist is registered so that referring doctors can avoid sending cases to out-of-state practitioners. Telemedicine can be valuable for travellers and those working overseas. A company in Perth, Western Australia (Global Doctor. See www.globaldoctor.com.au) offers a videoconference-based telemedicine service in Asia, including dermatology. The clinics are staffed by locally registered doctors who obtain opinions from the GPs and specialists in Western Australia. They are patronized by expatriates and affluent locals. However, it seems unlikely that this method of healthcare delivery will become the standard in Asia in the near future.

Remuneration

This is a major dilemma for private practitioners. In the case of videoconferencing, the patient has spoken with the attending specialist and would normally expect a bill. However, remuneration for store-and-forward teledermatology is more complicated and this has not been solved in the Australian situation as yet. The lack of government reimbursement for teledermatology and the absence of direct contact between the patient and dermatologist are disincentives to payment. Australian patients seem happy enough to pay for medications but have an aversion to paying for services such as consulting medical practitioners. This was summed up by an ophthalmology colleague who informed me that he did not think that dermatologists would be likely to get a fee for 'just looking at a few pictures'.

Billing practices

It has been the practice following standard face-to-face consultations in Western Australia to bill patients either at the consultation or subsequently by mail, but not to expect payment on the day. However, this is changing. It would be possible to bill patients after a teledermatology consultation by including their addresses in the referral data but I suspect that there would be problems with bad debts.

Another approach would be to hold the response to the referral on the server until payment is received.

The referring doctor could be asked to collect the fee but they would have no incentive to collect the money. Collecting fees for specialists is unlikely to be met with much enthusiasm by GPs. Demands for payment from colleagues could cause ill feeling and have the effect of reducing the number of referrals.

E-commerce and the teledermatologist

E-commerce is becoming more prevalent both between businesses (B2B) and between business and consumer (B2C). The increasing acceptance of e-commerce and improved techniques for collecting payment may help to overcome problems currently encountered by teledermatology practitioners. The obvious method would be to bill patients by credit card on the website prior to accepting the referral for transmission. However, not all patients have credit cards and many people are still uncomfortable about entrusting their credit card details to the Internet. The absence of a direct connection with the patient makes the operation more difficult.

Online teledermatology will necessitate some changes in the customary relationships between specialist and patient. Dermatologists could be thought of as wholesalers of dermatological expertise, which can be sold to the retailer, the referring doctor (GP or primary-care physician). The GP could then add a mark-up and 'sell' the product to the consumer. The relationship between the dermatologist and the referring doctor would be effectively B2B. The dermatologist would receive payment by credit card at the commencement of the store-and-forward encounter and the GP would recover the dermatologist's fee plus the mark-up on the patient's fee. An advantage is that only one fee is raised and, presumably, this would be quoted prior to the consultation.

Consent

Patients need to know that another practitioner has entered the doctor–patient relationship for privacy reasons, as well as to allow them to control the direction of their management. The health consumer movement appears to be driving this desire for control by patients of their management. If expense is to be incurred, there clearly needs to be financial consent as well.

Competition legislation

This could cause problems in jurisdictions where such legislation exists. In Australia, price setting collusion between doctors could contravene the Trade Practices Act.

Pigmented lesions

There is a high incidence of malignant melanoma in Western Australia. Melanomas are generally diagnosed early because of extensive education of the general public. There is a high risk of litigation concerning failure to diagnose. At least until epiluminescent images are transmitted routinely,[20,21] it would not be considered safe to give a teledermatology opinion about a pigmented lesion in Western Australia. The doctor dealing with the patient needs to decide whether to biopsy, but our advice is to err on the safe side and biopsy any lesion about which there is uncertainty.

Next steps

Artificial intelligence

Store-and-forward teledermatology may be enhanced by the use of artificial intelligence (AI). AI has enjoyed only relatively limited success in medicine in the past. Excessively ambitious aims may have been part of the problem. When used to assist in obtaining a more complete history and the best images, AI may be more effective.

Graphic representations and improved images

A useful addition will be graphical representations of the body to allow recording of the exact location of tumours and the overall distribution of rashes. Greater resolution and colour fidelity are likely to result from continued technical development.

Bandwidth

Bandwidth will increase allowing the transmission of larger files. This will allow more images at higher resolution than is feasible with telephone modem connections.

Convergence with the electronic health record

A decision has been taken by the State Health Ministers of Australia to proceed with a national electronic health record (EHR). This will probably be a centrally held database, although smart cards remain a possibility. Private practitioners will be major stakeholders in such a system. By July 2001, GPs in Australia will be starting to prescribe electronically. A GP will generate a prescription and send it to the central database that already links all pharmacists. The patient will be able to go to any pharmacist and obtain the pharmaceutical supplies.

Teledermatology systems will need to integrate with a national or even locally based EHR. It may be necessary to interrogate the system for demographic and medical data. This may pose problems with confidentiality.

Data protocols

Standard systems for coding diagnosis and treatment are becoming increasingly important with the increase in financial control over the practice of medicine and EHRs. It will be prudent to build support for these systems into teledermatology systems. The systems will need to be technologically compatible.

Technological developments

Various technological developments appear likely:

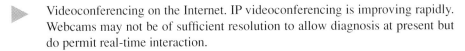 Videoconferencing on the Internet. IP videoconferencing is improving rapidly. Webcams may not be of sufficient resolution to allow diagnosis at present but do permit real-time interaction.

Attached text or video files. In my conventional dermatology practice, I give patients written instructions regarding their medications using previously stored text in my word processor. This is personalized with the patient's name and date, and is printed on my letterhead at the reception desk via a local area network. It may be possible to do the same over the Internet by attaching a text document to an email message sent directly to the patient or to the referring doctor. A video file could also be sent. Alternatively, the patient could be given a web site address to access the appropriate video and/or written instructions.

Dermatopathology

Laser confocal microscopy and other technologies will enable effective teledermatopathology.

Screening

Various types of screening could eventually be done via teledermatology possibly over the Internet. This is more likely to be the domain of public institutions and will probably depend on the development of more sophisticated and effective technology. One possibility would be melanoma screening (see Chapter 22).

Holography

Using holography, it may be possible to transmit a three-dimensional image of large areas of the unclothed body, enhancing appreciation of the distribution of widespread rashes in the future. This may permit 'virtual examination' of the patient by a distant dermatologist.

Image processing

Artificial intelligence to process an image of a rash and make a comment about the possible cause is likely in the future.

Conclusion

Although much of the early impetus for telemedicine including teledermatology has come from institutions such as the military and medical services to remote regions, there is a place for private teledermatology. This is most likely to flourish where small populations are sparsely distributed over large areas. Where large populations are underserved, the value of teledermatology is less obvious as it does not overcome the problem of available time other than reducing travel by doctors.

In addition to all of the usual problems associated with telemedicine, there are particular problems relating to payment. The solution to this problem depends on the technical sophistication of the population, attitudes to online payment and methods of payment for medical services. The most important factor is the local medical insurance arrangements both private and public.

References

1   Glaessl A, Schiffner R, Walther T, Landthaler M, Stolz W. Teledermatology – the requirements of dermatologists in private practice. *Journal of Telemedicine and Telecare* 2000;**6**:138–141.
2   High WA, Houston MS, Calobrisi SD, Drage LA, McEvoy MT. Assessment of the accuracy of low-cost store-and-forward teledermatology consultation. *Journal of the American Academy of Dermatology* 2000;**42**:776–783.
3   Federman DG, Concato J, Kirsner RS. Comparison of dermatologic diagnoses by primary care practitioners and dermatologists. A review of the literature. *Archives of Family Medicine* 1999;**8**: 170–172.
4   Wagner RF Jr, Wagner D, Tomich JM, Wagner KD, Grande DJ. Diagnoses of skin disease: dermatologists vs. nondermatologists. *Journal of Dermatologic Surgery and Oncology* 1985;**11**: 476–479.
5   Federman D, Hogan D, Taylor JR, Caralis P, Kirsner RS. A comparison of diagnosis, evaluation, and treatment of patients with dermatologic disorders. *Journal of the American Academy of Dermatology* 1995;**32**:726–729.
6   Perednia DA, Wallace J, Morrisey M, et al. The effect of a teledermatology program on rural referral patterns to dermatologists and the management of skin disease. *Medinfo* 1998;**9**:290–293.
7   Zelickson BD, Homan L. Teledermatology in the nursing home. *Archives of Dermatology* 1997;**133**: 171–174.
8   Burgiss SG, Julius CE, Watson HW, Haynes BK, Buonocore E, Smith GT. Telemedicine for dermatology care in rural patients. *Telemedicine Journal* 1997;**3**:227–233.
9   http://www.aad.org/Members/telemedicine.html [only available to members of the American Academy of Dermatology].
10 Clarke M, Jones RW, Lioupis D, George S, Cairns D. Teledermatology – UK experience of setting up an integrated teledermatology service. *Studies in Health Technology and Informatics* 1999;**68**: 274–277.
11 Loane MA, Bloomer SE, Corbett R, et al. A randomized controlled trial to assess the clinical effectiveness of both realtime and store-and-forward teledermatology compared with conventional care. *Journal of Telemedicine and Telecare* 2000;**6**(suppl 1):1–3.
12 Carlos ME, Pangelinan SI. Teledermatology in Department of Defense Health Services Region 10. *Journal of Healthcare Information Management* 1999;**13**:59–69.
13 Tait CP, Clay CD. Pilot study of store-and-forward teledermatology services in Perth, Western Australia. *Australasian Journal of Dermatology* 1999;**40**:190–193.
14 Vidmar DA, Cruess D, Hsieh P, et al. The effect of decreasing digital image resolution on teledermatology diagnosis. *Telemedicine Journal* 1999;**5**:375–383.
15 Krupinski EA, LeSueur B, Ellsworth L, et al. Diagnostic accuracy and image quality using a digital camera for teledermatology. *Telemedicine Journal* 1999;**5**:257–263.
16 Kvedar JC, Edwards RA, Menn ER, et al. The substitution of digital images for dermatologic physical examination. *Archives of Dermatology* 1997;**133**:161–167.
17 Whited JD, Hall RP, Simel DL, et al. Reliability and accuracy of dermatologists' clinic-based and digital image consultations. *Journal of the American Academy of Dermatology* 1999;**41**:693–702.
18 Wallace S, Sibson L, Stanberry B, et al. The legal and risk management conundrum of telemedicine. *Journal of Telemedicine and Telecare* 1999;**5**(suppl 1):8–9.

19   Telemedicine. Creating virtual certainty out of remote possibilities. An International, Comparative Analysis of Policy, Regulatory and Medico-legal Obstacles and Solutions. Report prepared by Robert Milstein, Consultant, January 1999. Available at http://www.telehealth.org.au/ [last checked 23 July 2001].

20   Piccolo D, Smolle J, Wolf IH, et al. Face-to-face diagnosis vs telediagnosis of pigmented skin tumors: a teledermoscopic study. *Archives of Dermatology* 1999;**135:**1467–1471.

21   Provost N, Kopf AW, Rabinovitz HS, et al. Comparison of conventional photographs and telephonically transmitted compressed digitized images of melanomas and dysplastic nevi. *Dermatology* 1998;**196:**299–304.

21

Mobile Teledermatology

Heikki Lamminen and Ville Voipio

Introduction

Ageing of the population will prove an enormous challenge to healthcare systems in industrialized societies. Telemedical home-care systems may provide improved home-care services at reduced cost. A few theoretical studies have been carried out concerning the need for home telecare. Preliminary data suggest that in the USA approximately 45% of home nursing visits could be carried out using telemedicine, while the figure is lower in the UK, about 15%.[1] Practical experience of home telecare includes the home telecare programme in Kansas, USA, which provided nursing services to patients in their homes in four towns in Kansas. On the whole, patients perceived telecare as a valuable resource that offered great potential, although many saw no immediate health benefits for themselves.[2] Other pilot trials of an analogue videotelephone in Kansas City and Belfast suggest that even relatively low-quality compressed video may be useful for home nursing. The effectiveness of videophones in home healthcare service has been found to be significant.[3] In Japan, a Personal Health Data system has been used to collect patient data such as ECG and health complaints, at the patient's home and send the information to staff at medical facilities.[4]

On the basis of the experience to date two telecare subsystems can be distinguished. One has the function of gathering, recording and transmitting data from elderly patients, such as ECG, physical activity and oxygen saturation rate in arterial blood. The other collects and sends visual information (images) from the patient's home. There is thus evidence to suggest that telemedicine may have a role in the delivery of home health care.[1]

Mobile telemedicine

Mobile communication devices have been of special interest in telemedicine for obvious reasons even though there have been few trials to date. The relevance of mobile systems for telemedicine in the third world has also been noticed.[5] Ricke and co-workers carried out a trial in which cooperation between physicians was investigated using desktop videoconferencing linked via satellite.[6] The major disadvantage of satellite systems is their high cost. However, mobile satellite systems have been utilized for US military operations during peacekeeping operations in Bosnia to obtain specialist medical advice from the USA.[7]

We have used wireless telemedical consultation for teledermatology. Primarily we have concentrated on the applicability and usefulness of the system in consultations between a nurse at a patient's home and a general practitioner. This kind of system is likely to be cost effective, because it can be used for purposes other than teledermatology consultations; most of the savings come from reduced travelling expenses.

Mobile healthcare processes

New telecommunication devices can offer new solutions for prevention, where a patient's role can be more active. Information technologies can then be used in more efficient and effective ways to reorganize work processes. Medicine is heavily dependent on technology, the main focus of which is cure rather than prevention.[8] Prevention is about improving the quality of life, not just preventing disease.[9] Approaches to prevention can be classified into three levels: primary, secondary and tertiary.[10] Primary prevention is the most basic and aims at preventing the onset of disease. Secondary prevention consists of the early detection and treatment of disease. Tertiary prevention seeks to minimize the disability and handicap following a disease that cannot be cured or leaves some loss of function. For these processes telemedicine and especially image transfer has much to offer. Changes in the environment of health care encourage greater patient participation and control, but at the same time patients realize that there is so much medical knowledge that many specialists are often needed to solve a particular medical problem. We have investigated a system which enables the transfer of wound pictures and information from home to healthcare centre. The resulting image database helps nurses to follow up the patient's care. Such applications are especially suited to tertiary prevention.

In planning structures and resources for health care, information about the changes in demand for healthcare services is essential. Also the condition, i.e. the transmitted information relating to a single home healthcare patient, often changes rapidly, which has effects on the frequency of visits. If telemedical systems are implemented without corresponding changes in healthcare processes, then the major effect will be increased expenditure. Working practices of healthcare professionals have to change and patients will have more control than before, but they will also have more responsibilities. To benefit from new telemedical solutions in health care, many cultural and social problems need to be solved. We need to support and activate the individual patient and decision-makers to realize these non-technical aspects. These tools aim at empowering the patient, and at the same time reduce the demand for health care. Training must be given to all participants of the systems in order to gain acceptance, but their future use depends on the perceived long-term benefits of the system to the users. Also the system must be implemented properly.

Mobile teledermatology

Visual information in medicine is important for making diagnoses, deciding on treatment and follow-up. The addition of visual information to an ordinary telephone call consultation is likely to improve the quality of home healthcare services, save costs and reduce the need for visits by patients and/or doctors. Although the techniques for transferring the information needed in these consultations are still developing and the standards of image processing and presentation are lacking, the usefulness and restrictions of these techniques requires evaluation now.

We have tried to find a low-cost method for teledermatology consultations. There are essentially two different approaches to teleconsultation. The older, and until now, more popular technique is videoconferencing which employs a two-way, real-time video connection. A newer application is store-and-forward, where data are first captured and then sent as an email attachment. The store-and-forward approach is readily applicable to teledermatology as most acute cases can be treated without real-time responses and dermatological conditions are rarely emergencies. There are also some encouraging reports about store-and-forward teledermatology in the literature.[11-13]

Even though videoconferencing equipment may have reasonably good image quality under ideal conditions, several studies indicate dissatisfaction with the image quality.[14,15] Store-and-forward telemedicine is cheaper and provides superior picture quality. However, if poor image quality occurs in videoconferencing it is more easily adjusted, because the specialist can advise the camera operator in real time. The operating costs of a store-and-forward system are negligible if an email connection is already available. Also, the acquisition cost of a store-and-forward system is very low if a suitable PC exists. One important reason for the slow adoption of store-and-forward-systems is the relatively large amount of technical expertise required to set them up. A videoconferencing system is often truly 'plug-and-play', and not significantly more difficult to operate than a video camera or a telephone. Store-and-forward telemedicine does not offer the real-time conferencing capability, which may make it less useful for educational purposes.

In order to prevent incompatibility in the future, it is important to use standard file formats, such as JPEG or TIFF. This is easy since most digital cameras use these formats anyway. For data protection, public encryption algorithms are considered safe. Public algorithms are also easy to decrypt later on, whereas proprietary algorithms tend to become obsolete and hence encrypted files may become unreadable eventually. One useful algorithm is PGP (Pretty Good Privacy), which can be easily integrated into most popular email systems.

Our experience

The purpose of our research project was to evaluate the usefulness, proper method of use, cost-effectiveness, technical reliability and restrictions of a mobile communication device in the transfer of voice, images and text between nurses visiting the homes of home-care patients and general practitioners in medical centres or specialists in university hospitals.

Setting

The study was conducted in the small Finnish town of Ikaalinen. Ikaalinen has a population of 8000 and an area of 840 km^2. The referral hospital is the Tampere University Hospital (TAUH). The distance between these two units is 55 km. The primary healthcare centre in Ikaalinen employs five GPs and one resident doctor as well as seven nurses for home health care. The total number of personnel is 97. The seven nurses make about 6000 house calls a year. One of them also carries out administrative work and one performs part of his work among children and pregnant women.

Five of the nurses are located in the centre at Ikaalinen and most of their visits are fairly close to the office. Two nurses work from a rural office, which is located 25 km from the centre. The study included all the visits made by four nurses during the test period (Table 21.1).

Table 21.1. The annual number of house calls made by the seven nurses in Ikaalinen

Nurse no.	Participant in the study?	Office location	House calls per year	Performs administrative work or holds child or maternity welfare clinic?
1	No	Centre	563	Yes
2	No	Centre	1213	
3	No	Centre	1230	
4	Yes	Centre	1234	
5	Yes	Centre	914	
6	Yes	Rural	691	
7	Yes	Rural	274	Yes

We analysed the results after two nurses had had the telemedicine equipment for a 2-month period. This included a 2-week training period during which they were taught to use the equipment. The study took place during the summer, when there are generally fewer home nursing visits.

During the first two months, a total of 71 house calls were made for 79 reasons; in eight visits the nurse had more than one task to do. The average age of the patients was 76 years (range 22–112); 13 patients were male and 58 were female. The reasons for a nurse's visit are shown in Table 21.2.

Telemedicine equipment

The system was set up using standard office equipment without any hardware modifications (Fig. 21.1). The mobile system included a digital still camera (Casio QV-7000SX) and an advanced mobile phone (Nokia 9110 Communicator). Photographs were taken with the digital camera and were then transferred wirelessly

Table 21.2. Reasons for home nursing visits

Reason for home visit	Visits (no.)
Wound care	5
Ventipress treatment	1
Injections	11
Blood tests	10
Product services delivery (e.g. napkins)	5
Respiration rate measurement	8
Medication and other service delivery	34
Blood sugar measurement	3
Bathing	1
Doctor's visit	1
Total	**79**

using the IrTran-P protocol to the mobile phone before being transmitted as email attachments to a server at the medical centre. Transmission from the mobile phone was via a Global System for Mobile Communications (GSM) network (at 9.6 kbit/s). The system did not utilize an open network, and there was a firewall installed at the Internet server.

Digital camera

The digital still camera (Casio QV-7000SX) (see http://www.casio.com/cameras/ [last checked 29 July 2001]) measured 141 (w) $\times$ 75 (h) $\times$ 53 (d) mm and weighed 280 g without batteries. The camera was powered by batteries or by an AC power adapter. Pictures could be taken using automatic operation of shutter and flashlight. The camera offered telephoto and wide-angle options as well as movie recording for 3.2 seconds. The latter allowed five frames per second and four images per frame (there were also 6.4- and 12.8-second options).

The exposure time was controlled electronically. Shutter speeds ranged from one-quarter to one-thousandth of a second. The camera included a built-in flash for dim or dark conditions. The camera operated with an automatic white balance control, which could be switched to manual (a fixed white balance to compensate for incandescent, fluorescent or daylight lighting). The automatic white balance setting worked well in most circumstances and the incandescent setting provided a much more neutral cast under incandescent lighting. The camera had a 2$\times$ optical zoom (5–10 mm focal length) and a 4$\times$ digital zoom. The images were stored as JPEG files. The size of one compressed image was approximately 200 kByte.

Communication device

We used a Nokia 9110 Communicator mobile phone (see http://www. nokia.com/phones/9110/index.html [last checked 29 July 2001]). The dimensions of the Communicator were $158 \times 56 \times 27$ mm, weight 253 g, and it was equipped with a back-lit monochrome display with a screen size of 640×200 pixels. Zooming was available when viewing the pictures. The Communicator's software included email, web browser, fax, SMS (short text messages) and other applications. The Communicator had an alphanumeric (QWERTY) keyboard. The email software allowed the user to select messages. The phone could be connected to the digital still camera via an infrared link. It could also be connected to a desktop or laptop PC through an infrared link or cable. Other features such as a calendar, notebook and address book helped nurses in their daily routines. The backlit screen could also be used for receiving visual information such as manuals, assignment lists, drawings, medical records or other documents, transferred via the infrared connection from the digital still camera to the Communicator.

The Communicator transmitted data using the GSM network. One of the advantages of the GSM system is that the same handset can be used widely: a mobile phone registered to a GSM network in Finland can also be used on a GSM network in Germany for example. This may be useful if the patient or the doctor is abroad. The GSM system provides users with several digital channels, and because the system encrypts the data, the transmission is relatively secure.

Digital camera connectivity

The digital still camera used an IrTran-P interface to transfer images to the Communicator. IrDA (see http://www.irda.org [last checked 29 July 2001]) offers protocols, such as the IrTran-P, for digital information exchange via wireless infrared connections. IrDA is used for high-speed, short-range, line-of-sight, point-to-point wireless data transfer – suitable for devices like digital cameras and handheld data collection devices for example. The IrDA data protocols consist of a mandatory protocol set and an optional protocol set. The mandatory protocols are: PHY (Physical Signalling Layer), IrLAP (Link Access Protocol), IrLMP (Link Management Protocol) and IAS (Information Access Service). The IrTran-P is an optional protocol. At present, IrDA connectors can be found in approximately 50 million electronic devices including desktop, notebook and palm PCs, printers, digital cameras, public phones/kiosks, mobile phones, pagers and other mobile devices. The theoretical transmission speed is 115 kbit/s for data transferred from the camera to the Communicator. In practice, however, the speed is a little lower.

Image transfer

Pictures taken by the nurses were sent as email attachments to a server of the municipality of Ikaalinen supplied by the local telephone company (IPP). Consulting doctors were then able to view the images and read the email messages using commercially available browser software (e.g. Internet Explorer or Netscape Navigator) or have a telephone conversation. If the GP could not provide an answer, he or she could either transfer the image to a specialist, or ask the patient to visit the healthcare centre or consult a specialist (at the TAUH).

Study design

During the study period, two nurses (nos 4 and 7) took a digital still camera and a Communicator with them on their visits. When required, the nurse took pictures and sent them by email to the healthcare centre in Ikaalinen. The nurse then made a telephone call, or sent an email or SMS message to the doctor, who could display the images on his computer screen (Fig. 21.1).

The two control nurses (nos 5 and 6) had GSM phones but no Communicator or digital camera for their visits. In order to assess the usefulness, technical reliability and restrictions of the system, all the nurses (nos 4, 5, 6 and 7) filled out a questionnaire after every visit to a patient's home during the test period. All nurses attended a short training session where they learned how to use the Communicator and digital camera. The control group needed to know about the Communicator and the digital camera in order to fill out the questionnaire.

Nurses filled out a questionnaire for each house call during the test period. The questionnaire included mainly closed questions. The questions were divided into three parts. In the first part the questions were concerned with the usefulness and reliability of the equipment. Nurses were asked whether they were able to use the equipment and if the equipment functioned reliably.

The second part of the questionnaire concerned the potential cost savings. Nurses were asked to evaluate the potential need for the patient in question to visit the healthcare centre. They were also asked to evaluate the potential need for

Mobile teledermatology system

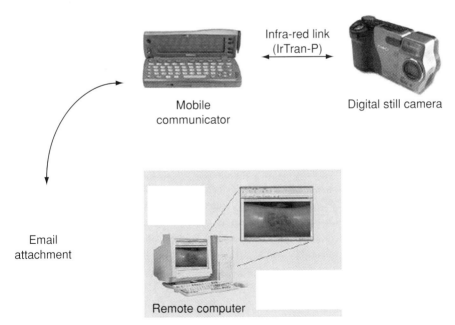

Fig. 21.1. The mobile teledermatology system.

transportation in each case and whether or not an attendant would be needed. Furthermore, the nurses were asked to estimate the travelling distance to the healthcare centre. The third part of the questionnaire dealt with the patients' opinions on the treatment.

Early results

In 68 out of 71 cases (96%) the patient did not need to visit the healthcare centre. In three of the control group visits (7%), having the ability to take a picture would have saved an appointment with a doctor. Table 21.3 shows the results based on the questionnaires.

Table 21.3. Preliminary study results

Question	Observed data for visits by two control group nurses in 2 months	Estimated data for visits by seven nurses in a year
Number of visits	43	6119
Picture transfer would have saved appointment with doctor	3 (7%)	420
Average length of a trip saved, one way (km)	30	30
Total length of trips saved, two ways (km)	180	25 200

Clinical aspects

In addition to the final diagnosis the teleconsultation may determine whether it is necessary to send the patient for further tests. In the questionnaire, the local practitioner and the consulting specialist were asked about the necessity for in-person consultation. A teleconsultation system justifies its acquisition if it can help the local practitioner send the right patients for further examinations. This saves resources and prevents unnecessary travelling.

To study the technical quality of photographs, the specialist answered questions concerning the subjective image quality. The aim was to identify situations where the image quality is not good enough.

The subjective image quality was good enough in most cases (Fig. 21.2). The image quality depends very much on the photographer's skills. Usually several photographs are required from one patient to give enough information. Lighting is the single most important factor affecting the image quality, especially colour. This is especially true with colour-sensitive tumour diagnoses.[16] The final evaluation of diagnoses has not yet been performed, so the diagnostic capability remains uncertain.

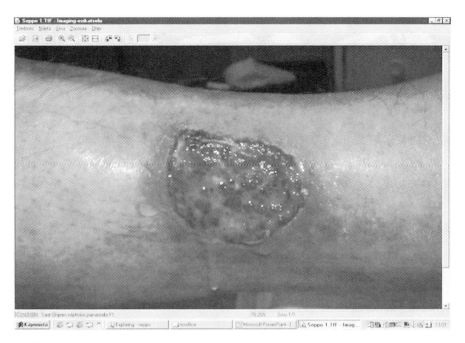

Fig. 21.2. A chronic ulcer on the leg of a home healthcare patient.

As found in other studies, the patients had positive or very positive attitudes towards teleconsultation. They felt it would improve the quality of treatment and save time. The greatest value seems to be for follow-up. Tertiary prevention, based on the nurses' experience, has proved to be the most promising (Fig. 21.2).

Economic aspects

The final economic analysis cannot be carried out yet as we only have results from the 2-month trial period, which was held in the summer at vacation time. Substantial savings will be achieved if the number of visits to the healthcare centre can be reduced. The key factor is travelling costs. Older people normally need transportation, which in most cases will be a taxi. Moreover, in many cases the patient will need an attendant. A visit to the healthcare centre often means extra effort. Elements such as the ease and comfort of treatment must be taken into consideration.

In this study the average cost of a one-way visit to the healthcare centre by taxi was about 65 euro. Nurses visit patients' homes in Ikaalinen 6119 times a year. According to the preliminary results we estimate that teleconsultation will save a round trip to the healthcare centre in 7% of the cases, so the potential savings amount to 55 683 euro per year in travelling costs. From that we have to subtract the price of the telemedicine equipment and the transmission costs. This gives a net yearly saving of 44 000 euro.

From previous economic studies carried out in telemedicine we know that costs may vary enormously, so the above-mentioned figures are simply estimates based on the preliminary results.

Future prospects

The preliminary results from the present study suggest that standard digital camera equipment may be used beneficially in teleconsultations for home health patients, especially for tertiary prevention. The actual operation of the camera was more critical than it is in videoconferencing. However, the cost was a fraction of that of videoconferencing, the static image quality was an order of magnitude better, and the method was more easily adaptable to remote field conditions.

The image resolution of the digital camera was high, and since there was no need to use extensive magnification, there was no need to use higher resolutions, although macro-imaging capability is advisable. With current digital photography equipment the image quality approaches that of conventional photography. Some studies carried out with conventional photographs[17] suggest that a photograph is a valuable diagnostic tool. Another benefit of using digital still pictures is the patient image archive thus formed. If the archive system is properly constructed it should be easy to find reference cases and research material. Some work is still required to find the most efficient workflow in this process.

The effective use of store-and-forward teleconsultation in dermatology requires training of the personnel[5] and new working methods at both the local unit and the central hospital to obtain the best results. The past few years have seen mobile phones become commonplace; in the next few years, it can be expected that smart mobile phones will be able to transfer live images. This will certainly have an effect on communication in general and will offer new possibilities in telemedicine.

According to our experience, teleconsultation in its present form, using commercially available equipment, is feasible. For home health care, a communications package including a digital camera and an advanced communication device can be used for consultations between nurses and general practitioners. Persons inexperienced in either taking photographs or using computers can learn to use the equipment in a couple of days. Based on our experience, people will adopt new technologies quickly when they are motivated to learn. In the future, people will be more familiar with these technologies and the devices will be easier to use.

Teleconsultation can produce cost savings for the healthcare sector. The key factors are reduced travelling costs and time savings. In Finland, travelling expenses are mainly paid for by the healthcare system. To enable a more detailed calculation of the cost savings, a longer time period of experimentation is required, with a large number of nursing visits.

The value of our mobile home health-telecare system was rated highly by the nurses, especially for dermatology and ophthalmology cases, in which visual information is of great importance for diagnosis, treatment and follow-up. Moreover, the photo library sent via email provided a good way to monitor diseases. For example, nurses could share information concerning wound healing better. An opportunity to transfer the images allowed further consultation between the GP and a specialist.

To summarize, information technology is one way of enhancing the sharing of knowledge and so it represents a possible way of increasing the efficiency of healthcare delivery.

References

1   Wootton R, Loane M, Mair F, et al. A joint US–UK study of home telenursing. *Journal of Telemedicine and Telecare* 1998;**4**(suppl 1):83–85.
2   Whitten P, Collins B, Mair F. Nurse and patient reactions to a developmental home telecare system. *Journal of Telemedicine and Telecare* 1998;**4**:152–160.
3   Nakamura K, Takano T, Akao C. The effectiveness of videophones in home healthcare for the elderly. *Medical Care* 1999;**37**:117–125.
4   Inada H, Horio H, Nakazawa K, et al. A study on development of a home health care support information system. *Medinfo* 1998;(9 Pt 1):269–271.
5   Wootton R. The possible use of telemedicine in developing countries. *Journal of Telemedicine and Telecare* 1997;**3**:23–26.
6   Ricke J, Kleinholz L, Hosten N, et al. Telemedicine in rural areas. Experience with medical desktop-conferencing via satellite. *Journal of Telemedicine and Telecare* 1995;**1**:224–228.
7   Macedonia CR, Littlefield RJ, Coleman J, et al. Three-dimensional ultrasonographic telepresence. *Journal of Telemedicine and Telecare* 1998;**4**:224–230.
8   Davies C. Hospital centred health care: policies and politics in the NHS. In: Atkinson P, Murcott A (eds). *Prospects for the National Health.* Beckenham: Croom Helm, 1979: 25–29.
9   Kemm J, Close A. *Health Promotion. Theory and Practice.* London: Macmillan Press, 1995.
10 Locker D. Prevention and health promotion. In: Scambler G (ed). *Sociology as Applied to Medicine*, 3rd edn. London: Baillière Tindall, 1991: 35–41.
11 Vidmar DA. The history of teledermatology in the Department of Defense. *Dermatologic Clinics* 1999;**17**:113–124.
12 Vassallo DJ. Twelve months' experience with telemedicine for the British armed forces. *Journal of Telemedicine and Telecare* 1999;**5**(suppl 1):117–118.
13 High WA, Houston MS, Calobrisi SD, et al. Assessment of the accuracy of low-cost store-and-forward teledermatology consultation. *Journal of American Academy of Dermatology* 2000;**42**:766–783.
14 Lowitt MH, Kessler II, Kauffman CL, et al. Teledermatology and in-person examinations: a comparison of patient and physician perceptions and diagnostic agreement. *Archives of Dermatology* 1998;**134**:471–476.
15 Gilmour E, Campbell SM, Loane MA, et al. Comparison of teleconsultations and face-to-face consultations: preliminary results of a United Kingdom multicentre teledermatology study. *British Journal of Dermatology* 1998;**139**:81–87.
16 Provost N, Kopf AW, Rabinovitz HS, et al. Comparison of conventional photographs and telephonically transmitted compressed digitized images of melanomas and dysplastic nevi. *Dermatology* 1998;**196**:299–304.
17 Harrison PV, Kirby B, Dickinson Y, Schofield R. Teledermatology – high technology or not? *Journal of Telemedicine and Telecare* 1998;**4**(suppl 1):31–32.

22

Automated Melanoma Diagnosis

Greg R. Day and Hugues Talbot

Introduction

Melanoma, the most aggressive of skin cancers, is increasing in incidence around the world, with white-skinned populations especially at risk. Unlike most other cancers however, melanoma often gives visible signs of its presence and progress, allowing suitably trained medical personnel to detect and treat the disease. If the cancer is detected early enough, it is simple to treat by limited excision. Friedman[1] has stated that '...The current death rate from malignant melanoma can be reduced to nearly zero through early detection coupled with prompt surgical removal'.

However, medical practitioners have often been frustrated with the difficulty of recognizing the visible indicators of melanoma. These indicators are often vague, and can display an enormous amount of variation, firstly within the types of melanoma, and secondly within the life of the lesion itself (for examples, see Fig. 22.1). Because the speed of detection is perhaps the single biggest factor in deciding disease prognosis, medical practitioners are forced to predict which lesions may become malignant in the future.

Recognition of melanoma is primarily based on the visual appearance of the lesion. Size, shape and colour have been shown to be important indicators for malignancy.[2] A visual inspection may take place at two levels. Traditionally, lesions are inspected unaided, by the naked eye. This level of inspection is known as the 'clinical view'. In recent years, however, epiluminescent microscopy (ELM) has become an increasingly popular method of inspecting lesions. This technique usually involves covering the surface of the lesion in transparent oil, and viewing it through an illuminated, low-magnification hand lens. Alternatively, a polarized lens without oil immersion can be

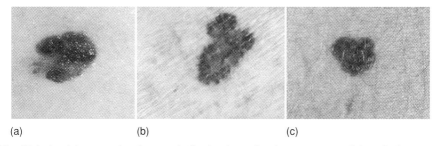

(a)   (b)   (c)

Fig. 22.1. (a–c) Images of melanoma, indicating the variety in appearance of these lesions.

used. Figure 22.2 shows a melanoma in the clinical view and using ELM. ELM has been shown to produce more accurate diagnosis than clinical-view inspection.[3-5]

The assessment of skin lesions for malignancy is subjective, and is very dependent on the clinician's experience.[6] There are few appropriately trained medical specialists. A number of rule systems to simplify identification of melanoma have been developed. The purpose of such systems is to improve recognition of melanoma versus benign lesions by less experienced clinicians.

The rule systems are for clinical-view use or for lesions viewed with ELM. One clinical-view rule set, the ABCD criteria (Asymmetry, Border irregularity, Colour variegation and Diameter) of Friedman et al[2] has become widely known, and is a mainstay for public education schemes around the world. For ELM, both Stolz et al[4] and Menzies et al[7] have developed well-known rule-systems.

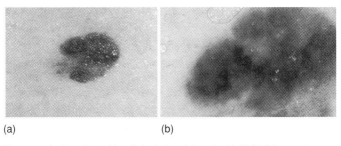

(a)   (b)

Fig. 22.2. The same lesion viewed in clinical view (a) and with ELM (b).

Although such systems are undoubtedly useful, a completely objective set of rules for recognizing melanoma from visual inspection of the lesion has not yet been developed. This lack of objectivity makes dissemination of knowledge concerning melanoma recognition difficult. In principle, an automated system could quantify the characteristics of a lesion, and then diagnose the lesion based on these characteristics. If such a system could be developed, and it could perform to the standard of expert clinicians, the rate of detection of melanoma could increase, and the death rate of melanoma could fall.

Automated melanoma diagnosis and telemedicine

An automated melanoma diagnosis system is any computer-based system that primarily uses computer processing as the method of distinguishing between benign and malignant lesions. It is generally considered that the system should be able to distinguish lesions at least as well as an experienced clinician. There is also potential for such systems to *outperform* experienced clinicians.

Figure 22.3 shows the general structure of all automated melanoma diagnosis systems. Information concerning the lesion is used as input to the automated system

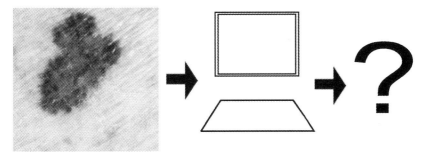

Fig. 22.3. The general structure of an automated melanoma diagnosis system. An image is input to a computer, which then analyses it and produces a diagnosis.

which examines the information for characteristics that distinguish malignant lesions from benign. A diagnosis is made based on these characteristics. In general, the system attempts to replicate the diagnostic process of human clinicians. The ultimate goal is to use the ability of computers to measure and classify large amounts of data and to outperform human clinicians.

Telemedicine

Current telemedicine applications allow examination and diagnosis to take place at a distance. Telemedicine means that the clinician and patient do not have to be in the same physical location. Hence, access to scarce knowledge is facilitated. This book contains many examples of such systems.

The medical knowledge being accessed is still scarce. Automated diagnosis systems are intended to encapsulate a small part of human specialist knowledge, and package it into a form that can be sent and used anywhere.

Although the ability to diagnose melanoma automatically is a specialized case of encapsulating medical knowledge (such a system would not be expected to recognize psoriasis for example), it illustrates many of the techniques and difficulties of recognizing disease through analysis of images. The techniques discussed here may be applicable to a wider range of dermatological conditions and hence may become an important component of dermatological practice in the future.

Review

Research into automated melanoma diagnosis has been underway for about 15 years. Major papers in the field are summarized in Table 22.1. There have been two significant periods in automated melanoma diagnosis system development. The first occurred prior to 1995, and systems developed at this time were concerned with diagnosis of clinical-view (i.e. macroscopic) images. Since then diagnosis systems have been mainly based on analysis of ELM images.

Table 22.1. Summary of automated melanoma detection system research

Author	Date	Sensitivity	Specificity	Images	Melanoma	Image type
Cascinelli et al[10]	1992	83	60	169	45	CV
Schindewolf et al[11]	1993	94	88	353	215	CV
Schindewolf et al[12]	1993	Accuracy=81(CV)*		320	194	CV
		Accuracy=78(ELM)*		320	194	ELM
Green et al[13]	1994	83	82	164	18	CV
Ercal et al[14]	1994	96	approx 62	399	135	CV
Menzies et al[15]	1997	93	67	170	75	ELM
Gutkowicz-Krusin et al[16]	1997	100†	61	104	30	ELM
Bischof et al[17]	1999	80–100	80-84	221	45	ELM
Binder et al[18]	1998	90	74	120	39	ELM
Seidenari et al[19]	1999	100	92	424	37	ELM

*Schindewolf et al compared CV and ELM images.
†Gutkowicz-Krusin et al fixed sensitivity at 100%.
CV = clinical view; ELM = epiluminescent microscopy.

Clinical images

Systems based on clinical images concentrated on reproducing the ABCD criteria of Friedman et al[2] in an effort to provide useful image analysis results for classification. However, relatively few published studies have investigated whether or not their algorithmic approach actually captured this specialist knowledge.

Epiluminescent microscopy

In the early to mid 1990s, the emphasis of work shifted from analysis of clinical-view images to analysis of ELM images. This move appeared to be based on the relative success of ELM images in clinical situations, and in particular, the ability to recognize melanoma earlier. It is hoped that similar benefits will be apparent for computer-based systems, although no evidence for such an outcome has been presented.

Despite the length of time that research has been conducted, there have been few developments of interest to the medical community as a whole. Although Table 22.1 indicates a number of very good results on large image sets, no automated diagnosis tool is in standard clinical use. Most developments have been concerned with the ability to take, store and retrieve images of skin lesions. However, it is possible that this situation may change in the next few years.

Techniques

Automated recognition of melanoma is a problem of image analysis. In general, the process is to obtain an image of the lesion, and analyse the image for characteristics that are indicative of malignancy. Once these characteristics are obtained, it should be possible to make some determination of the malignancy of the lesion.

Although the general description may sound straightforward, in practice, diagnosis of disease through image analysis is difficult. Few useful systems for automatic disease diagnosis exist in any medical discipline, although computers in medicine are commonplace. The three major techniques used in automated melanoma diagnosis research are: segmentation, which looks at identifying the lesion in the image; analysis, which obtains relevant measurements from the image; and classification, which attempts to provide a diagnosis based on these measurements.

Segmentation

At the start of the process, there is an image of a skin lesion (Fig. 22.1). To human observers, lesions are quite clearly identifiable in these images. From the point of view of a computer however, each image is simply a large array of numbers, representing the colours of each pixel in the image (Fig. 22.4). Somehow, the computer also needs to recognize that the image consists of two major areas, the lesion and the rest.

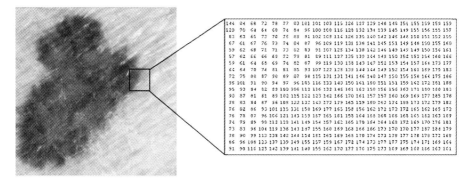

Fig. 22.4. To a computer, an image is simply a collection of numbers, representing the 'colour' of the pixels. The goal of segmentation is to decide which colours belong to which object in the image.

Segmentation is the separation of a digitized image into different areas based on their appearance. In the case of melanoma recognition, there are two major areas of interest, the lesion area, and 'everything else' (Fig. 22.5). 'Everything else' is primarily the skin component of the image, although a number of other areas may also exist. For example, lesions may be obscured by hair; this feature of the image is not of interest in the recognition process. Artefacts of the image-capture process itself may also occur, such as air bubbles and flash artefacts in ELM images. These artefacts are discussed more fully below, in the section 'Image acquisition'.

Segmentation is a familiar problem in image analysis generally, and a large literature exists describing different techniques. The size of the literature can be taken as an indication of the difficulty of the problem. Clearly, there is no 'universal' segmentation method that is applicable in every context, and most techniques rely on context-specific knowledge.

The problem of segmentation, already difficult in the simplest case, is further complicated by the context of the problem. In the case of skin lesions, even the human visual system may have difficulty separating the lesion area from the irrelevant skin

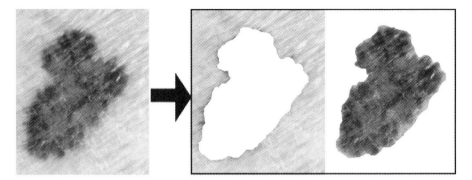

Fig. 22.5. Segmentation is the process of identifying different parts of an image (e.g. lesion and skin parts), based on their visual characteristics.

component. Indeed, Stolz et al[4] used the amount of border contrast as an indicator for malignancy when lesions are viewed under ELM. Lesions with more border contrast are considered more likely to be malignant, while those with less border contrast are considered more likely to be benign. If benign lesions are expected to have borders that are difficult to differentiate from skin, this suggests that segmentation of all epiluminescent skin lesion images will indeed be difficult.

Analysis

Once segmentation has taken place, using whichever technique is considered suitable, the lesion area can be analysed for characteristics of interest (Fig. 22.6). These characteristics are the values on which the system will base its classification of the lesion, either malignant or benign. Therefore, it is essential to choose characteristics that allow such discrimination to be made.

There are generally two approaches to selecting these characteristics. The first bases them on guidelines developed by human experts. For example, the system may use

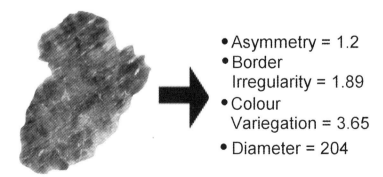

- Asymmetry = 1.2
- Border Irregularity = 1.89
- Colour Variegation = 3.65
- Diameter = 204

Fig. 22.6. Analysis is the process of measuring aspects of the image, which can then be used to obtain a diagnosis.

measures of lesion asymmetry, border irregularity and colour variegation (the ABCD criteria[2,4]). Ercal et al[8] and Gutkowicz-Krusin et al[15] have described systems for clinical view and ELM respectively.

The obvious advantage of this approach is that experienced human practitioners have already chosen the characteristics considered relevant for system developers to implement. An automated diagnosis system then follows (Fig. 22.7). However, reproducing human perception algorithmically is a notoriously difficult problem in computer science. Few computer applications in any context have performed this task well, and even those that appear to, such as computer chess programs, owe more to the ability of the computer to process huge quantities of data quickly than any actual reproduction of human knowledge.

The second approach ignores human guidelines and concentrates on using the abilities of the computer to measure large numbers of characteristics that may have little meaning to humans. This approach avoids the difficulty of reproducing human knowledge by concentrating on algorithms that are simple to implement. However, as can be seen by inspection of any image-processing textbook, the number of potential algorithms is extremely large, and some method must be provided for selecting those that are relevant.

Both of these approaches have advantages and disadvantages. Some studies that use a large number of characteristics seem to converge on those that in some way attempt to duplicate human perception. However, there is still a relevant difference in the way the analysis will be used. In the case where human perception is used as a more strict guideline, an expert system or AI (artificial intelligence) approach seems to be warranted, whereas in the case where a large number of characteristics are used, a more 'black box' approach to classification (i.e. where the reasons for classification are decided automatically and are unlikely to be interpretable by humans) is almost a necessity.

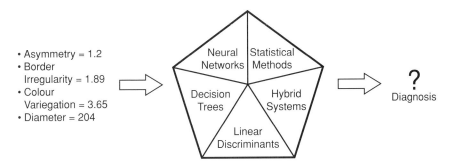

Fig. 22.7. Classification is the process of using the measurements obtained through analysis to assign a label or class to an image. From this, the classifier can assign a diagnosis to a lesion image.

Classification

Following the analysis stage, the measurements can be used to construct a classifier, or decision-maker regarding the malignancy of the lesion. The process of examining the results previously obtained, and assigning the underlying data source (in this case, the lesion) a class based on those results is called classification. Again, classification is a well-researched problem in computer science and statistics. An increasing number of techniques have been described. These include expert systems, statistical techniques, machine-learning algorithms and neural networks.

The classification problem can be further refined for an image-based diagnosis system, using a set of images with known diagnoses. The classifier is required to examine this set, and infer a model that will match set members (images) to their class (malignant or benign). Once this model is produced, new images can be presented to the classifier, which will infer the class of the lesion.

The goal of the classifier is to infer the model that adequately describes the lesion population as a whole. Unfortunately, the classifier never has access to the entire lesion population. The only thing that can be used to develop the classifier is a subset of this population with the best diagnosis that can be achieved in practice. The classifier will *infer* diagnoses on new lesions based on the composition of this subset. How does one know whether the model describes the lesion population as a whole? That is, how does one know whether the system will be useful in a real situation?

There is no simple answer to this question. Techniques such as cross-validation[9] allow us to be more confident in the ability of the model to generalize to the lesion population as it is described by the dataset used. However, there is no certainty that the results obtained from testing will be successful when used prospectively on real data.

These three areas represent the major components of an automated diagnosis system based on image analysis. As has been indicated, provision of these components is difficult, and each can only be an approximation to what may be achieved with human perception. However, given the abilities of computers to assess a large number of different characteristics, and to produce reliable weightings for each of the characteristics, it is plausible that the computer may eventually be able to outperform even expert human clinicians. In general, that is the goal for most automated melanoma diagnosis systems.

Image acquisition

Although the above three components represent the core of image-based automated diagnosis systems, there is an often-overlooked prior step, how the images are obtained. Because computer analysis is based completely on the data contained in the image, image-based diagnosis systems are extremely susceptible to failure due to poor quality images. In the case of melanoma diagnosis systems, the problem is compounded as often non-professional photographers take the images.

There are several areas of concern with image acquisition. First, there is the problem of the quality of the images. The photograph may be out of focus or incorrectly exposed. In clinical practice, these drawbacks may not be vital for archiving and teaching. But for computer analysis, it is essential that artefacts be as few as possible, and that the image characteristics are consistent from lesion to lesion.

Other areas of concern are image lighting and colour balance. The former refers to the ambient lighting and how the lesion is illuminated. Colour balance refers to the distribution of colours within the image. Both of these image characteristics should ideally be uniform in different images, otherwise significant difficulties with image segmentation and analysis will occur. These characteristics may be difficult to control.

Images used in computer-based analysis systems should be obtained under identical conditions, and to be of as high quality as possible. Such image sets are very difficult to obtain, and are the result of a large investment in time. Medical practitioners often take images of interesting cases but a broad representation of all types of lesions is required for these systems. Because there are no easily accessible image sets, it is difficult to compare automated diagnosis systems.

The comparison problem

The three major components of an image-based automated diagnosis system, segmentation, analysis and classification, are all difficult to achieve in practice. There are no clear guidelines as to suitable techniques, and to date at least, most research has been performed in an ad-hoc manner. Each research project has used different techniques, and comparison of these techniques has been impossible.

Being unable to compare different research projects, the results of each project cannot be identified. A large number of techniques for automated melanoma diagnosis have been tried, but there is no way of identifying those of most benefit. The major reason is that the image sets used for each of the research projects are different. Because the variability in lesions is so enormous, each image set is likely to represent a very small portion of the potential lesion population.

Consider two melanoma diagnosis systems, A and B. Each of these systems has been tested on a different set of lesion images, image set A and B. Imagine that system A can identify 90% of lesions using image set A, while system B can diagnose 80% of image set B. Because it is extremely unlikely that either image set A or B is representative of the entire population of lesions, we cannot conclude that system A is in fact more useful with real data than system B. To compare the results of system A with system B would require each of the systems to be run on the other image set. The difficulty in obtaining and transferring image sets, differences in image quality requirements, together with confidentiality and other legal issues, have meant that no comparisons between systems have been performed to date.

The overall effect of this situation is twofold. First, it means that much of the research to date is of limited value, as useful techniques cannot readily be identified. Second, new research projects are required to collect their own images, and develop their own techniques more or less from scratch. The basic foundation of research, that of building on previous work, cannot be performed effectively in this context.

Commercial tools

The situation for commercial ELM systems, either currently available or in development, is not very clear. At the time of writing, no fully diagnosing system can be purchased, but a number of 'monitoring' tools, with high-quality digital image capture, image archival and retrieval, comparison with a database of images of typical lesions and some diagnosing capability have been announced. Perhaps the most promising of these instruments is the Skin SolarScan (ex-Polarprobe) being developed jointly between Polartechnics Ltd, the CSIRO and the Sydney Melanoma Unit at the Royal Prince Alfred Hospital in Sydney. However, very little public information is available about this product (http://www.polartechnics.com.au/ [last checked 27 July 2001]). This situation is typical. Melafind (http://www.melafind.com/ [last checked 27 July 2001]) and MoleMaxII (http://www.molemaxii.com/ [last checked 27 July 2001]) are two other systems being developed.

It appears that even though research into automated diagnosis of melanoma using image analysis has shown that the concept is feasible, the production of a commercially viable diagnosing instrument is a significant undertaking and has not truly been achieved yet. In addition to the technical difficulties, such as good quality image capture and calibration, lesion segmentation, artefact removal, feature extraction and model building, a host of design, production, marketing and governmental hurdles have to be overcome. Finally, such a medical instrument will have to gain acceptance from the medical community and the patients.

The future

It is likely that research in automated melanoma diagnosis will continue for some time. The challenge remains tantalizingly near, yet frustratingly out of reach. Many researchers have produced excellent results on a limited subset of images, but the techniques fail when attempts are made to generalize to the lesion population. Part of the difficulty is the immense variability of melanoma and benign lesions. Not only that, but the temporal factor of defining when a lesion will become malignant or not adds another layer of complexity. For example, a pathologist may classify an excised lesion as benign. However, if the lesion is not excised, there is no guarantee it will remain benign throughout its lifespan.

Even though interesting monitoring instruments such as the Skin SolarScan are becoming available, it appears that truly diagnosing instruments are still in the future. From the technical standpoint, published research shows that an instrument that can diagnose better than most GPs is feasible. Some recent research suggests that with a large enough lesion image pool and sufficiently well designed camera, feature extraction and reasoning model, an instrument with excellent accuracy, comparable to the best specialists, might be feasible. However this says nothing of the practical feasibility of such instruments, as outlined above. Monitoring systems are already available. These instruments may become the basis of truly diagnosing instruments of the future.

Hurdles to be overcome by a potential melanoma diagnostic tool include:

1. availability of a large set of lesion images (comprising thousands of images) covering all the known cases in all skin types

2. design of a good image capture device for high resolution with true colour, colour calibration and flat lighting

3. design of a good set of characteristics for diagnosis

4. design of reliable automated image analysis

5. design of a credible, open reasoning model

6. design of a simple and powerful user interface

7. design able to incorporate software upgrades

8. demonstration of convincing results in real-life conditions

9. approval by the regulatory authorities (such as the FDA), based on clinical trials

10. acceptance by the medical community and the community at large.

None of these points are trivial, and the sum of them amounts to a formidable undertaking. Designing a monitoring tool corresponds to points 2, 6, 7, 8 with an emphasis on 6, so that doctors can see the benefits of such instruments over the simple hand-held dermoscope. It is heartening to see that such instruments are very close to becoming available, and if well designed, they have the potential to achieve point 10. There has been a great deal of research into points 1, 3, 4 and 5 from different perspectives. A successful instrument will require a more open style of research.

Discussion

It is clear that automated melanoma diagnosis will continue to attract considerable research efforts. This is in part due to the continuing rise in the incidence of melanoma, and the corresponding requirement for specialized knowledge concerning recognition of the disease to be more available. If an automated diagnosis system that was clinically useful could be developed, access to medical specialists would be less vital. However, it appears that developing such a system may still be some way in the future.

This topic has important implications for telemedicine. Automated diagnosis tends to epitomize what is required from a telemedicine system, namely the ability to improve access to scarce medical knowledge. Because dermatology is such a visual discipline, automated image-based analysis and diagnosis may be fundamental to the practice of dermatology in the future.

References

1   Friedman R, Rigel D, Silverman M, Kopf, A, Vossaert K. Malignant melanoma in the 1990s: the continued importance of early detection and the role of physician examination and self-examination of the skin. *Ca – A Cancer Journal for Clinicians* 1991;**41**:200–226.

2   Friedman R, Rigel D, Kopf A. Early detection of malignant melanoma: the role of physician examination and self examination of the skin. *Ca – A Cancer Journal for Clinicians* 1985;**35**:130–151.

3   Pehamberger H, Binder M, Steiner A, Wolff K. *In vivo* epiluminescence microscopy: improvement of early diagnosis of melanoma. *Journal of Investigative Dermatology* 1993;**100**:356S–362S.

4   Stolz W, Braun-Falco O, Bilek P, Landthaler M, Cognetta AB. *Color Atlas of Dermatoscopy.* Oxford: Blackwell Science, 1994.

5   Binder M, Schwarz M, Winkler A, et al. Epiluminescence microscopy: a useful tool for the diagnosis of pigmented skin lesions for formally trained dermatologists. *Archives of Dermatology* 1995;**131**:286–291.

6   Binder M, Kittler H, Steiner A, Dawid M, Pehamberger H, Wolff K. Reevaluation of the ABCD rule for epiluminescence microscopy. *Journal of the American Academy of Dermatology* 1999;**40**:171–176.

7   Menzies S, Crotty K, Ingvar C, McCarthy W. *An Atlas of Surface Microscopy of Pigmented Skin Lesions.* Sydney: McGraw Hill Book Company Australia Pty Limited, 1996.

8   Ercal F, Chawla A, Stoecker W, Lee H C, Moss R. Neural network diagnosis of malignant melanoma from colour images. *IEEE Transactions on Biomedical Engineering* 1994;**41**:837–845.

9   Witten IH, Frank E. *Data Mining.* San Francisco: Morgan Kaufmann Publishers, 2000.

10   Cascinelli N, Ferrario M, Bufalino R, et al. Results obtained by using a computerized image analysis system designed as an aid to diagnosis of cutaneous melanoma. *Melanoma Research* 1992;**2**:163–170.

11   Schindewolf T, Stolz W, Albert R, Abmayr W, Harms H. Classification of melanocytic lesions with color and texture analysis using digital image processing. *Analytical and Quantitative Cytology and Histology* 1993;**15**:1–11.

12   Schindewolf T, Stolz W, Albert R, Abmayr W, Harms H. Comparison of classification rates for conventional and dermatoscopic images of malignant and benign melanocytic lesions using computerized colour image analysis. *European Journal of Dermatology* 1993;**3**:299–303.

13   Green A, Martin N, Pfitzner J, O'Rourke M, Knight N. Computer image analysis in the diagnosis of melanoma. *Journal of the American Academy of Dermatology* 1994;**31**:958–964.

14   Ercal F, Lee H, Stoecker W, Moss R. Skin cancer diagnosis using hierarchical neural networks and fuzzy systems. In: *Intelligent Engineering Systems Through Artificial Neural Networks*, vol 4. New York:ASME Press, 1994: 613–618.

15   Menzies S W, Bischof L M, Peden G, et al. Automated instrumentation for the diagnosis of invasive melanoma: image analysis of epiluminescence microscopy. In: Altmeyer P, Hoffman K, Stucker M, Schwarze HP, Freitag M, eds. *Skin Cancer and UV Radiation,* Berlin: Springer-Verlag, 1997:1064–1070.

16   Gutkowicz-Krusin D, Elbaum M, Szwaykowski P, Kopf A W. Can early malignant melanoma be differentiated from atypical melanocytic nevus by *in vivo* techniques? Part ii: automatic machine vision classification. *Skin Research and Technology* 1997;**3**:15–22.

17   Bischof L, Talbot H, Breen E, et al. An automated melanoma diagnosis system. In: Pham B, Braun M, Maeder AJ, Eckert MP, eds. *New Approaches in Medical Image Analysis*, vol 3747. Bellingham, WA: SPIE, 1999: 130–141.

18   Binder M, Kittler H, Seeber A, Steiner A, Pehamberger H, Wolff K. Epiluminescence microscopy-based classification of pigmented skin lesions using computerized image analysis and an artificial neural network. *Melanoma Research* 1998;**8**:261–266.

19   Seidenari S, Pellacani G, Giannetti A. Digital videomicroscopy and image analysis with automatic classification for detection of thin melanomas. *Melanoma Research* 1999;**9**:163–171.

23

The Economics of Teledermatology in the UK and New Zealand

Maria Loane

Introduction

The clinical feasibility of teledermatology has been well documented throughout this book and this leads us to the final question – what are the costs? The widespread implementation of teledermatology services is unlikely to happen without solid evidence of cost-effectiveness. Economic evaluations, although difficult to conduct in the field of telemedicine generally, are essential if teledermatology is to progress to become an operational service.

No society has the resources to meet the demand for unlimited health care and healthcare providers are already straining to contain costs. Part of the problem specific to dermatology is that general practitioners (GPs) traditionally receive little dermatological training, which limits their ability to correctly diagnose and manage dermatological conditions. This shortfall in dermatological skill and knowledge in the primary care sector has been reported not only in the UK,[1,2] but also in the USA[3] and Australia.[4] Telemedicine techniques are often proposed as a potential solution for improving primary care dermatology services. However few studies have assessed the health economics of such interventions. Most of the work to date has taken place in the UK and Norway. Indeed the first randomized control trial (RCT) evaluating the costs of primary care teledermatology compared to hospital outpatient care was conducted in the UK.

The UK multicentre teledermatology trial

The UK multicentre teledermatology trial was carried out in three centres in the UK, Belfast, Craigavon, and Manchester, and one centre overseas in Hamilton in New Zealand (Fig. 23.1). The trial was conducted in three phases using low-cost equipment and low-bandwidth transmission: phases 1 and 2 evaluated the clinical feasibility and patient satisfaction of real-time teledermatology, while phase 3 measured the health economics.

In phases 1 and 2 diagnostic and management accuracy was compared between real-time teledermatology consultations and conventional face-to-face consultations in the same patients.[5–7] This is important, as the cost-effectiveness of healthcare

UK Multicentre Teledermatology Trial

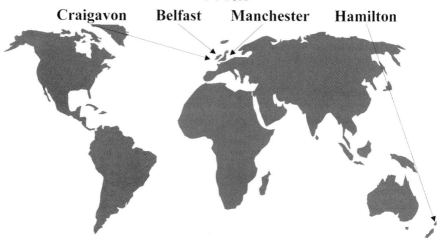

Fig. 23.1. The UK multicentre teledermatology trial was carried out in three centres in the UK (Belfast, Craigavon and Manchester) and one in New Zealand (Hamilton).

delivery depends on clinical effectiveness as well as the actual cost of providing care. As Perednia has pointed out 'higher failure rates can quickly erase any differential in the cost of clinic visits to general or specialty care providers'.[8]

In phase 3 of the UK trial, a societal cost analysis of teledermatology was conducted. An RCT assessed the costs and clinical outcomes of the initial real-time teledermatology consultation compared to the initial conventional alternative. The costs and clinical outcomes of store-and-forward teledermatology were also evaluated for a subset of the patients seen by real-time teledermatology.

Cost analysis of real-time teledermatology

An RCT is the preferred method for evaluating clinical outcomes of alternative interventions as it limits the inherent biases that are present in other study designs. This approach allows economic data to be collected simultaneously in order to assess the costs of providing health care.[9] In the UK trial the cost analyses were calculated from a societal perspective – that is costs and benefits borne by the hospital, the GP and the patient.

Two hospital dermatology departments and four health centres took part in the RCT in Northern Ireland. Each hospital allocated a weekly session for teledermatology and a similar session for conventional outpatient consultations. Patients were randomized at the point of referral to either the teledermatology consultation or the conventional hospital outpatient consultation. The dermatologist recorded the clinical outcome of the consultation as well as the length of clinician time involved. Patients were asked to complete an anonymous questionnaire detailing expenditure incurred by attending the appointment. The dermatologists and GPs involved in the study were interviewed to quantify the costs and benefits to the healthcare team.

Clinical outcomes recorded at the time of consultation do not necessarily reflect accurate utilization of healthcare resources. For instance, a patient may be discharged from hospital care but may return to their GP and seek a re-referral if the skin complaint has not been satisfactorily resolved. A follow-up review of patient records was carried out to determine the true picture of healthcare activity.

Over one year, 204 patients participated in this phase of the trial – 102 were randomized to the teledermatology consultation and 102 to the hospital outpatient consultation. The average age of the patients studied was 39 years (SD 24) and there were more females (58%) than males (42%).

The reported clinical outcomes of each consultation were similar. The dermatologist recommended a further hospital appointment for 46% of patients seen by real-time teledermatology and 45% of patients seen conventionally.[10] The review of patient records showed that 41% of real-time teledermatology patients and 40% of conventional patients were *actually* seen again by the dermatologist. These findings indicate that real-time teledermatology is clinically feasible compared to conventional outpatient care, as almost the same proportion of patients in both groups required additional consultations with the dermatologist.

Cost calculations

All costs were grouped into fixed and variable costs. The fixed costs described the equipment, depreciation and telecommunications costs, while the variable costs included the clinicians' time, the patients' time and the patients' travel costs. In the UK National Health Service (NHS) the purchase of capital equipment incurs a standard interest charge of 6% while the period of depreciation for electronic equipment is seven years. All calculations were based on actual costs observed in the trial. This is an important consideration as the equipment used in the trial was purchased in 1995, but the trial took some years to complete. Variable costs were calculated based on information from the consultation records and patient questionnaires. The daily rate charged for clinician time in our calculations was intended to cover overhead costs of the healthcare provider.

Benefit calculations

The GPs involved in the study estimated that dermatology outpatient referrals could be reduced by an average of 20% in one year as a result of the learning benefits and increased confidence obtained from being present at the joint videolink consultation. This means that the costs of consultant time, patient time and patient travel could have been avoided in 20% of cases. In addition, the GPs estimated that it would take an average of six training days to gain the same level of dermatological experience. This represents a further benefit to the practice, as the GP did not need to be away from the practice for the six days or pay for attending a training course.

Total calculations

The net societal cost per patient of the teledermatology consultation was £132.10 compared to £48.73 for the conventional consultation.[10] Two key factors need to be taken into account when interpreting these results.

First, four health centres and two hospitals were equipped with the videoconferencing equipment, yet only 102 patients were randomized to the teledermatology arm of the trial. This means that an average of 25.5 patients were seen by teledermatology at each health centre over the 12 months of the study. The high capital cost of the equipment combined with low usage did not render the system economically viable in this instance. Furthermore, the equipment used in the study was purchased in 1995 and these prices were used in the analysis. Current market prices for similar equipment have fallen by 40%, which clearly would have an effect on overall costs.

Second, the trial was conducted under somewhat artificial circumstances in order to minimize patient inconvenience and encourage participation. The health centres that participated in the trial were deliberately chosen because of their close proximity to the hospital. The average patient round-trip travel distance was 10 km for patients seen by teledermatology and 26 km for patients seen conventionally. In a real-life scenario it is likely that the distances between healthcare providers and specialist hospitals would be greater. A sensitivity analysis can be used to examine the effect on the calculations of basing the analysis on more realistic assumptions.

Sensitivity analysis

A sensitivity analysis showed that if each health centre devoted one morning session a week to teledermatology, the average cost per patient of the teledermatology consultation decreased substantially. If current equipment prices (year 2000) were used in the calculations and the average round-trip travel distance to hospital increased from 26 km to 74 km, the average cost of the two consultations would have been equal (£67.23).

Cost analysis of store-and-forward teledermatology

Clinical outcomes and costs of store-and-forward teledermatology were also investigated. In the trial, patients seen by store-and-forward teledermatology had instant photographs of their skin lesion taken by the GP, which were forwarded to the hospital dermatologists along with a standard referral letter. The clinical outcome of the store-and-forward consultation was recorded by a different hospital dermatologist to avoid possible recall bias from the videolink consultation.

Instant photographs were available for 96 patients. The dermatologists reported that 69% of patients seen by store-and-forward teledermatology needed an outpatient appointment compared to 45% of those seen in real-time.[11] Poor photographic image quality and inadequate information on the referral letter made treatment recommendations impossible. This suggests that store-and-forward teledermatology is not as clinically effective as real-time teledermatology or conventional outpatient consultation, because more patients need to be seen by the dermatologist in person.

Cost calculations

The fixed costs of the store-and-forward consultation covered the equipment cost of purchasing a camera and film for each of the four health centres involved in the study. The variable costs included the clinicians' time, patient time and patient travel costs. The net societal cost per patient of the store-and-forward consultation was £26.90[11]

Store-and-forward teledermatology was much cheaper than real-time teleconsultations and also cheaper than conventional outpatient consultations, due mainly to the speed of the consultation and the fact that the equipment costs were low. The dermatologist knew within minutes of looking at a photograph and referral letter if a diagnosis and management plan were possible without seeing the patient in person. However a drawback of the store-and-forward technique is that there is no interaction

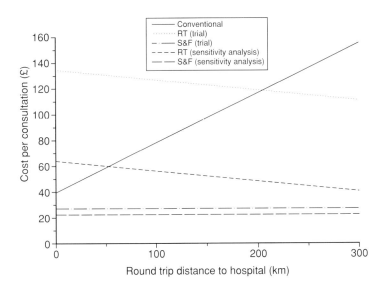

Fig. 23.2. The average consultation cost of the different techniques for delivering care.

between the dermatologist and the GP, so that the GP gains little or no educational or training knowledge that could be applied to the benefit of other patients within the practice.

Figure 23.2 shows the average consultation cost of the different techniques for delivering care.

Cost analysis using total and marginal costs

The economic evaluations carried out in the early stages of phase 3 described average societal costs per patient. Average costs of a real-time teledermatology consultation are affected by workload – the more the equipment is used to see patients, the lower the average cost. However this does not necessarily reflect the true picture. Fixed equipment costs remain the same regardless of how often the equipment is used. If a health centre invested in equipment and used it on a limited number of patients, the fixed costs would be the same as those for a health centre that purchased the same equipment and used it to its maximum potential. A more rigorous approach to assessing the economics therefore is to calculate both the *total* costs of the consultations and the *marginal* cost of doing an additional consultation (assuming that the fixed costs remain the same).

An RCT was carried out to assess the total and marginal costs of real-time teledermatology compared to conventional outpatient care. Clinical outcomes of each consultation were also evaluated. Over two years, one urban and one rural health centre referred patients to a specialist hospital. A total of 274 patients took part in the study – 46% were randomized to the teledermatology consultation while 54% were randomized to the conventional outpatient consultation. As before, there were slightly more females than males (56% vs 44%). The average age was 40 years (SD 25). Two-thirds of the patients were registered with an urban practice, while one-third were registered with a rural practice.

The clinical feasibility of real-time teledermatology was once again demonstrated.[12] The cost analysis was conducted from a societal perspective and compared the total societal costs and benefits of the two methods of delivering specialist dermatology care. As before, fixed costs described the actual equipment costs and the ISDN line installation and rental costs. The variable costs covered the total cost of the clinicians' time, patient time, patient travel and ISDN call costs. The total benefits were a reduction in the number of outpatient referrals with concurrent savings in dermatologist time, patient time and patient travel costs. GP educational and training benefits derived from being present at the joint videolink consultations were *not* included in the analysis.

Observed total and marginal costs

Table 23.1 shows the total *observed* costs and benefits of the consultations to society. It is evident that the costs of the telemedicine consultation (as observed in the trial)

Table 23.1. Total consultation costs

Type of cost saving	Telemedicine (£)		Conventional (£)	
	Urban (n = 77)	Rural (n = 49)	Urban (n = 105)	Rural (n = 43)
Variable costs				
Consultant time	2441.70	1696.35	4091.73	1314.58
GP time	1855.69	1289.23	0	0
Patient travel	113.35	45.72	197.73	350.05
Patient time	335.08	174.35	659.71	432.36
Call costs	65.63	45.60	0	0
Total variable costs	**4811.46**	**3251.25**	**4949.17**	**2096.98**
Fixed costs				
Cost of capital	1606.88	1240.63	0	0
Depreciation	3825.90	2953.89	0	0
Telecommunications costs	1777.44	1699.48	0	0
Total fixed costs	**7210.21**	**5894.00**	**0**	**0**
Total fixed + variable costs	**12021.68**	**9145.25**	**4949.17**	**2096.98**
Savings: non-referrals due to GP learning benefits				
15% of conventional consultant cost	613.76	197.19	0	0
15% of patient travel cost	29.66	52.51	0	0
15% of cost of patient time	98.96	64.85	0	0
Total savings	**742.38**	**314.55**	**0**	**0**
TOTAL SOCIETAL COST	**11279.30**	**8830.70**	**4949.17**	**2096.98**
Marginal cost	52.85	59.93	47.13	48.77
Unit cost	146.48	180.22	47.13	48.77

were higher than the conventional alternative for both the urban and rural patients. This was due mainly to the additional costs of equipment and GP time.

From a hospital perspective, the observed total cost of the teledermatology consultation was £6865 (marginal cost per patient was £26.41) compared to the conventional total cost of £5406 (marginal cost per patient was £36.53). This indicates that in the circumstances of the trial, teledermatology was dearer than conventional outpatient care. However, if the hospital workload was increased it was actually cheaper to see additional patients by teledermatology.

From a general practice perspective, the observed total cost of the teledermatology consultation was £6973 in urban areas (marginal cost £24.95) compared to £5849 in rural areas (marginal cost £27.24). The GP does not normally incur costs after referring a patient to hospital for an outpatient consultation.

From a patient perspective, the observed total cost of the teledermatology consultation was £448 in urban areas (marginal cost £5.82) and £220 in rural areas (marginal cost £4.49). The observed total cost of the conventional outpatient consultation was £857 in urban areas (marginal cost £8.17) and £782 in rural areas (marginal cost £18.20). From the patient's perspective, telemedicine was cheaper than conventional care as it involved less travel and time costs.

A study of the educational interaction between GPs and specialists reported that GPs preferred teaching based on clinical cases and liked to use referrals as a two-way learning process.[13] Real-time teledermatology enables this kind of learning opportunity. The increased educational benefits and experience apply to all patients presenting to primary care with dermatological conditions and not only those requiring referral. It represents a benefit to the GP alongside the savings to society obtained from the reduction in actual hospital referrals. This benefit was not included in our cost analysis.

Sensitivity analysis on total and marginal costs

The sensitivity analyses were based on more realistic assumptions and assumed that:

▶ equipment is purchased at current (year 2000) prices;

▶ depreciation costs are paid over the lifetime of equipment (7 years);

▶ ISDN line rental is paid for 7 years;

▶ 10 patients are seen per morning session, 45 working weeks per annum = 450 × 7 years = 3150 patients;

▶ observed patient travel distance increased threefold, i.e. urban patients travelled 26 km, rural patients travelled 18 km (telemedicine) and 155 km (conventional);

▶ the hourly rate of clinician time is £67.00 for GP and £89.00 for dermatologist;

▶ there is a 20% reduction in outpatient referrals;

▶ all remaining variables are as observed in the trial.

The analysis showed that the unit cost of the urban consultation was £41.41 (telemedicine) and £41.27 (conventional). The unit cost of the rural consultation was £39.32 (telemedicine) and £67.15 (conventional). The marginal costs of telemedicine were £36.09 for urban patients and £34.57 for rural patients. By contrast, the marginal costs of conventional care were £41.27 for urban patients and £67.15 for rural patients.

The sensitivity analysis showed that teledermatology was an economically viable alternative to conventional outpatient care when more realistic assumptions were applied to the data. In urban areas, the unit or average cost of both the teledermatology and conventional consultation was almost the same, while the marginal cost of seeing additional patients was lower for the teledermatology consultation. In rural areas both the unit and marginal costs were less for teledermatology compared to conventional outpatient care.

Conclusion

Assessing the economics of new healthcare interventions is a notoriously difficult task, not least in deciding which type of economic analysis is most appropriate and whose perspective to take, i.e. a societal perspective, healthcare provider's perspective or patient's perspective. The costs of providing a real-time teledermatology service are no longer prohibitive, although at present the financial benefits are more likely to accrue to the patient (especially in rural areas) rather than the health service provider. This finding is consistent with other studies that have reported similar economic benefits for patients seen by teledermatology.[11,15] However the healthcare team benefits from teledermatology in other ways. GPs can apply the educational and training knowledge gained from being present at the teledermatology consultations to the benefit of *all* patients in the practice. Specialist hospitals benefit, since patients who do not need hospital facilities or resources are managed effectively within primary care, thus freeing up valuable hospital resources.

The net result is that GPs do not always have the necessary skills and expertise to manage dermatological conditions effectively and efficiently. It has been shown that non-dermatologists are more likely to use expensive, less effective combination products to treat common fungal skin disorders while dermatologists use more effective and thereby cost-effective treatment products.[16] In addition dermatologists are better at recognizing and managing skin lesions – one study showed that dermatologists were twice as likely to diagnose seborrhoeic keratoses correctly compared to GPs.[17] If unnecessary procedures are being carried out in primary care as a result of incorrect diagnosis, then this affects the overall cost of delivering care. Both real-time and store-and-forward teledermatology techniques enable dermatological expertise to be more widely available within primary care, which should improve the overall standard of healthcare delivery and provide a better quality and more effective service to patients.

References

1   Basarab T, Munn SE, Russell-Jones R. Diagnostic accuracy and appropriateness of general practitioner referrals to a dermatology out-patient clinic. *British Journal of Dermatology* 1996;**135**:70–73.
2   Harlow ED, Burton JL. What do general practitioners want from a dermatology department? *British Journal of Dermatology* 1996;**134**:313–318.
3   Ramsey DL, Benimoff-Fox A. The ability of primary care physicians to recognize the common dermatoses. *Archives of Dermatology* 1981;**117**:620–622.
4   Hornsey A. (personal communication).
5   Loane M, Corbett R, Bloomer S, et al. Diagnostic accuracy and clinical management by realtime teledermatology: results from the Northern Ireland arms of the UK Multicentre Teledermatology Trial. *Journal of Telemedicine and Telecare* 1998;**4**:95–100.
6   Oakley AMM, Astwood DR, Loane M, *et al.* Diagnostic accuracy of teledermatology: results of a preliminary study in New Zealand. *New Zealand Medical Journal* 1997;**110**:51–53.
7   Gilmour E, Campbell SM, Loane MA, et al. Comparison of teleconsultations and face-to-face consultations: preliminary results of a UK multicentre teledermatology study. *British Journal of Dermatology* 1998;**139**:81–87.
8   Perednia DA. Fear, loathing, dermatology, and telemedicine. *Archives of Dermatology* 1997;**133**: 151–155.

9   Barber JA, Thompson SG. Analysis and interpretation of cost data in randomized controlled trials: review of published studies. *British Medical Journal* 1998;**317**:1195–1200.

10 Wootton R, Bloomer SE, Corbett R, et al. Multicentre randomized control trial comparing real-time teledermatology with conventional outpatient dermatological care: a societal cost–benefit analysis. *British Medical Journal* 2000;**320**:1252–1256.

11 Loane MA, Bloomer SE, Corbett R, et al. A comparison of real-time and store-and-forward teledermatology: a cost effectiveness study. *British Journal of Dermatology* 2000;**143**:1241–1247.

12 Loane MA, Corbett R, Eedy DJ, et al. A randomized control trial assessing the health economics of real-time teledermatology compared with conventional care: an urban versus rural perspective. *Journal of Telemedicine and Telecare* 2001;**7**:108–118.

13 Marshall MN. Qualitative study of educational interaction between general practitioners and specialists. *British Medical Journal* 1998;**316**:442–445.

14 Oakley AMM, Kerr P, Duffill M, et al. Patient cost–benefits of realtime teledermatology – a comparison of data from Northern Ireland and New Zealand. *Journal of Telemedicine and Telecare* 2000;**6**:97–101.

15 Stensland J, Speedie SM, Ideker M, House J, Thompson T. The relative cost of outpatient telemedicine services. *Telemedicine Journal* 1999;**5**:245–256.

16 Smith ES, Fleischer AB, Feldman SR. Nondermatologists are more likely than dermatologists to prescribe antifungal/corticosteroid products: an analysis of office visits for cutaneous fungal infections, 1990–1994. *Journal of the American Academy of Dermatology* 1998;**39**:43–47.

17 Sowden JM, Lewis-Jones MS, Williams RB. Who best manages seborrhoeic keratoses? *British Journal of Dermatology* 1996; **135**(suppl 47):47.

24

The Economics of Teledermatology in Northern Norway

Trine S. Bergmo

Introduction

Economic assessments of new healthcare technologies are needed by decision-makers to determine cost-effective resource allocations. Resources, such as people, time, facilities, equipment and knowledge, are scarce. Choices must be made concerning their deployment, and methods such as 'gut feeling' and 'educated guesses' are not always the best way to reach a decision. An economic evaluation can be defined as the comparative analysis of different courses of action in terms of both their costs and consequences. Economic analyses serve to identify, measure, value and compare the costs and consequences of the alternatives being considered.[1] When evaluating telemedicine, the costs of providing the service may be easily identified and measured compared to the benefits of the service. The benefits can be measured in terms of avoided costs, or the costs of the alternative method of providing health care, rather than the health benefits gained for the patients involved. Assuming that the health outcome for the patient is not affected by the intervention, a cost-minimization analysis or a cost comparison can be used to determine the most cost-effective alternative.

Few economic analyses that have been carried out have been based on field trials. The costs of providing telemedicine services may be known from an existing service and compared to the costs that might have been incurred without telemedicine. Estimating the costs of alternative methods of providing care based on what the patients used to do before the implementation of telemedicine is difficult and is associated with a high degree of uncertainty. The economic assessments of teledermatology described in this chapter have been based on assumed possible alternative ways of providing dermatology care to rural clinics.

The major referral centre in northern Norway, the University Hospital in Tromsø (UHT), has been involved in telemedicine services since the late 1980s.[2] One of the first telemedicine applications to become a routine service was teledermatology, which linked the dermatologists at the UHT to patients and a general practitioner (GP) in Kirkenes. An economic analysis of this service has been carried out[3] and will be outlined below. First, the Norwegian healthcare funding is briefly described, then, a cost-minimization analysis of the service in Kirkenes is presented. The relationship between the cost of investing in teledermatology, the actual distance and patient workloads are highlighted. This is in order to assess, from a health-service perspective, how many of the health clinics in the region might potentially save money by investing in real-time teledermatology. Then, the potential for still image teledermatology is presented.

The results from one economic evaluation should not be generalized. This is because most analyses of telemedicine use the avoided travel costs to measure the benefit of the implementation. Such cost estimations make the results dependent on the actual distances involved. The annual workload is another crucial variable that will differ from setting to setting and will influence the results. Other aspects that will be discussed are the effect teledermatology might have on referral patterns and other benefits that are usually not accounted for in most telemedicine research. Finally the financial principles for reimbursing telemedicine are discussed.

Healthcare funding

The Norwegian healthcare system is primarily funded by taxes, with the government paying for most services. Patients pay a small user fee for each visit. Averaged over a patient's lifetime, approximately 95% of all healthcare expenses are paid for by the government. The government also covers the travel costs associated with receiving health services.

Specialists are paid a salary for the duties they perform at the hospital. A few specialists provide services that are not a part of their hospital duties, in which case they charge a fee for service. GPs are either salaried or capitated, i.e. paid a basic salary which depends upon the number and type of patients they serve, and then are paid a little more per patient seen in their clinic. Fewer than 2% of physicians charge their patients privately.

An economic evaluation of a real-time teledermatology service

Real-time teledermatology has been a routine service provided by the University Hospital of Tromsø to Kirkenes, since 1989. Kirkenes is a rural community of about 10 000 people approximately 800 km from Tromsø (a 12-hour drive). In 1989 a pilot project was carried out to determine whether the quality of a teleconsultation was sufficient for diagnostic purposes compared to a face-to-face consultation. This showed 100% agreement between the two.[4] The hospital dermatologists were satisfied and they decided to put the teledermatology system into routine use. In 1993 the hospital in Kirkenes purchased a phototherapy unit, thus enabling patients to receive phototherapy without having to travel to Tromsø.[2]

Previous studies have documented the reliability of diagnoses made over a videoconferencing link compared with the conventional face-to-face diagnoses.[5-10] However, avoiding patient travel also requires the ability to treat the condition locally.

Some patients require face-to-face consultation for procedures, tests and treatment that are not available at their local health clinic. Most studies have examined the success of teledermatology by assessing the diagnostic accuracy of videoconferencing, rather than telemedicine as a tool to examine, test and treat patients at their local health clinic, and with that avoid travel. If avoided travel, rather than health outcomes, is used to quantify the benefits of investing in telemedicine, the GP must be able to provide tests and treatment locally as well.

In 1998, there were 375 patient consultations with the hospital dermatologist by real-time teledermatology in Kirkenes (there were 372 patient consultations in 1997). Sixty per cent of the patients were new and the remainder were follow-up patients (Fig. 24.1). In addition, 100 Kirkenes patients were referred to the hospital outpatient clinic in Tromsø for special clinical conditions, such as dermatological scalp problems, problems in or around the genital area and possible cancer. Thus, the teledermatology service was a suitable form of consultation for 79% of the total patients in the Kirkenes area, given that local phototherapy and bath facilities were available.

Cost assessment

A cost-minimization analysis assesses the cost difference between two or more techniques, given that the health outcome for the patients involved does not differ between the alternatives.[1] The cost of the teledermatology service was compared to the costs of other methods of treatment assuming a similar health outcome. These were a combination of a visiting service and patient travel; patient travel to the nearest secondary-care centre (UHT); and a locally employed dermatologist.

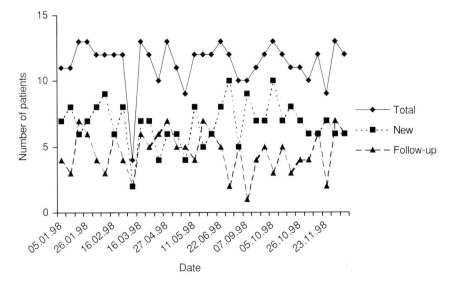

Fig. 24.1. Numbers of patients seen at the weekly teledermatology clinic in Kirkenes during 1998.

Equipment used for real-time teledermatology

The participating sites used commercial videoconferencing units (Master Vision, Tandberg), including two extra monitors, connected by ISDN lines at 384 kbit/s. A three-chip video camera with motorized zoom lens (Sony, DXC 930) was connected to the videoconferencing unit at the local health centre to enable the GP to transmit close-up real-time images to the hospital dermatologist. A phototherapy machine (Waldman, UV 700 1K) and bathroom facilities were also available locally. Phototherapy was provided by a specially trained nurse, supervised by the GP.

Procedure

Patients with dermatological conditions requiring a specialist consultation were referred to the dermatology outpatient clinic in Tromsø. The specialists then decided, based on the information in the referral letter, whether the patients should attend the GP in Kirkenes or travel to the dermatology clinic. The patients who attended their local clinic were, together with the GP, seen by a hospital dermatologist over the video-link. An interactive consultation ensued – first, the GP gave a brief medical history, the specialist then viewed close-up video-pictures of the skin area under examination and interviewed the patient, as in a normal consultation; and finally all three discussed a suitable treatment plan.

Before the real-time teledermatology service, the specialist used to travel regularly to the local health clinic to conduct outpatient consultations. With the observed workload a visiting service alone would be insufficient to meet the demand for dermatological consultations. A combination of a visiting service and patient travel would therefore be required to provide a practical alternative method of providing care. An upper limit of 240 patients per year was the maximum the visiting specialist could handle. The remaining patients were assumed to travel to the clinic at the UHT. The costs included in this option were the relevant travel costs and salary and allowance for a specialist and a nurse. The costs of patient travel to the central clinic were based on the price of airfares and transport to and from the airport.

Another possible way of providing the required service would be to employ a dermatologist in Kirkenes. The cost of employing a dermatologist locally was based on an annual salary for a medical specialist including employment costs.

Assumptions about costs

The costs considered were those falling on the public health service. Costs borne outside the social and healthcare sector were excluded. Lost production and lost working time due to absence from work were not included. Capital items were assumed to have a 5-year lifetime, a discount rate of 6% and an annual maintenance cost of 5% of the equipment's purchase price, except for the phototherapy machine and the bath facilities. The latter items were assumed to have longer lifetimes of 10 and 20 years, respectively. Average wages (including employment costs) were used to reflect the consumption of resources. All figures and prices had a 1998 basis to facilitate cost comparison.

In 1998, 100 patients travelled to Tromsø for an outpatient consultation at the hospital in addition to the patients seen over the video-link. The cost of this patient travel to the outpatient clinic was not included, neither were costs common to all methods such as treatment costs, that is costs of drugs and hospitalization, since it was assumed that these would not differ between the methods. This implies that the cost components included were incremental resource use, that is, only the costs that differed between the methods.[11] This approach means that nothing can be concluded about the total cost (i.e. total resource commitment) of any method.

Costs and break-even values

The annual fixed and variable costs of the alternatives evaluated are shown in Table 24.1. Total annual fixed costs that enabled patients to receive phototherapy locally were common to real-time teledermatology, a visiting service and a locally employed specialist. These costs included the phototherapy unit, bath facilities and a full-time nurse. Other costs differed between the alternative methods, such as the cost of investing in videoconferencing, travel and salaries.

Figure 24.2 shows the total costs of treating patients with dermatological conditions at a local health clinic. At the actual 1998 workload of 375 patients, teledermatology cost less than the other options: teledermatology cost NKr470 780, while the visiting service and patient travel to the hospital cost NKr880 530, patient travel to the nearest secondary-care centre cost NKr 1635 075 and a locally employed dermatologist cost NKr958 660 (1NKr is 0.12 euros, US$0.11). As shown in Figure 24.2, the result depended on the annual workload. If the annual workload had been below 85 cases,

Table 24.1. Annual costs (in NKr) for providing dermatology care to the local clinic by four different methods

Type of cost	Real-time telemedicine	Visiting service/ patient travel	Patient travel	Locally employed dermatologist
Fixed costs				
Phototherapy and bath facilities	30 810	30 810		30 810
Personnel costs at the clinic	277 300	277 300		917 300
Videoconference unit and camera	56 975			
Telecommunications costs (rental)	12 450			
Maintenance costs	21 250	10 550		10 550
Total fixed costs	**398 785**	**318 660**		**958 660**
Variable costs (per patient)				
GP, specialist, technician time and call costs	192			
Average costs of visiting service		603*		
Travel costs and consultant costs		3090	3090	
Treatment costs for phototherapy at the central hospital‡			3840 × 0.33†	
Total variable costs	**192**	**603* then 3090**	**4360**	**0**

* For the first 240 patients.
†Accommodation for a two-week stay in Tromsø for one-third of the patients.
‡A total of 126 patients received phototherapy treatment in 1998.

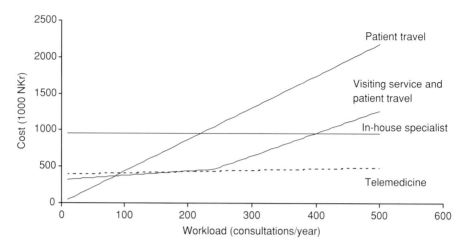

Fig. 24.2. Total costs of the alternatives analysed.

then patient travel would have been the cheapest method. A visiting service was the cheapest method for workloads above 85 and below 195 consultations per year. Telemedicine was the cheapest alternative for workloads higher than 195 patients per year.

Real-time teledermatology and cost-effectiveness in general

Generalization of the results from one setting to another, given the assumptions stated, depends on the workload, whether the visiting service is an available option and the actual travel costs. Key success factors for the service in Kirkenes are a combination of experienced medical doctors, the long distance and the high annual workload.

The results from the service in Kirkenes have been generalized to other rural sites. The costs of introducing a real-time teledermatology application (including phototherapy) in each municipality in the two northernmost counties in Norway were compared with patient travel to the nearest secondary care centre. The results for 40 rural health clinics were analysed and the same method was used as in the evaluation of the teledermatology service in Kirkenes.

It was assumed that 70% of the patients could be managed locally. The costs of using teledermatology at the local clinics were based on the experience of the real-time service in Kirkenes, the actual travel costs and the registered number of referrals from the rural district. The costs of personnel at the local sites were an estimated average based on patient workloads and the need for nurses and technical support. The savings were the avoided travel and consultation costs at the outpatient clinic in Tromsø.

Figure 24.3 shows the unit cost curve for real-time teledermatology including local phototherapy. The triangles represent the different health clinics (assuming one teledermatology application in one healthcare clinic in each municipality). Only four out of 40 healthcare clinics analysed had a sufficient patient workload for teledermatology to be considered cost-effective. The triangles located below the cost curve represent situations that were not cost-effective, because of a short distance and/or too low patient workloads. The triangles above the cost curve represent health clinics where teledermatology would be cost saving.

If real-time teledermatology were implemented without investing in a phototherapy unit and bath facilities, the cost would be lower, but this service would not necessarily be more cost-effective for the health sector. Fewer patients would be able to receive treatment locally and because of that, less money would be saved through avoided travel.

Shared investment

Intermunicipal cooperation seems to be a possibly cost-effective way of providing a real-time teledermatology service to patients living in remote areas of northern Norway. The patients then travel to a dermatology centre in their own or in a neighbouring municipality, instead of all the way to Tromsø. The telemedicine centre would probably be situated in the most populous area in the region. Such a telemedicine centre would save several hours of travel time for each specialist consultation and 75–90 % of the travel costs, depending on the distance between the shared centre and the patient's home. Such a cooperation could make teledermatology

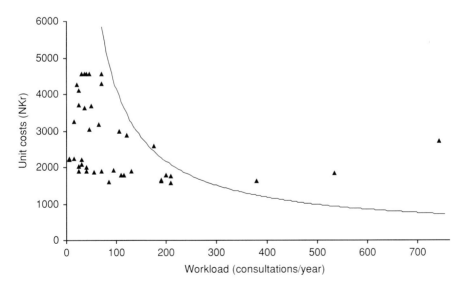

Fig. 24.3. Unit costs of teledermatology (including local phototherapy and patient travel) for 40 local health clinics in northern Norway (▲).

a cost-saving service for several of the sites that are not cost-effective, i.e. those located below the unit cost curve in Figure 24.3.

Still image teledermatology

Pre-recorded telemedicine using still images in an electronic referral requires less investment than traditional real-time videoconferencing. GPs can use a digital camera, a computer with appropriate software and ordinary email to transmit close-up still images of skin problems and text messages to a specialist. It is likely that such a technique will be cost-effective for more remote clinics than a real-time telemedicine service. However, this does not imply that still image telemedicine as a basis for reaching a diagnosis and suggesting a treatment plan will be cost-effective in general. Still images of a dermatological problem are less suitable for treatment purposes than videoconferencing.[12,13] This allows the GP to treat fewer patients locally than if videoconferencing is used and consequently the travel savings will be less.

A financial assessment of the potential cost-effectiveness of using still images in one healthcare clinic in each municipality showed that on average one-third of the clinics analysed in the two northernmost counties had a cost-saving potential.[12] If more than one health clinic in each municipality invested in still image equipment, even less would be cost-effective, because of the reduction in avoided patient travel per site.

Assuming that 30% of the total annual workload can be handled locally using still image teledermatology without having to travel to a specialist consultation, 23% of the total health clinics in northern Norway have a cost-saving potential. Assuming that 50% of the total annual workload can be handled locally, 41% of the local clinics will save money by investing in still image telemedicine.[12] This result shows that teledermatology in general is not cost-effective, even if the healthcare clinics invest in low-cost, store-and-forward equipment. The main reason for this is the strong relationship between the type of technology, the number of avoided journeys and the distance from the specialist clinic. However, teledermatology may be justified because it may provide more information in the referral for the specialist to decide the level of urgency and save time for the patients if they avoid travel.

Validity of economic evaluations of teledermatology

Several factors are important in assessing whether teledermatology is a cost-saving method of examining and treating patients at a local health centre. The most important one is the annual workload, but other factors that influence the result are equipment prices, the costs of the alternative methods, geographical distance and assumptions about the cost structure. Several simplifying assumptions were made in the present economic evaluations of different methods of providing dermatology care to local health clinics. All cost figures are to some extent the product of the assumptions made in their calculation. Therefore they must be interpreted in the light of their local circumstances. What is cost-effective in one location may not be cost-effective in another. The key issue is to determine the relevant economic aspects that will aid decision making when it comes to resource allocation within the healthcare sector.

Methodological issues

An important part of any economic evaluation is to identify critical methodological assumptions or areas of uncertainty, and to employ different assumptions or estimates in order to test the sensitivity of the results and conclusions.[1] A sensitivity analysis tests the robustness of the evaluation and if variations in the underlying assumptions do not significantly alter the results, this will increase one's confidence in them.

In the present study the choice of the discount rate had little effect on the results, because of the relatively short equipment lifetimes. The equipment lifetime will, however, affect the magnitude of the costs. A shorter lifetime for the equipment, such as that for local phototherapy, will not alter the ranking between the alternatives, but simply make the cost curves for teledermatology, a visiting service and a locally employed dermatologist shift outward, and make patient travel relatively less expensive (Fig. 24.2). A shorter lifetime for videoconferencing equipment will shift the cost curve for telemedicine outward: for example, a 4-year lifetime would make real-time teledermatology in Kirkenes cheaper than the other methods for patient workloads above 224 patients per year, instead of 195. Assuming an annual maintenance cost of 10% instead of 5% will also cause an outward shift in the cost curve for the teledermatology service. A sensitivity analysis showed that the results of the present evaluations were robust to changes in these assumptions about the cost structure.

The alternative methods of providing dermatology care to the local clinics and their accompanying costs are important considerations when evaluating the implementation of telemedicine. Conventionally, patients travel to the nearest secondary-care centre. But a locally employed dermatologist and a visiting service are also options, at least in principle, with different costs. In addition to cost considerations, this is often a resource policy issue depending on whether specialist time is scarce, i.e. whether there is a shortage of specialists or not. The distance between the sites is another crucial variable. In the Kirkenes situation, the distance of about 800 km makes aeroplane travel the only practical option. Travel by bus, private car or boat would imply additional accommodation and time costs, and therefore these have not been accounted for in this evaluation.

If the alternative way of providing care is a visiting service, telemedicine will save specialist time spent on travelling. In terms of opportunity costs this is a 'health benefit foregone', that is, the specialist could otherwise have spent time producing health benefits for other patients – since the specialist spent the time on a plane, the potential benefits are foregone. Whether the introduction of telemedicine will make consultants' time more or less available is ambiguous. This would depend on the effect telemedicine has on the referral pattern.

Referral pattern

An important factor when evaluating telemedicine is its effect on the referral pattern. Some research suggests that some patients who should have been referred are not referred, and that more knowledgeable GPs have higher referral rates.[14] However, Wootton et al[7] estimated that the dermatology referrals were reduced by 20% as a result of the learning effect of telemedicine. At the same time they found a higher recorded GP follow-up rate in the telemedicine alternative than the conventional way of providing care. Whether the GP can handle more patients due to the learning effect, and whether the follow-up rate increases in general or not is unknown. If the referrals increase as a result of teledermatology the specialist would have to manage more patients and the overall cost of telemedicine would then be underestimated. In northern Norway there is a shortage of dermatologists[13] and this effect might have a negative effect on the provision of dermatology care.

Experience from the teledermatology service in Kirkenes indicates that increased access to dermatology care increases the demand for specialist consultations.[13] The number of patients referred to the specialist by videoconferencing from Kirkenes increased considerably (over threefold) over the years with teledermatology. This might have something to do with increased demand as a result of increased supply, but it is a complicated issue with several possible explanations. The effect has also been mentioned elsewhere.[15] To provide healthcare services for more patients will increase expenditure. This implies that telemedicine will increase healthcare costs, but hopefully will also produce better health for those who get treatment that they otherwise would not have received. This depends on the fact that the increased demand meets an actual need in the population. Both the extra costs and benefits of such increased supply should be accounted for. This is an interesting and important topic for further research in telemedicine.

Non-monetary benefits

A teledermatology service may have an effect on a number of other variables besides a reduction in the costs of providing services. Such variables should also be assessed in order to allow a full economic evaluation. A cost-minimization analysis is a partial evaluation measuring only the costs and not the benefits of the intervention.[1] Outcome measures such as health benefits and benefits related to the process of the telemedicine setting compared to conventional medicine may also be relevant to include in an over-all evaluation. Teleconsultations between Kirkenes and Tromsø have reduced the waiting period for the patients. More rapid diagnosis and treatment may improve patient recovery and thus health outcome. Earlier recovery, however, has not been documented in the teledermatology service in Kirkenes. The benefits reported for the patients involved were principally reduced waiting time and avoided travel. But reduced absence from work has been reported by our patients to be the most important benefit, especially for those who avoid a longer stay at the central hospital for phototherapy.

Reduced waiting time

The waiting time for a consultation with the dermatologist for the patients in the Kirkenes area is at most three weeks.[13] The waiting period for patients who have access to telemedicine is much lower than for patients requiring dermatological care living in areas without telemedicine. On average, the waiting period at the hospital in Tromsø, for non-priority patients is six months. The reduced waiting time for patients in the Kirkenes area is not a result of the telemedicine service per se, but rather a result of how the service is organized with a fixed weekly time quota allocated to telemedicine for the Kirkenes area. As long as videoconferencing takes just as much time for the specialist as ordinary face-to-face consultations, it is difficult to see that this service will improve overall access to a finite number of dermatologists. What seems to have happened with the dermatology link between Tromsø and Kirkenes is that the distribution of specialist time has been altered in favour of patients in the Kirkenes area. If GP referral rates were reduced due to a long-term learning effect of telemedicine, one would expect overall access to dermatologists to improve. But given the way that telemedicine services are organized in northern Norway, new telemedicine implementations might make the waiting period for those who do not have access to the specialist via telemedicine even longer.

Patient satisfaction

Several studies have measured the attitude of patients to the use of telemedicine with various results.[14] Of the patients who saw the specialist over a video-link in Kirkenes, only 10% were dissatisfied while the rest of the patients were very satisfied.[13] Other research confirms this tendency.[5,16,17] The reason for this could be that the patients have a true preference for a teleconsultation, or they might value other benefits like avoided travel, a reduction in the waiting time, reduced absence from work and the presence of two doctors discussing their problems.[18]

Fifty-six patients living in the Kirkenes area took part in a survey of attitudes to teledermatology. These patients were participating in a trial comparing the use of still images to real-time videoconferencing with respect to diagnostic accuracy. The patients were asked to rank the use of still images and videoconferencing in relation to a visiting service and patient travel. The results showed that 36% (20 patients) would prefer still image teledermatology performed by their local GP. Thirty-nine per cent (19 patients) would prefer a visiting specialist service in Kirkenes, 13% (seven patients) would prefer travelling to the specialist at the secondary care hospital in Tromsø and 11% (six patients) would prefer real-time videoconferencing in Kirkenes. According to the patients, the benefits of using still image teledermatology were a familiar local GP, reduced absence from work, avoided travel and the opportunity to consult a specialist in an acute phase of their skin problem.[18]

Reimbursement

Teledermatology became reimbursable in Norway in 1996. The hospital that allocates the time of their dermatologists to teleconsultations has the right to bill the National Health Insurer NKr411 per telemedicine consultation that they perform. Most of the activity in hospital outpatient clinics is reimbursed the amount depending on the type of consultation and intervention performed. Telemedicine is reimbursed on the same principle as any other healthcare service performed by outpatient clinics.

The primary healthcare institutions are not reimbursed yet for telemedicine consultations. Telemedicine increases costs for the GPs, so reimbursement will be necessary to increase the use of telemedicine in this sector.

Reimbursement for telemedicine services should theoretically be based on cost-effectiveness. To give healthcare personnel an incentive to use telemedicine where it is not cost-effective might produce some undesirable effects for the healthcare system as a whole. An overall reimbursement schedule might not be possible as long as telemedicine is only cost saving in specific areas where the annual workload and travel costs to a secondary-care centre are high.

Conclusion

Healthcare costs have increased considerably over the last decade. Prior to implementing new services, decision-makers should ensure that such investments do not increase healthcare costs any further, especially if the intervention does not produce better health for the patients. Whether telemedicine has an effect on the patients' health outcome is largely unknown.[19,20] More research is needed to document the overall effect of telemedicine.

Whether teledermatology is a cost-saving method of examining and treating patients at a local health centre depends on a number of different factors. The most important one is the annual workload, but also equipment prices, costs of the alternative methods, geographical distance and assumptions about the cost structure will influence the result. Caution must therefore be exercised in generalizing results from one setting to another. Each decision about whether to implement teleconsultation based on financial arguments must be made in the light of the local circumstances.

Real-time teledermatology has a cost-saving potential in a few of the rural communities of northern Norway. One of the reasons for this is that the region is scarcely populated. With a few exceptions, the population ranges from 1000 to 4000 inhabitants in each municipality. This seems to be too low to base teledermatology services in these rural areas on purely economic grounds.

References

1   Drummond MF, Stoddard GL, Torrance GW. *Methods for the Economic Evaluation of Health Care Programmes*. Oxford: Oxford University Press, 1994.
2   Elford RD. Telemedicine in northern Norway. *Journal of Telemedicine and Telecare* 1997;**3:**1–22.
3   Bergmo TS. A cost-minimization analysis of a real-time teledermatology service in northern Norway. *Journal of Telemedicine and Telecare* 2000;**6:**273–277.
4   Nymo B, ed. Telektronikk, special edition – 1994 'Telemedicine'. *Telektronikk* 1993;**89:**(1).
5   Loane MA, Corbett R, Bloomer SE, et al. Diagnostic accuracy and clinical management by real-time teledermatology. Results from the Northern Ireland arms of the UK Multicentre Teledermatology Trial. *Journal of Telemedicine and Telecare* 1998;**4:**95–100.
6   Oakley AMM, Astwood DR, Loane MA, Duffill MB, Rademaker M, Wootton R. Diagnostic accuracy of teledermatology; results of a preliminary study in New Zealand. *New Zealand Medical Journal* 1997;**110:**51–53.
7   Wootton R, Bloomer SE, Corbett R, et al. Multicentre randomised control trial comparing real-time teledermatology with conventional outpatient dermatological care: societal cost–benefit analysis. *British Medical Journal* 2000;**320:**1252–1256.
8   Phillips CM, Burk WA, Shechter BA, et al. Reliability of dermatology teleconsultations with the use of teleconferencing technology. *Journal of the American Academy of Dermatology* 1997;**37:**398–402.
9   Lowitt MH, Kessler II, Kauffman CL, et al. Teledermatology and in-person examinations. *Archives of Dermatology* 1998;**134:**471–476.
10 Lesher JL Jr, Davis LS, Gourdin FW, et al. Telemedicine evaluation of cutaneous diseases: a blinded comparative study. *Journal of the American Academy of Dermatology* 1998;**38:**27–31.
11 Bergmo TS. An economic analysis of teleradiology versus a visiting radiologist service. *Journal of Telemedicine and Telecare* 1996;**2:**136–142.
12 Bergmo TS. [Will still image telemedicine save costs?] *Tidsskrift for den Norske Laegeforening* 2000;**120:**1777–1780. [In Norwegian.]
13 Moseng D. [Teledermatology – the north Norwegian experiences.] *Tidsskrift for den Norske Laegeforening* 2000;**120:**1893–1895. [In Norwegian.]
14 Taylor P. A survey of research in telemedicine. 2:Telemedicine services. *Journal of Telemedicine and Telecare* 1998;**4:**63–71.
15 Perednia DA. Fear, loathing, dermatology, and telemedicine. *Archives of Dermatology* 1997;**133:** 151–155.
16 Loane MA, Bloomer SE, Corbett R, et al. Patient satisfaction with real-time teledermatology in Northern Ireland. *Journal of Telemedicine and Telecare* 1998;**4:**36–40.
17 Jones DH, Crichton C, Macdonald A, et al. Teledermatology in the Highlands of Scotland. *Journal of Telemedicine and Telecare* 1996;**2:**(Suppl 1):7–9.
18 Arild E, Ekeland AE. [Teledermatology – still images: patient responses.] *Working paper. Hustrykkeriet, Regionsykehuset i Tromsø*, 1999. [In Norwegian.]
19 Kristiansen IS, Poulsen PB. [Saving billions with telemedicine: fact or fiction?] *Tidsskrift for den Norske Laegeforening* 2000;**120:**2305–2311. [In Norwegian.]
20 Aavitsland P. [Telemedicine – medicine at distance.] *Tidsskrift for den Norske Laegeforening* 2000;**120:**2245. [In Norwegian.]

25

Conclusion

Richard Wootton and Amanda Oakley

Introduction

As the experience in this book shows, teledermatology can be used in a variety of different ways for a broad range of purposes, basically clinical or educational. So far as clinical work is concerned, there are two fundamentally different approaches, which offer their own pros and cons[1] (Table 25.1). Which approach is to be preferred depends on the context in which the teledermatology service is to be operated. A current research question of some interest is whether email messages with still pictures attached will be a better choice for clinical teledermatology than real-time videolinks. Email has the advantage of being cheaper and more convenient for the doctors involved than a videoconsultation, but seems to have a lower diagnostic accuracy.[2] If a higher proportion of patients referred by email require a face-to-face consultation in the end, then the overall cost-benefits may be rather finely balanced. Indeed, the ideal teledermatology technique will probably turn out to be a hybrid, combining the best of both approaches.

When technology is simple and advantageous it is rapidly adopted. Equally, unwanted or inappropriate technology has frequently proved to be an expensive white elephant. In the last decade successful telecommunications advances have included mobile phones, the World Wide Web and electronic mail. If it can be seamlessly incorporated into the daily routine, telemedicine will become as normal a part of medical practice as conducting a Medline search or making a mobile phone call is today. The widespread adoption of telemedicine would have radical consequences for the organization and structure of health services.

The successes of teledermatology include the technology and the ability to make an accurate diagnosis. Educational success for both the health professional and consumer has been mainly due to the rapid spread of the Internet as a communication tool and information resource.

Current problems

Telemedicine can in principle be as easy as making a telephone call or selecting a television channel. However processes remain cumbersome in most health systems, since they usually lack integrated electronic medical records and secure telecommunications between primary care and specialists. The full cost of

Table 25.1. Summary of advantages and disadvantages of teledermatology (adapted from Eedy and Wootton[1]) (a) teledermatology in general

For	Against
Management plans are as good as those in a conventional consultation	Some patients will always require an outpatient appointment
An equitable service can be provided, especially to remote areas	There is a tendency to focus on the presenting lesion, instead of the patient as a whole
GPs can refer to a centre of their choice	The diagnosis may be uncertain or incorrect
The technique is generally highly acceptable to patients	A minority of patients prefer to see a dermatologist in person
Costs to patients are decreased, e.g. travel and time off work	Teledermatology should only be one facet of a dermatology service and not a 'quick fix' for the deficiencies of the health service
Dermatologist time could be saved, particularly in doing frequent remote clinics	There may be professional resistance to change
Equipment costs are steadily decreasing; in addition image quality is steadily increasing	There are security, privacy and legal liability concerns (although none are insuperable)
Teledermatology could result in shorter waiting lists for conventional consultation	

(b) real-time videoconferencing

For	Against
The interactive consultation enables a three-way discussion between patient, GP and dermatologist	Not cost effective over short distance
Diagnostic and management accuracy are effective (and better than store-and-forward)	May be less favoured by elderly, shy or young patients
Greater clinical information is available compared with store-and-forward techniques	Lower static picture resolution when compared with store-and-forward
There is significant educational value to the GP	It is difficult to synchronize patient, GP and dermatologist to be present at the same time
Useful for monitoring treatments at a distance, e.g. phototherapy	Equipment failure leads to wastage of expensive medical time
Cost effective over long distance and/or using a specialist nurse to take images	Videoconferencing is as time consuming as a conventional consultation.

(c) store-and-forward

For	Against
Cheap and effective way of giving diagnosis and management plans	Dermatologists find it repetitive and boring
Accuracy shown to be adequate	Unable to get information directly from GP and patient
Good triage tool for those who may need hospital-based appointment or treatment	Loss of rapport with the patient
A large number of images can be reviewed at a time convenient to the dermatologist	Loss of educational component for GPs
Health problems may be processed more quickly than by conventional referral	Images may be mistakenly identified as belonging to another patient
Data can be accessed from any location where there is Internet access	Time consuming for the GP to supply comprehensive data and manage digital image transfer
Easy to obtain further opinions from local or international experts	Data may be widely distributed without the patient's knowledge or consent

telemedicine is rarely reimbursed. Thus clinical teledermatology has yet to become an integral part of health care.

Physicians need reassurance about the legal aspects of telemedicine because they are understandably nervous about the risk of misdiagnosis. As a previous book in this series has explained, there are not likely to be major traps for physicians who practise by telemedicine in a prudent manner.[3] However we await effective international laws and standards of practice for telemedicine.

It is not easy to demonstrate economic benefit from teledermatology to a health funder's satisfaction. In general the patient's savings are not budgeted for, and it is rare that a dermatology problem would otherwise require an expensive helicopter transfer (Fig. 25.1). Consultations with prisoners or those living on isolated islands and other remote locations represent a special case, since other factors than the strict economic issues may determine adoption.[5] Equipment and administration costs can be more easily justified if the telemedicine system is multipurpose and used extensively.

Teledermatology research projects have not always (often?) resulted in a continuing clinical teledermatology service. Some of the most successful have been described in this book. The novelty factor of telemedicine rapidly loses its appeal if the equipment is unreliable and complicated, if referral data (history and images) are inadequate or if there are structural impediments to effective practice, such as scheduling conflicts, overwork, lack of reimbursement or other disincentives.

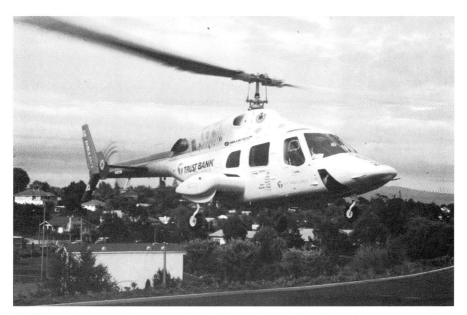

Fig. 25.1. Emergency helicopter transfer at Waikato Hospital, New Zealand. In some specialties, for example neurosurgery, emergency transfer is common. If telemedicine can reduce the numbers of emergency transfers, there may be significant economic benefits.[4] However, it is rare that emergency transfer is required for dermatology patients, so the economic benefits may be less striking.

What do users think of teledermatology?

What do the users think of teledermatology? On the whole, users like teledermatology. Unsurprisingly patients are generally enthusiastic about teledermatology;[6-8] after all, they benefit directly from reduced travel and less time off work. Most patients are pleased that their condition is being diagnosed and treated quickly and when asked directly, almost 90%[8] agreed that a teleconsultation saved time and expenditure in travelling to hospital. In general, younger patients were more accepting of the new technology than the elderly.[9] Patients who are less tolerant or do not do so well include the elderly, small infants, those who are shy and embarrassed at being videoed, and those with genital rashes.[10]

The medical profession is perhaps less enthusiastic than patients about tele-dermatology, since the advantages to the individual practitioner are not usually significant. In this respect, teledermatology is no different from much of the rest of telemedicine. GPs seem to report greater satisfaction with teledermatology than do their dermatologist colleagues.[7,11,12] In the UK, GPs reported very high levels of satisfaction (>80%) with real-time consultation and stated that 75% of teleconsultations were of educational benefit.[13] In a larger study, GPs estimated that the knowledge transfer effect of real-time consultation was equivalent to six days' training per year.[11] By comparison, dermatologists' criticisms were usually concerned with picture quality, lack of rapport with patients, inability to palpate lesions or carry out diagnostic tests and that the systems were time-consuming to use and unsatisfying.[7,12,14] In a study using high-bandwidth videoconferencing, where image quality would have been better, dermatologists were highly satisfied with the interpersonal aspects of videoconsultations and tended to be more certain of their diagnoses.[6]

The future

Improving access to expert health care is likely to produce increased demand and to strain inadequate health budgets. Governments have other, equally deserving healthcare priorities. We do not yet have enough experience with telemedicine in general, or teledermatology in particular, to be able to predict confidently the circumstances in which it will succeed. What this book shows however is that the technology is not a limiting factor in teledermatology. The important (and largely unsolved) problems concern how teledermatology can be used to best advantage and how it can be integrated into day-to-day practice. As the experience reported in this book demonstrates, there are many unanswered questions about teledermatology. We therefore need research. Without proper research trials, of adequate size and power, teledermatology will remain a niche application.

In the meantime, we must plan systems with better security, the development of internationally accepted standards, careful research programmes and improved health outcomes for our patients. We should strive to incorporate templates into practice management systems for ease of referral and data retrieval, and encourage the adoption of broadband telecommunications systems. Any implementation of telemedicine should involve an evaluation, since without the evidence that a particular technique is cost-effective, it is unlikely to be sustainable.[15]

Teledermatology in the future may employ advanced technology, such as three-dimensional imaging, the ability to 'palpate' the skin from a distance and tele-robotic surgery. Smart systems may diagnose melanoma from an image and hierarchical queries may provide dermatological expertise to the man in the street. The dermatologist's role may change from hands on clinician to one of facilitator or information broker, guiding the patient through the information overload.

The ideal in dermatology is likely to remain interactive and face-to-face; we will always welcome patients to our hospital clinics and we will always enjoy meeting our colleagues at conferences. Teledermatology has resulted in the development of close online friendships so that some face-to-face encounters will have increased in number – patients travel to congresses arranged by their online support group, doctors to conferences to meet their online mailing list colleagues. Enhanced knowledge improves the relationship between provider and patient and ultimately should improve their health.

The art of successful telemedicine lies in finding situations in which the advantages of practice at a distance outweigh the disadvantages.

We hope you have enjoyed this book.

References

1   Eedy DJ, Wootton R. Teledermatology: a review. *British Journal of Dermatology* 2001;**144**:696–707.
2   Loane MA, Bloomer SE, Corbett R, et al. A comparison of real-time and store-and-forward teledermatology: a cost–benefit study. *British Journal of Dermatology* 2000;**143**:1241–1247.
3   Stanberry BA. *The Legal and Ethical Aspects of Telemedicine*. London: Royal Society of Medicine Press, 1999.
4   Maass M, Kosonen M, Kormano M. Transportation savings and medical benefits of a teleneuroradiological network. *Journal of Telemedicine and Telecare* 2000;**6**:142–146.
5   Wootton R, Hebert MA. What constitutes success in telehealth? *Journal of Telemedicine and Telecare* 2001;**7**(suppl 2):3–7.
6   Lowitt MH, Kessler II, Kauffman L, Hooper FJ, Siegel E, Burnett JW. Teledermatology and in-person examinations: a comparison of patient and physician perceptions and diagnostic agreement. *Archives of Dermatology* 1998;**134**:471–476.
7   Phillips CM, Burke WA, Allen MH, Stone D, Wilson JL. Reliability of telemedicine in evaluating skin tumors. *Telemedicine Journal* 1998;**4**:5–9.
8   Loane MA, Bloomer SE, Corbett R, et al. Patient satisfaction with real-time teledermatology in Northern Ireland. *Journal of Telemedicine and Telecare* 1998;**4**:36–40.
9   Lesher JL Jr, Davis LS, Gourdin FW, English D, Thompson WO. Telemedicine evaluation of cutaneous diseases: a blinded comparative study. *Journal of the American Academy of Dermatology* 1998;**38**:27–31.
10 Elford DR. Teledermatology. *Journal of Telemedicine and Telecare* 1997;**3**: 4–6.
11 Wootton R, Bloomer SE, Corbett R, et al. Multicentre randomised control trial comparing real time teledermatology with conventional outpatient dermatological care: societal cost–benefit analysis. *British Medical Journal* 2000;**320**:1252–1256.
12 Pak HS, Welch M, Poropatich R. Web-based teledermatology consult system: preliminary results from the first 100 cases. *Studies in Health Technology and Informatics* 1999;**64**:179–184.

13   Gilmour E, Campbell SM, Loane MA, et al. Comparison of teleconsultations and face-to-face consultations: preliminary results of a United Kingdom multicentre teledermatology study. *British Journal of Dermatology* 1998;**139**:81–87.

14   Loane MA, Gore HE, Corbett R, et al. Effect of camera performance on diagnostic accuracy: preliminary results from the Northern Ireland arms of the UK Multicentre Teledermatology Trial. *Journal of Telemedicine and Telecare* 1997;**3**:83–88.

15   Wootton R. Telemedicine in the National Health Service. *Journal of the Royal Society of Medicine* 1998;**91**:614–621.

▶ Index

Page numbers in **bold** refer to boxes, figures and tables